Bedside Cardiology

Bedside Cardiology

THIRD EDITION

Jules Constant, M.D.

Clinical Associate Professor of Medicine,
State University of New York at Buffalo School of Medicine;
Director of Clinical Cardiology, Buffalo General Hospital, Buffalo, New York

Little, Brown and Company
Boston / Toronto

To Elizabeth, my wife

Preface

The Third Edition of *Bedside Cardiology*, like the first two editions, is designed for those who wish to learn how to diagnose cardiovascular disorders by means of history and physical examination. However, it encourages the use of phonocardiograms and pulse tracings for teaching and self-training. This edition continues to try to teach at three levels. An asterisk (*) before a statement denotes material for the trainee in cardiology (or for reference). Terms appearing in **boldface** type are for use by those in the first three years of medical school (these boldface terms are included in the Glossary following the text, which explains their meaning in detail). The rest of the material is for the senior student, family physician, or internist.

The question-and-answer method has been continued as a stimulus to clear thinking (as well as to concise writing). However, material particularly for the cardiologist has been presented as much as possible in narrative form under the subheading *Note*.

The many advances in the understanding and diagnosis of cardiological conditions made over the nine years since the second edition are reflected by the hundreds of additional references. Much of this new knowledge has been brought about by developments in echocardiography. In this Third Edition, besides many new illustrations, such as tables for the x-ray diagnosis of cardiomegaly, the patient history checklist has been considerably updated, the section on prolapsed mitral valves and papillary muscle dysfunction has been almost completely replaced, and there is a new section on how to tell ejection fraction by physical examination.

J. C.

Acknowledgments

For their criticism of the manuscript and for their donation of many of the illustrations, I would like to thank Dr. Graham J. Leach, London, England; Dr. Narasimha Ranganathan, Toronto, Canada; Dr. Tsuguya Sakamoto, Tokyo, Japan; Dr. James A. Shaver, Pittsburgh, Pennsylvania; and Dr. John Wanamaker, Sayre, Pennsylvania.

J. C.

Contents

Bedside Cardiology

1. *The Evolving Checklist in History-Taking*

GENERAL ADVANTAGES OF A CHECKLIST

Traditionally, students have learned to take a history by memorizing a standard checklist and have been warned that a checklist should not be used in front of a patient. It is my contention that not using a detailed checklist in front of a patient can lead to poor diagnosis and that ultimately computerized questionnaires may have to be used because of this inadequate approach.

At the inception of our elective training program in cardiology, a general checklist was drawn up to be certain that at least the important questions would be asked. It was surprising to find how good a history could be taken with this aid, but it became apparent that students and house staff did not know what subsequent questions to ask if the patient responded affirmatively to a more general question. This prompted the incorporation of further questions to be asked when the patient says yes.

It became apparent also that cardiological diagnosis could be taught to students by listing the relevant questions under the differential diagnosis. For example, if the patient admitted to having edema, an asterisk could be placed beside the question, indicating that the student should turn to a separate sheet outlining the differential diagnosis of edema, with a list of further questions to elicit each possible cause. The checklist then became a teaching tool—that is, the student learned the differential diagnosis of cardiac symptoms while taking a history.

As we learned more about the relation between symptoms and diagnoses, the checklist evolved further. For example, when we learned that excess perspiration is found in almost all patients with pheochromocytomas, this question went into our new checklist on the sheet for "If the Patient Says Yes to Hypertension" as a question under the subtitle "Pheochromocytoma."

Many students are resistant to the idea of reading questions to patients, thinking that patients might consider them incompetent or their memories faulty. They fear that the patient's image of the physician as an omniscient, godlike figure will be lost if they are seen reading questions like a clerk in a bank. In fact, just the opposite impression seems to be conveyed to the patient. When we solicited patient opinion, we found that the patient usually did not even recall a few days later that a checklist had been used or expressed amazement at the tremendous amount of thought that must have gone into the preparation of such a detailed questionnaire. The commonest reaction we have found in patients who have had other physicians take histories from them is delight that this physician cared enough about them to try to get a good history.

Another argument against the checklist is that it prevents the physician from noticing a patient's facial expression, which may reveal the true meaning behind the answer. This objection implies that the physician's eyes are glued to the questions. However, it is easy to keep a finger on the place as one looks up at the patient during questioning.

To the objection that the list gives the patient no opportunity to be spontaneous or to associate freely, it has been found that, on the contrary, one of the checklist's strengths is that should the patient wish to enlarge on a point or go to another complaint spontaneously, the physician can keep to his organized line of questioning merely by noting where he is on the checklist. Without a checklist, a physician may object to the patient's getting off the subject for fear he may forget his place in his memorized list.

Another major objection to a printed checklist is that it does not allow the addition of new diagnostic symptoms that are learned from the literature. Physicians often say that they have a thousand sheets of a checklist that was made up when they first went into practice, which can no longer be used because it is not applicable to what they have since learned. The checklist proposed here is not to be used as a "checkoff list" but as a "reminder list." This checklist does not use yes or no answers. A checkoff list may not have enough room beside each question to write down all the details when the patient says yes to a question or when there is a lengthy history of present illness. These objections are overcome here because our histories are written on separate blank sheets. This is the only way to make the history form flexible, because there is only a slight relationship between the headings on the checklist and the way in which the final history may be written. When a physician learns of a new question or a new differential diagnosis, he has only to make up one new reminder list or add merely a word or two to the present one. We believe a checklist with a place beside each question for the answer is very unsatisfactory because it does not allow for changes in organization. The answers from the checklist are put down in an unorganized form and are then rewritten or dictated under a few headings. (A simplified method of organizing the history from the answers written on scrap paper will be found later.) We believe this checklist serves as an example of the kind of checklist that the physician should make up for himself no matter what specialty he practices, because of the following advantages:

1. No negative findings need be written down. If the checklist has been followed, you know which questions have been asked. This makes the final history much shorter and easier to read.
2. If in retrospect a diagnosis was missed because a certain question was not asked, it goes down on the checklist for all future history-taking. No errors of omission in history-taking need ever be made twice.
3. You may utilize new information gained from experience, reading, and lectures as efficiently as a computer merely by inserting into your checklist any new symptom that for the first time you have learned is part of a certain diagnosis. You are in effect programming your own computer by the built-in memory in your checklist. Thus, the reminder list grows with your increase in knowledge.
4. There is no feeling of insecurity on leaving the bedside that you may have forgotten to ask something.
5. You can actually take a history much faster because there is no hesitation while you try to recall your place in your memorized checklist, especially if the patient rambles. If your histories are longer with a written checklist than with a mental checklist, then your mental checklist was inadequate. The checklist presented in this chapter is not actually as long as it appears at first glance because many questions are repeated under different headings in order to complete a differential diagnosis.
6. The checklist helps the physician who must, during the first visit at least, take a

good chief complaint history. If, for example, the patient complains of chest pain, one turns to the sheet headed "If the Patient Says Yes to Chest Pain," which shows the complete differential diagnosis of chest pain and serves as an organized outline for the present illness.

Write the facts on scrap paper and organize them as follows:

Name, Date, Age, Address, and Telephone Number

Orientation

Why patient came or was referred, and who referred. Marital state and occupation.

History of Chief Complaint or Complaints

For example, if the patient has chest pain, write the complete story of chest pain from the checklist.

Chamber Enlargement Possibilities

This is the place for palpitations.

Other Etiologies

Not pertinent to chief complaints. These headings should contain the word *possibilities* (e.g., if the patient has known valvular heart disease, Rheumatic Heart Disease Possibilities would be an appropriate heading).

Note: a) Do not record negative answers. The checklist makes them unnecessary.

  b) Do not repeat symptoms under separate headings.

  c) Do not give your opinions on diagnoses or symptoms in the history.

REMINDER LIST HISTORY: HEART FAILURE POSSIBILITIES

Left Ventricular Failure or High Left Atrial Pressure Possibilities

+ 1. Dyspnea on exertion (DOE) on the level or on climbing either hills or steps? If not, is it because the patient is too limited in his exertion by chest or leg pains (p. 11)?

+ 2. Orthopnea (because of dyspnea, the patient must raise head *and shoulders* in order to sleep) (p. 12)?

+ 3. Paroxysmal nocturnal dyspnea (PND) (p. 13)?

+ 4. Pulmonary edema (sudden shortness of breath [SOB] and wheezing or cough at rest in the daytime)?

  5. Cardiovascular symptoms in pregnancy? If yes, which trimester? (Dyspnea in the first trimester is a recognized phenomenon thought probably to be caused by a

---

+ before a question indicates that when the patient answers yes, follow-up questions are available on the page number given in parentheses.

placental product; in the last trimester, although it may be cardiac in origin or due to a high diaphragm.)

6. Cough or wheeze on exertion or on assuming a supine position? (May mean high left atrial pressure of early heart failure.)

7. Therapy with
    a) Low-salt diet?
    b) Drugs? For all drugs, give the dose and when the drug was begun. Ask if the drug helped, how long it was taken, and why it was stopped.
       If the patient is on digitalis: tablet, capsule, or elixir? What side effects have been noted?
       1) Gastrointestinal: diarrhea, anorexia, nausea, vomiting?
       2) Muscle weakness [17].
       3) Cerebral: dizziness (e.g., faintness, vertigo, or loss of balance), hallucinations, irritability?
       4) Visual: blurring or inability to focus? Needs change of glasses? Color illusions?
       5) Cardiotoxicity: palpitations, skipping, or "flip-flops"?
       If the patient is on diuretics, what side effects have been noted?
       1) Weakness due to hypokalemia?
       2) Muscle cramps or pains due to low intracellular potassium or magnesium? Were any potassium-retaining agents or supplements used? How were potassium supplements tolerated? How was low-salt diet tolerated? Was it strict?

Is the patient taking preload and afterload-reducing drugs? Were drugs taken that could precipitate borderline heart failure (i.e., beta blockers, quinidine, disopyramide, verapamil, or reserpine)?

Peripheral Venous Congestion or Pseudo Right Heart Failure Possibilities[1]

+ 1. Peripheral edema? Maximum and minimum weight? Reasons for any weight gain or loss (p. 13).

2. Abdominal swelling? (If this occurs before or simultaneously with orthopnea or dyspnea, consider tamponade.)

3. Upper abdominal pain, especially on exercise? (This suggests increased stretch of liver capsule due to hepatomegaly.)

4. Bending or stooping discomfort? (Suggests hepatomegaly.)

Low Output State Possibilities

1. Weakness and fatigue? Do these occur only in the morning (depression)? Is afternoon nap necessary? If these signs occur only in the afternoon, they suggest low

---

[1] Conventionally called right heart failure, although the right ventricle may not have actually "failed." The term *failure* should be avoided because it has two meanings. It may mean symptoms or signs resulting from a high venous pressure and peripheral edema, which are almost always caused by left-sided myocardial or valvular damage alone. The other meaning refers to true right ventricular failure. The right ventricle rarely fails except with severe pulmonary stenosis, severe pulmonary hypertension, a massive pulmonary embolus, or right ventricular infarction. **Tamponade*** causes a biventricular failure, due mainly to restriction of diastolic filling.
*Boldface type indicates that the term is explained in the Glossary.

blood sugar or hypothyroidism. Is the patient on drugs that could cause weakness (e.g., digitalis, diuretics, beta blockers, or tranquilizers)? Is there a psychoneurotic basis (relationship to family, spouse, work supervisor)? Is the patient taking a contraceptive pill, diphenylhydantoin, or spironolactone (suggests folic acid deficiency)?

2. Coldness of extremities? For how long?
3. Excess perspiration? (A common sign of failure in infants. If recent in an adult and not due to hyperthyroidism or neurosis, it suggests severe failure. With warm hands, it suggests thyrotoxicosis; with cold hands, it suggests psychoneurosis [*neurocirculatory asthenia*] or heart failure.)
4. Insomnia due to hyperpnea on going to sleep or dozing (**Cheyne-Stokes respiration**)? Ask spouse if he or she noticed this.
5. Nocturia with polyuria (due to daytime failure compensated at rest)?

Fixed Output State Possibilities

+1. Syncope, faintness, or dizziness (p. 14)?
+2. Chest pain, tightness, pressure, or discomfort (p. 16)?

Chamber Enlargement Possibilities

  1. Trepopnea (certain positions in bed cause discomfort or SOB not due to failure)?
+2. Palpitations or awareness of heartbeat (p. 19)?
  3. Has patient been told of an enlarged heart? When was he first told? If yes, was it after an ECG or x-ray or echocardiogram? If x-ray was done in hospital, was it portable?
  4. Has an x-ray examination been done? When and where were first and last ones done?

Past Cardiac Surgery

1. Date and place of surgery? Type of operation or prosthesis? Name of surgeon?
2. Heart failure or other cardiac symptoms present before surgery? Which symptoms were helped, and for how long?
3. Was patient catheterized before or after surgery? Was he told about the results of the studies?
4. Complications after surgery: embolic phenomenon, infections, or other?
5. What treatment was given after surgery (anticoagulants, digitalis, diuretics)? For how long?

ETIOLOGIES

Rheumatic Heart Disease Possibilities

History of Rheumatic Fever

1. Chorea ("St. Vitus' dance"), twitches, or clumsiness for a few months in childhood? Epistaxis? Frequent sore throats? Tonsillectomy and adenoidectomy? When?
2. Growing pains (i.e., *nocturnal* pains or aches in the legs)? (Arthritis or other joint involvement in the daytime suggests rheumatic fever.)

Boldface type indicates that the term is explained in the Glossary.

3. Was the diagnosis of rheumatic fever based merely on signs of fever and murmur, or were there actually red, swollen, painful joints and rash? Hospitalized?
4. What therapy was given: aspirin, steroids, prophylactic penicillin, prolonged bed rest?
5. Is there a family history of rheumatic fever? (This is almost as suggestive of a rheumatic origin of a patient's murmur as a history of rheumatic fever in the patient.)

History of Rheumatic Heart Disease

1. Murmurs heard on previous examination (school, pre-camp, operation, hospitalization, insurance, military service)?
2. Results of cardiac catheterization? When and where was it done?

Complications of Rheumatic Heart Disease

1. In the presence of mitral disease:
   a) Hemoptysis? Is it mixed or pure? Quantity, color, frequency? (If this occurs with dyspnea or pleuritic pain, consider pulmonary infarction. If it arises from the submucosal bronchial veins, the blood is dark, and the cause is usually high left atrial pressure due to mitral stenosis.)
   b) Hoarseness without obvious upper respiratory infection? (This is Ortner's syndrome or the cardio-vocal syndrome, due to the pressure of a large left atrium on an enlarged pulmonary artery, which in turn may press on the peribronchial lymph nodes to compress the recurrent laryngeal nerve. Dysphagia may be due to both pressure by a large left atrium and stretch of the autonomic fibers to the esophagus [6, 8, 22].
   c) Winter bronchitis or wheezing?
   d) Ruptured chordae tendineae (suggested by sudden worsening of dyspnea, orthopnea, or PND)?
   e) Embolic phenomena: hematuria, pleurisy, unilateral weakness? Sudden loss of vision or loss in one visual field of one eye (calcium emboli from aortic valve [3])?
2. In the presence of aortic stenosis: angina, exertional syncope, or dyspnea (a classic triad)?
3. In the presence of aortic regurgitation (AR): nocturnal angina (but a sign of vasospastic angina if no AR)? Awareness of large pulsations in arms, neck, or chest?
4. Epilepsy (increased incidence with mitral stenosis)?
5. Possible infective endocarditis:
   a) Fever and night sweats (enough to require change of pajamas)?
   b) Tooth extraction or cleaning or other possible causes of bacteremia?
   c) Prolonged treatment with penicillin or other antibiotic?
   d) Embolic phenomena: hematuria, back pain, petechiae, tender finger pads, or cerebrovascular accident (unilateral weakness, paralysis, or speech difficulty)?

Ischemic Heart Disease Possibilities

+1. Chest pains or tightness (p. 16)?
 2. Previous myocardial infarction? If yes, what were the symptoms and hospital course? What was patient told about site and severity? What hospital? Was the patient put on long-term drugs (e.g., beta blockers)?

3. Risk factors:
   a) Major: Hypertension, high cholesterol, heavy smoking, or family history of infarction or angina at an early age.
   b) *Minor:* Diabetes, artificial or premature menopause, intermittent claudication, or sedentary occupation.
   Diet or drugs to lower cholesterol level?
   High uric acid level or gout (patient tends to be hypertensive or obese [9]).
4. Marked postprandial somnolence? (Suggests severe hyperlipidemia.)

HYPERTENSIVE HEART DISEASE POSSIBILITIES

+1. Hypertension (p. 19)?

HIGH OUTPUT FAILURE POSSIBILITIES

1. Anemia:
   a) Has patient been ever been told he has anemia? Pins and needles? Bleeding from menorrhagia, hemorrhoids, or ulcers (causing occult blood or melena)? Is anemia being treated?
   b) Bone marrow or metabolic disorders: upper gastrointestinal surgery in the past (causing vitamin B_{12} deficiency), sickle cell disease in self or family, contact with lead or radiation?
2. Thyrotoxicosis: heat intolerance, weight loss, polyphagia, polyuria, excessive sweating, frequent stools, nervousness, irritability, restlessness, muscle weakness on climbing? Palpitations? Thyroid surgery or treatment? Goiter?
3. Beriberi: alcoholism with poor eating habits while drinking, occupation bartender, diet fads, upper gastrointestinal surgery in the past? Peripheral neuritis, syncope on exercise in hot weather? Marked daily or weekly fluctuation of symptoms?

COR PULMONALE POSSIBILITIES

1. Chronic obstructive pulmonary disease: pulmonary function tests? Easier to breathe leaning forward? Smoking history? Told of emphysema? Chronic cough and sputum?
2. Asthma, wheezing, or dyspnea relieved by bronchodilators?
3. Ever work with beryllium or in a soft or hard coal mine?
4. Pulmonary emboli? History of phlebitis? Marked diuresis with diuretics? On contraceptive pill? Ever experience sudden dyspnea at rest, with palpitations, pleurisy, faintness, cold sweat, or hemoptysis? Recurrent stabbing groin pain [21]? Recent trauma or surgery? Pregnancy or long automobile trip?
5. History of lung infiltrate or tuberculosis?
6. Primary pulmonary hypertension? **Raynaud's phenomenon** [30]? (Occurs in about a third of patients with primary pulmonary hypertension.)

PERICARDITIS, EFFUSION, CONSTRICTION, OR TAMPONADE POSSIBILITIES

Etiologies

1. Chest trauma, recent heart surgery? (The postcardiotomy syndrome—fever, pleurisy, pericarditis, and polyserositis—may occur as long as 2 months after heart surgery.) Myocardial infarction (Dressler's syndrome, which is the same as postcardiotomy syndrome but follows myocardial infarction, now extremely rare), radiation to chest in past few months, uremia, metastatic cancer, lymphoma, leukemia, myxedema, scleroderma, lupus, rheumatoid arthritis, contact with tuberculosis, or recent viral infection? Is patient taking drugs that would produce lupus erythematosus syndrome: procainamide, hydralazine, penicillin, isoniazid? Is he on minoxidil?

Symptoms of Pericarditis

1. Chest pain on motion, swallowing, or deep breathing?
2. Joint symptoms? (With face rash, symptoms suggest possible lupus erythematosus; with rash on limbs or body, rheumatic fever.)
3. Past history of pericarditis? (In about one-fourth of cases idiopathic pericarditis is recurrent.)
4. Epigastric pain for 1 to 3 days before the chest pain? (This is the initial manifestation in one-third of patients with acute idiopathic pericarditis.) Pain may occur solely in the abdomen [25].

Symptoms of Tamponade

1. Dyspnea on exertion (DOE)?
2. Edema or abdominal swelling preceding dyspnea? Abdominal swelling before or simultaneous with edema (highly suggestive of tamponade)?
3. Does DOE stop immediately when the patient stops moving (rare sign)?

MYOCARDITIS, ENDOCARDITIS, AND OTHER HEART DISEASE POSSIBILITIES

1. Acute myocarditis: recent influenza-like illness with myalgia [19]?
2. Infective endocarditis: Has patient ever been told of murmur? Drug addiction, fevers, surgical or dental cause of bacteremia, prolonged penicillin treatment, hematuria, back pain, petechiae, strokes?
3. "Collagen" disease: Raynaud's phenomenon, dysphagia, arthritis, or arthralgias, tight skin, epistaxis, rash in sunlight?
4. Ankylosing spondylitis: Pain in the hip or sciatic region, or low back pain? Does the pain awaken patient in the early morning hours? Morning back stiffness? Pain increased on coughing?
5. Carcinoid heart disease: diarrhea, bronchospasm, flushing of the upper chest and head that lasts from minutes to days?
6. Parasitic disease (trichinosis or Chagas' disease): rare meat? Foreign travel?

7. Hypophosphatemia: high intake of phosphorus-binding antacids, aluminum hydroxide gel? Acute alcohol excess [7]?

8. Atrial myxoma: embolic phenomena, recurrent fevers, arthralgias, or skin lesions of a vasculitis type? Paresthesias in hands? Pulsations in neck (giant A waves, as in tricuspid stenosis)? Syncope or faintness on changing body position?

9. Hemochromatosis: history of diabetes, especially if patient is insulin resistant? Skin color changes? Liver failure and enlargement symptoms: upper abdominal pain, sexual impotence, or gynecomastia? Arthritis? Frequent transfusions?

10. Sarcoidosis: syncope (due to complete atrioventricular block)? Known bundle branch block? Abnormal chest radiograph? Cough? Kidney stones or eye symptoms (uveitis)?

11. **Hypertrophic subaortic stenosis:**
    a) Family history of sudden death?
    b) Angina or syncope after but not during exercise?
    c) Intermittent murmur?
    d) Do symptoms become worse on digitalis?

12. Amyloid heart disease: postural hypotension with peripheral neuropathy? Skin plaques or lesions, especially if there is bleeding on scratching?

13. Luetic aortic regurgitation or aneurysm? History of venereal disease or positive serology ("bad blood")? Hoarseness due to recurrent laryngeal nerve compression by aneurysm [29].

14. Traumatic causes. Chest injury in the past? (Traumatic tricuspid regurgitation may not cause cardiac symptoms for up to 3 years after the accident [20].)

CONGENITAL HEART DISEASE POSSIBILITIES

A. To be asked only if patient is an infant.
   1. Growth and development? (Compare with siblings.) High birth weight suggests **transposition of the great vessels.**
   2. Mother's pregnancy:
      a) Stilbestrol in pregnancy has been linked to transposition of great vessels.
      b) Viral illness. (In the last trimester, may produce myocarditis in newborn.)
      c) Diabetes in pregnancy suggests transposition if combined with high birth weight.
   3. Frequent pneumonias? (Suggests either large left-to-right shunts with increased pulmonary blood flow or severe pulmonary stenosis with decreased pulmonary blood flow.)
   4. Excessive sweating? (Sign of failure in infants.) Asthmatic attacks in newborn? (Suggests pulmonary edema.)
   5. Has mother been aware of infant's heart beating against chest wall or the vibrations of a thrill?

B. To be asked if patient is a child or adult.
   1. Mother's pregnancy: rubella in first trimester? (Suggests **patent ductus arteriosus, ventricular septal defect, atrial septal defect, tetralogy of Fallot,** supravalvular aortic stenosis, or pulmonary artery stenosis. Deafness and cataracts are the common noncardiac lesions.)
   2. Family history: congenital heart disease or murmur in family?

3. Cyanosis: When did it begin? (Cyanosis either from birth or within a few days of birth suggests transposition.) Delayed for years and associated with palpitations suggests **Ebstein's anomaly,** especially if present with little DOE. If delayed until adolescence or middle age, suggests atrial septal defect with **Eisenmenger's reaction** or [syndrome]. Does it occur with crying, feeding, or warm bath or only with syncope? (Suggests **tetralogy.**) **Differential cyanosis** and **clubbing**? (Suggests patent ductus arteriosus with Eisenmenger's syndrome, especially if there is unexpectedly little DOE.) Frequent phlebotomies?

4. Syncope or faintness? Do these signs occur on exposure to cold or only during effort or excitement? (Suggests **primary pulmonary hypertension.**) With straining after a long sleep and with cyanosis? (Suggests tetralogy of Fallot or *complete* **atrioventricular block.**) Only with effort? (Suggests severe aortic stenosis, pulmonary stenosis, or primary pulmonary hypertension.)

5. Angina? (Suggests severe aortic or pulmonary stenosis.)

6. Exact day the murmur was first heard? (Stenotic murmurs are heard in newborn nursery; left-to-right shunt murmurs are often delayed a few weeks.) Was it discovered by a physician who had seen the patient before or by a physician seeing the patient for the first time?

7. Squatting or knee-chest position frequent? (Suggests decreased pulmonary flow due to tetralogy of Fallot or, more rarely, due to tricuspid atresia.)

8. Headaches, epistaxis, leg fatigue or aches after exercise, cold legs, or claudication? (Suggests coarctation. Epistaxis alone suggests rheumatic fever.)

9. When and where was cardiac catheterization done? What were parents told of findings?

10. Dysphagia? (Consider coarctation, with the right subclavian artery passing behind the esophagus.)

11. Awareness of pulsations in the neck? (Consider coarctation, aortic regurgitation, thyrotoxicosis, or the venous pulsations of giant A waves in primary pulmonary hypertension or severe pulmonary stenosis.)

12. Strokes? (Consider emboli from endocardial fibroelastosis if patient is an infant, or emboli from idiopathic cardiomyopathy if patient is a child. May be due to paradoxical emboli or cerebral abscess if patient is cyanotic. Somnolence with cyanosis suggests cerebral abscess.)

13. Hoarseness? (Suggests primary pulmonary hypertension or large patent ductus arteriosus [14].)

14. Surgery? When, where, and by whom? What were the symptomatic results?

15. Mental retardation? (Consider **Down's syndrome** or supravalvular aortic stenosis.)

16. Swelling, pain, warmth, and tenderness of lower extremities? (Hypertrophic osteoarthropathy suggests patent ductus arteriosus with Eisenmenger's syndrome.)

17. Recurrent bleeding from the nose, lips, or mouth, with hemoptysis or melena, multiple cerebral symptoms such as dizziness and visual disturbances, and a family history of epistaxis? (This complex of symptoms comprises hereditary hemorrhagic telangiectasia or Rendu-Osler-Weber disease, and suggests a pulmonary arteriovenous fistula, especially if the patient is cyanotic.)

18. Weakness and incoordination? (Suggests the cardiomyopathy of Friedreich's ataxia or muscular dystrophy.)

FOLLOW-UP QUESTIONS

If Patient Says Yes to Dyspnea on Exertion

Orientation

1. What does the patient mean by DOE? (Some confuse it with weakness.)
2. When did it begin? Did it suddenly become worse after being the same for years? (If the patient has rheumatic heart disease, consider atrial fibrillation, ruptured chordae tendineae, pulmonary embolus, or acute infarction due to coronary embolus or thrombus. If there is a prolapsed valve, consider ruptured chordae.

Severity

1. How far can the patient walk on the level, uphill, or upstairs at a fast, normal, or slow rate before DOE occurs?
2. Has it made him walk more slowly?

Etiology

1. Failure:
   a) Effect of digitalis, diuretics, low salt intake, afterload or preload treatment, or cardiac surgery?
   b) Does the patient also have classic orthopnea, paroxysmal nocturnal dyspnea, or cough and wheeze on exertion or on assuming a supine position?
2. Anginal equivalent (SOB instead of angina [13, 16]):
   a) Does it last as long as angina (10–20 minutes)?
   b) Is it sometimes associated with chest tightness, pressure, or pain?
   c) Does it occur at rest?
3. Arrhythmias:
   a) Has the patient ever been told he has an abnormal rhythm?
   b) Did the dyspnea begin suddenly one day and persist (e.g., as if from a persistent arrhythmia)?
   c) Does it occur with palpitations or begin and end suddenly while resting?
   d) Has he ever checked his pulse with the SOB?
4. Anxiety or unknown cause:
   a) Has the patient ever had a "nervous breakdown" or a need for tranquilizers or a psychiatrist?
   b) Has he ever been told of hyperventilation or noticed overbreathing?
   c) Is dyspnea associated with numbness, tingling, dizziness, pain near apex of heart, cold perspiration, or palpitations? (This suggests DaCosta's syndrome or **neurocirculatory asthenia** [15].
   d) Is it relieved by a few deep breaths or by further exercise?
   e) Is it worse if the patient is upset, and is he helped by sedatives?
   f) Are there days without any dyspnea on heavy exertion?
5. Pulmonary disease or dysfunction:
   a) Associated with much weight gain?
   b) Asthma? Ever wheeze, especially with intense exertion? Told of asthma? Does he have more difficulty breathing out than breathing in? Is he helped by bronchodilators?

    c) Chronic obstructive pulmonary disease: easier to breathe leaning forward, smoking history, chronic cough with sputum? Has the patient had pulmonary function tests, or been told of emphysema?

    d) Pulmonary embolism: SOB, faintness, or syncope combined with either palpitations, hemoptysis, general chest or pleuritic pain, cold sweats, or phlebitis? Is patient on the contraceptive pill? Has pulmonary embolism occurred during pregnancy? Varicose veins? Recent long trip sitting?

    e) Pneumothorax: sudden dyspnea and pleuritic pain of chest wall or shoulder, without radiating into the arm, but with dry cough?

6. Severe anemia: has patient ever been told of any bleeding from menorrhagia, hemorrhoids, or ulcers, either occult or with melena? Sickle cell disease, bone marrow, or metabolic disorders? Pins and needles? History of gastrectomy? Treatment for anemia such as vitamin B_{12} or iron?

7. Compression of pulmonary artery or bronchi [29]? Lung tumor known?

If Patient Says Yes to Orthopnea

Orientation

1. When did it begin?
2. Spontaneous, or has patient been told by physician to use more pillows?

Severity

1. How many pillows needed?
2. How soon after patient lies flat is dyspnea noted?

Etiology

1. Trepopnea: difficulty breathing in the horizontal position but not due to heart failure.
    a) Due to cardiomegaly? Is the discomfort really due to the patient's feeling the heart beat on the bed when lying on the left side?
    b) Musculoskeletal, chest wall, or neurological disorders: is the discomfort experienced when the patient is lying flat due to neck or shoulder girdle pain, backache, or dizziness?

2. *High left atrial pressure:*
    a) Does dyspnea occur whether patient lies on back, left side, or right side?
    b) Is it improved by digitalis or diuretics?
    c) Does dyspnea occur if patient slips off pillows accidentally?
    d) Does dyspnea begin within a half minute of lying flat?

3. Markedly decreased vital capacity:
    a) Not completely free of dyspnea at any chest elevation? (Often seen in severe mitral stenosis.)
    b) Is patient dyspneic for less than a minute in the supine position and then feels all right? (Suggests pulmonary hypertension.)

If Patient Says Yes to Paroxysmal Nocturnal Dyspnea

Orientation

1. When did PND first begin?
2. How frequent is it (number of times per night, week, month, or year)?
3. Longest and shortest time between attacks?

Is It Due to Left Ventricular Failure?

1. How long after patient is asleep does dyspnea occur? (It usually takes about 2–4 hours for tissue fluid to enter and fill the intravascular space enough to raise the left atrial pressure to a high level. If rapid accumulation occurs, the patient will awaken within 2–4 hours and may have a recurrence the same night. If accumulation occurs slowly, the patient may awaken after 4–6 hours; in this case, another episode within a few hours suggests that the cause of the PND is not cardiac failure.) Heavy or light sleeper? (If patient is a light sleeper, PND is likely to occur sooner after falling asleep; it may not be as severe and may recur the same night.)
2. What must patient do to get rid of it? (If it is due to left ventricular failure, the patient must dangle, get out of bed or take a rapid-acting nitrate.)
3. How long does it last? Shortest and longest time? (It takes at least 10–30 minutes for fluid to be redistributed into the extravascular space.)
4. Is it accompanied by cough? If there is sputum, is it frothy or pink? Which starts first, the cough or SOB? (Chronic bronchitis patients may be awakened by a cough.)
5. Wheezing? (Demonstrate what is meant by this.) Is there a history of asthma in the family? Is it relieved by treatment for asthma?
6. Does it ever occur during the day when the patient is sitting or walking? (This suggests that you are not dealing with true left ventricular failure PND, which requires the sleep physiology.)
7. Related to amount of work or fatigue during the day?
8. Effect of digitalis, diuretics, low-salt diet, and afterload or preload treatment?
9. Does patient awaken for some other reason (postnasal drip, nocturia, palpitations, or trepopnea) and then notice the dyspnea?
10. Chest pain or tightness with PND? (If so, it may be nocturnal angina.)

If Patient Says Yes to Peripheral Edema

Orientation

When was it first noted?

Severity

1. Shoes too tight because of it? Does edema extend up to knees?
2. Effect of digitalis, diuretics, low-salt diet, preload and afterload treatment? When did treatment begin?
3. Gone in the morning?

Etiology

1. Cardiac causes:
   a) Helped by digitalis or afterload reduction? (Edema may be decreased by diuretics or low-salt diet, no matter what the etiology.)
   b) Other symptoms of low cardiac output (fatigue, dyspnea, or cold extremities) or high left atrial pressure?
   c) Edema preceded dyspnea by days, weeks, or months? (This suggests constriction or tamponade, especially if abdominal swelling preceded the edema, because venous pressure may rise for days, weeks, or months before cardiac output falls.)
2. Stasis or obstructive edema: began with weight gain, obesity or pregnancy, tight panty girdle, varicose veins, or phlebitis history? Is it unilateral? Is collar becoming tight and face swollen (superior vena cava obstruction)?
3. Hormonal causes:
   a) Premenstrual: associated with breast fullness, headache, and mood changes?
   b) On estrogen or contraceptive pills?
   c) Aldosteronism: hypertension, weakness, tetany, paresthesias, or high licorice intake?
   d) Myxedema: voice change, dry skin, absent sweating, cold intolerance, unusual sluggishness, weight gain, constipation, sleepiness, menorrhagia, diminished hearing, watery or puffy eyes? Treated for hyperthyroidism? Effect of thyroid hormone? Results of thyroid tests?
4. Lymphatic obstruction: foot fungus, prostatic carcinoma symptoms, abdominal swelling or mass? (Consider ovarian cancer.)
5. Intermittent idiopathic edema of women: emotionally labile, unrelated to menses, history of menstrual disorders?
6. Drug-induced: Is patient taking antihypertensives such as clonidine, hydralazine or Rauwolfia derivatives? Is he on nonsteroidal anti-inflammatory drugs such as ibuprofen phenylbutazone or indomethacin? On calcium blockers, especially nifedipine?
7. Renal: facial and hand edema, worse on awakening? History of renal disease?
8. Cirrhosis: history of alcoholism, hepatitis, or jaundice? Anorexia, fatigue, weakness, or ascites? Bleeding from varices? (If polycythemia vera is present, consider hepatic vein thrombosis as a cause of ascites [Budd-Chiari syndrome].)

If Patient Says Yes to Syncope, Faintness, or Dizziness

Orientation

1. What does the patient mean by "dizziness" (faintness, loss of balance, lightheadedness, blurred vision, sinking feeling, floating, spinning, unsteadiness, swaying, swimming, turning, giddiness, or vertigo)?
2. When did it begin?
3. How often does it occur? What is the longest and shortest time between episodes?

Etiologies

1. Epilepsy: How long is patient unconscious? Mind clear or foggy after? Prodrome or aura before attack? Begins with twitch of extremity? Sore tongue or incontinence after? History of head trauma or family history of convulsions? Were convulsions

seen by observers? Ever had EEG? Ever seen by neurologist? What antinconvulsant therapy has been tried?

2. Acute infarction: preceded by chest or arm discomfort, dyspnea, or perspiration? Hospitalized with "heart attack" diagnosis after?

3. Hysterical causes: never occurs when alone? Associated with paresthesias of hands and face, or always with dyspnea and chest pain (suggestive of hyperventilation)? Never injured self despite absence of prodrome?

4. Orthostatic due to peripheral autonomic fault: relation to body position? History of diabetes or sympathectomy or use of antihypertensive agents? History of prolonged bed rest or recumbency, or occurrence only with micturition?

   Other autonomic disturbances: nocturnal diarrhea, impotence, sphincter disturbances, peripheral neuritis, absence of sweating, worse in hot weather or if fatigued? Occurs only during pregnancy? On dialysis? Prodrome of faintness? Large varicose veins? On diuretics?

5. Excess bleeding: piles, black stools, history of anemia, menorrhagia, use of anticoagulants plus trauma to abdomen? (Ruptured spleen may produce symptoms as late as a week after occurrence of trauma.)

6. Vertebral-basilar insufficiency (syncope not a feature): vertigo, tinnitus, diplopia, dysarthria, dysphagia, unilateral or bilateral transient blindness, face, arm, or leg weakness, numbness and tingling?

7. Subclavian steal: symptoms of vertebral-basilar insufficiency with repeated arm movements; occasionally associated with syncope, nausea, fatigue, and headaches [4, 31]. Has the patient undergone a Blalock-Taussig operation? Claudication of hand and arm [10]?

8. Carotid insufficiency (syncope may occur): unilateral blindness, weakness or paresthesias, dysarthrias, or aphasias (lasting a few minutes to a few hours)?

9. Vasovagal causes: Preceded by nausea, weakness, or "sinking feeling" in epigastrium? Associated with acute fear or anxiety? Skin wet after attack? Pallor before or after attack? Associated with tight collar, head turning, or hyperextension of neck? (Suggests hypersensitive carotid sinus.)

10. Obstruction of flow through heart: Fixed aortic stenosis or pulmonary hypertension or stenosis is associated with syncope on exertion or with palpitations secondary to ventricular tachycardia or fibrillation. Hypertrophic subaortic stenosis or hypertrophic hyperkinetic cardiomyopathy with cavity obliteration is suggested by posttussive or postural signs, or signs occurring immediately after cessation of exertion (disproportionate sympathetic tone to decrease in venous return). Atrial myxoma is suggested by repeated fevers, embolic phenomena, or dyspnea with changes of posture. Raynaud's phenomena may precede myxoma symptoms [28].

11. Adams-Stokes attacks: is patient flushed after attack, subjective or objective? Told of slow pulse? Are attacks unrelated to exertion?

12. Pulmonary embolism: preceded by lightheadedness, with or without dyspnea [12, 24]?

13. Cough syncope, with strenuous cough (occurs in supine as well as upright position) [1]?

14. Hypoglycemia: Signs occur with perspiration, on empty stomach? Ever had glucose tolerance test?

15. Hyperventilation: numbness and tingling of hands and around mouth? Dry mouth and smothering sensation?

16. "Drop attacks" (sudden loss of postural tone without losing consciousness): Patient is a dead weight when someone tries to raise him up. Requires pressure on soles of feet to rise by self.
17. Stroke: followed by unilateral weakness or slurred speech?
18. Cardiac syncope: preceded by palpitations? Occurs with prolonged Q-T syndrome (precipitated by quinidine, disopyramide, exercise, fatigue, anxiety, sudden loud noise, and preceded by nausea or headache).
19. Sick sinus syndrome: slow pulse history? Palpitations? On calcium or beta blockers? Ever had pacemaker?

If Patient Says Yes to Chest Pain or Tightness

Orientation

When did it first begin? Under what circumstances? How often does it occur? Longest and shortest time between episodes?

Site

1. Ask the patient to show you where the pain or tightness is. Do not ask the patient to point. (If patient voluntarily points with one finger, it suggests nonanginal chest pain. If he uses a fist or sweeps across the chest, the pain is characteristic of angina.) Is the site typical for angina (e.g., retrosternal, in the neck or jaw, across the upper chest, radiating to the inner surface of the left arm)? Is it atypical but still possibly anginal (e.g., in the xiphoid, epigastrium, upper chest, down the lateral aspect of the arm extending to the triceps, biceps, pectorals, upper paravertebral area or left scapular area, and radiating down the right arm, with a heavy or lifeless feeling in the arm; or is the pain localized in the wrist, elbow, or even the right shoulder, or simply in the teeth area, like a toothache)?
2. Is there more than one primary site?
3. Character of pain: is it typically anginal (i.e., tightness, pressure, constriction, or squeezing sensation), or is it atypical but still possibly anginal (e.g., sticking, burning, aching, cramping, sharp, gaslike, or like indigestion)? Is it deep inside and tearing?
4. Is the pain probably nonanginal?
   a) Where is the pain? Note whether the patient points with one finger (a nonanginal sign). Is it superficial, as if in the skin?
   b) is there more than one pain? If so, ask about each one separately.
   c) Does the discomfort last over 30 minutes? If yes:
      1) How many times has it occurred (may be infarction if only once or twice)?
      2) With palpitations?
      3) After lying down?
      4) Repeated stabs over 30 minutes?
   d) Does the discomfort last less than 5 seconds? If yes, tap out 5 seconds. Under what circumstances does it last only a few seconds (with exertion or at rest)? How long was it there before he stopped walking or other exertion?
   e) Does it increase with one deep inspiration?
   f) Can one movement of an arm or the trunk bring it on?
   g) Does it disappear immediately when the patient lies down? (Increased venous return aggravates angina.)

h) Does it reach its maximum level immediately and then decrease, or does it gradually increase before reaching its maximum point?

i) Is it cardiac causalgia (i.e., does it occur only after myocardial infarction on left side of chest and shoulder and with hoarseness)?

j) Does the patient seek relief by walking around the room [27]?

Anginal Equivalent Possibility

This term has two meanings:

1. To some, it means pain only in the referred area. This is atypical angina, not an anginal equivalent.
2. To most cardiologists, it means only dyspnea without the pain. (Dyspnea accompanies anginal chest pain or discomfort in about one-third of patients with true angina.) Does the patient have DOE or dyspnea at rest that lasts 10 to 20 minutes and is not helped by digitalis?

Precipitating Causes and Severity

Effect of exertion (arm or leg), cold air, emotion, food, changing weather, sexual activity, lying on left side? Are there palpitations, for instance, awareness of heartbeat with the pain? (Some angina occurs only with arrhythmias and some arrhythmias occur only with vasospastic angina.) Is patient on tachycardia-producing drugs such as atropine or hydralazine? How much exertion is needed to bring it on (i.e., is it mild, moderate, or severe)? Is it coming on more frequently or easily (unstable angina)? Emotional problems at work or at home? Is patient hypertensive?

Associated Signs or Symptoms

Pallor, dyspnea, flatulence, nausea, vomiting, or sweating?

Relieving Factors

Are symptoms relieved by rest, sedatives, long-acting vasodilators, surgery, anticoagulants, antithyroid treatment, quinidine, beta blockers, or calcium blockers? Are they helped by nitroglycerin? Is nitroglycerin taken prophylactically or for symptoms? Side effects of medication?

Etiology

CORONARY DISEASE
1. General indications of coronary disease: Risk factors include diabetes, hypertension, sedentary life, artificial menopause, contraceptive pill (especially with smoking), high cholesterol level, **intermittent claudication,** heavy smoking, previous infarction, or family history of cardiovascular disease. Ever had gout? (About 16 percent of patients with gout will develop ischemic heart symptoms within 8 years) [9].
2. Unstable angina (may signify impending infarction):
   a) Without apparent cause, is pain coming more frequently, with less provocation, lasting longer, or occurring at rest in the past few days or weeks?
   b) Is pain associated with sweating, faintness, or dyspnea for the first time?
3. Is the pain vasospastic angina, variant angina, or Prinzmetal's angina? Does it occur mostly at rest, especially at night? Precipitated mostly by cold air? Are there good

months and bad months? Does it tend to occur at the same time each day or night, especially toward morning?

4. What does the patient think is the cause of the pain?

NONCORONARY CAUSES

1. Pericarditis: Is pain worse in supine position, relieved by leaning forward, or increased with inspiration?
2. Congenital absence of pericardium: Is pain relieved by changing position in bed, or brought on by lying on the left side? Lasts a few seconds or minutes?
3. Esophagitis or spasm: Is there burning pain, brought on by eating or lying down? Acid reflux into mouth (water brash)? Relieved with antacids or hot drink? Hiatal hernia seen on x-ray? Dysphagia? Nitroglycerine takes at least 3 minutes to relieve pain.
4. Root neuritis: Is there a past history of herpes zoster or back injury? Does nitroglycerin relief wear off in a few minutes? Is pain relieved or precipitated by certain movements of the chest or arms? With a herniated cervical disc, pain radiates to radial side of hand. Cervical root compression is relieved by nitroglycerine and is precipitated by reaching to touch the contralateral scapula and turning head away from that scapula.
5. Scalenus anticus or thoracic outlet syndrome: Are there paresthesias and pain along the ulnar distribution? Aggravated by abduction of arm, lifting a weight, working with hands above the shoulders, sleeping on side, or turning head? Is pain more or less continuous [2, 26]?
6. Costochondritis, myositis, or local neuritis: Does local pressure bring on the pain? This etiology is suggested by a history of herpes zoster or chest injury, Tietze's syndrome (painful swelling of costal cartilage): Is pain worse on coughing, or unilateral or localized to one costochondral junction, or helped by salicylates [18]? Gout: Is there a history of attack of gout with first episode of chest pain or preceding chest pain by many years? No radiation from anterior chest? Relieved by colchicine and not by nitrates? Lasts from minutes to days [11]?
7. Fixed cardiac output state: Is there a history of murmur or valvular disease suggesting severe valvular aortic or pulmonary stenosis? (Pulmonary hypertension is thought not to produce anginal pain [33].)
8. Inadequate coronary flow or oxygen supply not due to coronary disease or fixed cardiac output: Is there a history suggesting anemia, arrhythmias, or severe aortic regurgitation? (Nocturnal angina suggests aortic regurgitation or vasospastic angina.)
9. Prolapsed mitral valve syndrome: Is pain associated with lightheadedness, fatigue, and palpitations?
10. Aortic dissection: Does pain reach peak severity at onset?
11. Acute infarction: Site of pain is similar to patient's chronic angina or lower on chest, but pain lasts longer and is associated with perspiration, faintness, or syncope [27]. (If pain is confined entirely to left side of chest, it suggests posteroinferior infarction. If it is symmetrical across chest, it suggests anterior infarction [23].)

Diagnostic Tests

1. Electrocardiogram, resting or with exercise? Type of exercise test and results?
2. Coronary angiograms and results?
3. Nuclear cardiac tests and results?

If Patient Says Yes to Palpitations

Orientation

1. When did they first begin? Shortest and longest duration? Shortest and longest time between episodes?
2. How much do they bother the patient (i.e., will he still need medical treatment if assured that palpitations are harmless)?

Types and Rates of Tachycardia

Distinguish paroxysmal tachycardia from premature contractions.

1. Is tachycardia continuous or is there only an occasional strong beat? Is it regular or irregular? Ask patient to tap out the rate and rhythm. Did patient ever take his own pulse rate or was he ever told what his heart rate was?
2. Was he ever told of abnormal rhythm? When was last ECG performed?

Distinguish ectopic tachycardia from sinus tachycardia.

1. Does tachycardia have a sudden onset and end? (Atrial tachycardias may start suddenly but often end gradually because sinus tachycardia follows them.)
2. Does onset occur while the patient is resting, sitting quietly? Is patient ever awakened by it?
3. Does it always occur with exercise? (Suggests sinus tachycardia.)
4. Do pulsations in neck come and go? (A giant A wave of pulmonary hypertension or tricuspid stenosis disappears with atrial fibrillation. Cannon A waves occur whenever there is AV dissociation or retrograde P waves.)
5. Do any maneuvers by either patient or physician stop it?

Etiology

1. Much tea, coffee, alcohol, or tobacco? Any known precipitating factors?
2. Drug: on digitalis? Dose and type? On diuretics without potassium-retaining agents? On tachycardia-producing drugs, such as hydralazine, or anticholinergic ulcer drugs?
3. Is thyroid disease present? (See p. 7 for questions.)
4. Does flushing, headache, or sweating occur with it? (Suggests pheochromocytoma.)
5. Are symptoms changed or helped by change of body position, drugs, or vagal stimulating maneuvers?
6. Has patient been told of abnormal ECG? (Suggests **Wolff-Parkinson-White syndrome**.)
7. Is sick sinus syndrome present, with faintness or syncope, weakness, or fatigue? Has the patient been told of slow pulse? (Suggests bradycardia-tachycardia syndrome.)

If Patient Says Yes to Hypertension

Orientation

1. When was patient first told? Under what circumstances was it discovered?
2. Has treatment been taken regularly? What drugs in what dosage have been taken?

Etiology

1. Renal: Has there been a previous kidney infection or nephritis, or back injury in sport or accident? Frequency of urination or nocturia, polyuria, prostatism, kidney x-rays, renal calculi, gout, severe diabetes (Kimmelstiel–Wilson)?
2. Essential hypertension:
   a) Family history of hypertension?
   b) At what age was patient first told? (Essential hypertension usually does not become manifest before the fourth decade.)
3. Coarctation of aorta: cold legs or intermittent claudication, nosebleeds, shoulder-girdle pain? Have angiocardiograms been done?
4. Pheochromocytoma: flushing with pounding headaches, dizziness, sweating, palpitations, nausea, chest pain, and paresthesias? Weight loss? Elevated blood sugar?
5. Eclampsia: edema, hypertension, albuminuria, or convulsions in pregnancy?
6. Aldosteronism: episodic or continual weakness, tetany, polyuria (mostly nocturnal), polydipsia, or headaches?
7. Cushing's syndrome: hirsutism, corticosteroid intake, easy bruising, slow wound-healing, acne, muscle weakness, kidney stones, emotional lability or depression?
8. Hormonal causes: on contraceptive pills?
9. Hyperparathyroidism: peptic ulcer (calcium stimulates gastric secretions), renal calculi, constipation, lethargy, or polyuria?

Severity

1. Past blood pressure reading?
2. Visual problems, convulsions, strokes, headaches, dyspnea on exertion, orthopnea, PND, or epistaxis?
3. X-ray or ECG abnormalities known?
4. Amount and success of medical or surgical therapy? Side effects of treatment: muscle aches and cramps (from electrolyte imbalance), weakness, sleepiness, postural hypotension, nausea, nasal stuffiness, impotence, or palpitations?

NEW YORK HEART ASSOCIATION
FUNCTIONAL AND THERAPEUTIC CLASSIFICATION

This functional classification [5] refers to fatigue, dyspnea, or angina. The original classification is too long to memorize, and a simplified one follows.

Class 1   The patient is asymptomatic, or symptoms occur on extraordinary exertion. (There is no class 0, or classification for a patient with a normal heart.)

Class 2   Symptoms occur on ordinary exertion.

Class 3   Symptoms occur on less than ordinary exertion.

Class 4   Symptoms occur at rest or on slight exertion.

Note: The functional classification is easily remembered if one simply remembers the words *ordinary exertion,* because Class 1 simply adds *extra* in front of ordinary, Class 2 adds no words in front of ordinary, and Class 3 adds *less than* in front of ordinary.

The therapeutic classification also refers only to patients with abnormal hearts.

Class A   No restriction.
Class B   Severe effort restricted.
Class C   Ordinary effort moderately restricted.
Class D   Ordinary effort markedly restricted.
Class E   Confined to chair.

REFERENCES

1. Aaronson, D. W., Rovner, R. N., and Patterson, R. Cough syncope: Case presentation and review. *J. Allergy Clin. Immunol.* 46:359, 1970.
2. Adson, A. W. Surgical treatment for symptoms produced by cervical ribs and the scalenus anticus muscle. *Surg. Gynecol. Obstet.* 85:687, 1947.
3. Brockmeier, L. B., et al. Calcium emboli to the retinal artery in calcific aortic stenosis. *Am. Heart J.* 101:1, 1981.
4. Conrad, M. C., Toole, J. F., and Janeway, R. Hemodynamics of the upper extremities in subclavian steal syndrome. *Circulation* 32:346, 1965.
5. Criteria Committee, New York Heart Association. *Diseases of the Heart and Blood Vessels; Nomenclature and Criteria for Diagnosis* (6th ed.). Boston: Little, Brown, 1964, p. 114.
6. Daley, R. Massive dilatation of the left atrium. *Br. Heart J.* 44:724, 1980.
7. Darsee, J. R., and Nutter, D. O. Reversible severe congestive cardiomyopathy in three cases of hypophosphatemia. *Ann. Intern. Med.* 89:867, 1978.
8. DeSanctis, R. W., Dean, D. C., and Bland, D. F. Extreme left atrial enlargement. *Circulation* 29:14, 1964.
9. Fessel, W. J. High uric acid as an indicator of cardiovascular disease: Independence from obesity. *Am. J. Med.* 68:3, 1980.
10. Folger, G. M., Jr., and Shah, K. D. Subclavian steal in patients with Blalock-Taussig anastomosis. *Circulation* 31:241, 1965.
11. Frank, M., DeVries, A., and Atsmon, A. Gout simulating cardiac pain. *Am. J. Cardiol.* 6:929, 1960.
12. Fred, H. L., Willerson, J. T., and Alexander, J. K. Neurological manifestations of pulmonary thromboembolism. *Arch. Intern. Med.* 120:33, 1967.
13. Hagman, M. Relationship between dyspnea and chest pain in ischemic heart disease. *Acta Med. Scand.* 644:16, 1981.
14. Hornsten, T. R., Hellerstein, H. K., and Ankeney, J. L. Patent ductus arteriosus in a 72-year-old woman. *J.A.M.A.* 199:148, 1967.
15. Jarcho, S. Functional heart disease in the Civil War (DaCosta, 1981). *Am. J. Cardiol.* 4:809, 1959.
16. Kennedy, H. L., and Underhill, S. J. Ischemic ST segment depression and dyspnea. *Am. Heart J.* 89:544, 1975.
17. Lely, A. H., and vanEnter, C. H. Non-cardiac symptoms of digitalis intoxication. *Am. Heart J.* 83:149, 1972.
18. Levey, G. S., and Calabro, J. J. Tietze's syndrome: Report of two cases and review of the literature. *Arthritis Rheum.* 5:261, 1962.
19. Lewes, D., Rainford, D. J., and Lane, W. F. Symptomless myocarditis and myalgia in viral and *mycoplasma pneumoniae* infections. *Br. Heart J.* 36:924, 1974.
20. Marvin, R. F., Schrank, J. P., and Nolan, S. P. Traumatic tricuspid insufficiency. *Am. J. Cardiol.* 82:723, 1973.
21. McIntyre, K. M., Belko, J. S., and Sasahara, A. A. Pulmonary embolism: Premonitory signs and recurrence after vena cava ligation. *Arch. Surg.* 98:671, 1969.
22. Morgan, A. A., and Mourant, A. J. Left vocal cord paralysis and dysphagia in mitral valve disease. *Br. Heart J.* 43:470, 1980.
23. Nissen-Druey, C. Localization of pain from myocardial infarction. *Z. Kardiol.* 63:320, 1974.
23A. Ortner, N. Recurrenslamung bei Mitral-stenose. *Wien. Klin. Wschr.* 10:753–755, 1897.

24. Oster, M. W., and Leslie, B. Syncope and pulmonary embolism. *J.A.M.A.* 224:630, 1973.
25. Powers, P. P., Read, J. L., and Porter, R. R. Acute idiopathic pericarditis simulating acute abdominal disease. *J.A.M.A.* 157:224, 1955.
26. Riddell, D. H., et al. Scalenus anticus symptoms: Evaluation and surgical treatment. *Surgery* 47:115, 1960.
27. Short, D. Diagnosis of slight and subacute coronary attacks in the community. *Br. Heart J.* 45:299, 1981.
28. Skanse, B., Berg, N. O., and Westfelt, L. Atrial myxoma with Raynaud's phenomenon as the initial symptom. *Acta Med. Scand.* 164:321, 1959.
29. Varkey, B., and Tristani, F. E. Compression of pulmonary artery and bronchus by descending thoracic aortic aneurysm. *Am. J. Cardiol.* 34:610, 1974.
30. Walcott, G., Burchell, H. B., and Brown, A. L., Jr. Primary pulmonary hypertension. *Am. J. Med.* 49:70, 1970.
31. Williams, C. L., Scott, S. M., and Takaro, T. Subclavian steal. *Circulation* 28:14, 1963.
32. Wood, P. Polyuria in paroxysmal tachycardia. *Br. Heart J.* 23:457, 1961.
33. Zimmerman, D., and Parker, B. M. The pain of pulmonary hypertension: Fact or fancy? *J.A.M.A.* 246:2345, 1981.

2. *Cardiac Clues from Physical Appearance*

EYES

1. How does infective endocarditis affect the eyes?

   ANS.: a) Conjunctival hemorrhages and petechiae (due to bleeding tendency plus minute emboli). Evert lids to see these lesions.

   b) Oval hemorrhages near optic disk with white spot in center (Roth's spots).

2. Which cardiac condition besides hypertensive heart disease is associated with papilledema?

   ANS.: Hypoxic **cor pulmonale** with hyperpnea. In this case, it is due to high cerebrospinal fluid pressure with little elevation of jugular pressure.

3. With which cardiac lesions are cataracts associated?

   ANS.: They may be part of the rubella syndrome, and a persistent **ductus arteriosus** (PDA) and pulmonary artery (not valve) stenosis are the most common cardiac lesions. Other features may include deafness and mental deficiency due to microcephaly. The rate of growth may be slow.

*4. Which cardiac abnormalities are associated with **hypertelorism**?

   ANS.: a) Pulmonary stenosis (PS), especially in association with an atrial septal defect (ASD). Hypertelorism also occurs in **Noonan's syndrome** and multiple lentigines syndrome [4].

   b) **Hurler's disease,** or gargoylism, with mitral regurgitation.

   c) Supravalvular aortic stenosis.

5. Which kind of corneal arcus (circumferential light gray or yellowish ring around the rim of the iris) is associated with hypercholesterolemia or coronary disease?

   ANS.: A thick band that begins inferiorly and is inside the limbus, allowing a thin rim of iris pigment to be seen between the arcus and the sclera.

   Note: a) The usual "arcus senilis" is not necessarily associated with hyperlipidemia or coronary disease. It begins superiorly and extends to the rim or limbus of the iris.

   *b) An arcus may be absent or diminished on one side if there is reduced blood flow to that side due to carotid occlusion or previous inflammation [8].

Boldface type indicates that the term is explained in the Glossary.

*Material marked with an asterisk is for reference and for advanced students in cardiology.

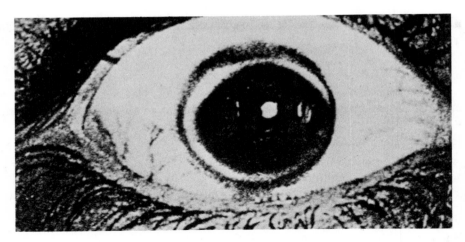

This type of arcus is a thick band of yellowish material surrounded by peripheral pigment and suggests a high serum cholesterol. It is not an arcus senilis, which has little known significance. (Courtesy Ayerst Laboratories.)

6. Which cardiac lesions are common in patients with the epicanthus of **Down's syndrome** (trisomy 21)?
   ANS.: **Endocardial cushion defects,** especially of the complete variety.
7. Which cardiac lesions should you suspect in the presence of an Argyll Robertson pupil (a pupil that reacts to accommodation but not to light)?
   ANS.: Luetic aortic aneurysm or luetic aortic regurgitation (AR) with coronary ostial stenosis.
8. Which cardiac condition besides thyrotoxic heart disease may be associated with exophthalmos?
   ANS.: Advanced congestive heart failure with high venous pressure and weight loss. The stare is probably due to lid retraction caused by the strong sympathetic tone accompanying the low cardiac output and exaggerated by the slight proptosis.
     *Note: Severe tricuspid regurgitation (TR) can even cause systolic pulsation of the eyes. A pulsatile exophthalmos also may be caused by a carotid-cavernous sinus arteriovenous fistula, in which case a murmur can be heard over the eyeball.
9. What cardiac lesions should you suspect if you see a tremulous iris (iridodonesis)?
   ANS.: This sign suggests Marfan's syndrome, in which the iris is not properly supported by the lens because of dislocation or weakness of the suspensory ligament. The cardiac lesions associated with it are aneurysms of the aorta or pulmonary artery and myxomatous degeneration of the aorta or mitral valve, with consequent regurgitation.
10. What are the retinal signs of various degrees of **arteriosclerosis** [18]?
   ANS.: Grade 1   The light reflex is increased in width (with minimal or no AV compression).
          Grade 2   Crossing abnormalities (arteriovenous nicking and right-angled crossings of the arteries over the veins).
          Grade 3   Copper-wire arteries (red color of artery is slightly brownish due to thick walls).

Grade 4   Silver-wire arteries (no red color is seen at all, only a whitish light reflex).

Note: a) The copper-wire sign implies that the light streak has become so wide that it occupies most of the surface of the vessel.

b) Hollenhorst plaques are flakes of cholesterol emboli seen as glinting spots, often seeming larger than the vessels in which they reside.

11. What are the retinal signs of different degrees of hypertension?

ANS.:   Grade 1   Generalized attenuation (arteriovenous ratio of less than 2:3 or 3:4).

Grade 2   Focal constriction or spasm.

Grade 3   Hemorrhages and exudates. (Exudates may either resemble cotton wool or be hard and shiny.)

Grade 4   Papilledema.

Note: Pure attenuation of the arterioles is best seen in toxemia of pregnancy or in young persons with rapid onset of hypertension. Minimal narrowing is most easily seen beyond the first or second bifurcation where the arteries actually become arterioles.

12. What is the significance of **xanthelasma**?

ANS.: Some (but not all) patients with xanthelasma have hypercholesterolemia [19].

*13. What three cardiac conditions are associated with blue scleras?

ANS.: a) Osteogenesis imperfecta is associated with AR.

b) Marfan's syndrome is associated with great-vessel aneurysms and mitral or aortic valve regurgitation.

c) Ehlers-Danlos syndrome, with its hyperelastic, fragile skin, hyperextensible joints and kyphoscoliosis, is associated with ASDs, tetralogy of Fallot, or regurgitant valves.

SKIN

General

1. Where should you look for tendon **xanthomas**? What do they signify?

ANS.: Achilles tendon, extensor tendons of hands, plantar tendons on soles of feet, and patellar tendons. Usually xanthomas in these sites indicate type II hyperlipoproteinemia (high cholesterol levels and premature coronary disease).

Note: Xanthomas in the palmar creases denote type III hyperlipoproteinemia.

*2. Which cardiac diagnosis is associated with the smooth, glossy, drum-tight skin on the fingers seen in scleroderma?

ANS.: Scleroderma may cause myocardial fibrosis or cor pulmonale due to pulmonary fibrosis.

3. What is the shoulder-hand syndrome?

ANS.: It is a sympathetic abnormality of the left (or occasionally both) upper extremities in which painful abduction of the shoulder is associated with swollen, painful hands and fingers. It occasionally follows infarction and coronary bypass surgery after several months. It has become rare now that long periods of immobility are no longer part of the treatment of infarction.

Skin Temperature

1. Which conditions besides thyrotoxicosis that affect the heart can cause warmer than normal skin?
   ANS.: a) Severe anemia.
   b) Beer drinkers' acute **beriberi.**
2. What cardiac conditions are suggested by cold hands or feet?
   ANS.: a) If hands and feet are moist, they suggest anxiety and may explain chest pains, palpitations, and fatigue as seen in **neurocirculatory asthenia** (Da Costa's syndrome).
   b) If only the feet are cold, and the patient has a history of **intermittent claudication,** peripheral arterial obstruction with poor collateral circulation is suggested.
   c) If cold extremities are relatively recent in onset (few weeks to a few years), a low output state is suggested.
   Note: The cold hands of the low output state can become warm when palmar erythema (liver palms) develop, secondary to cardiac cirrhosis.

Skin Color

1. How can you distinguish central from peripheral **cyanosis** clinically? What is the significance of this?
   ANS.: Central (blue or purple) cyanosis is seen in warm as well as cold areas. Have a nurse or colleague stand beside the patient and compare tongues. In black patients, the conjunctiva may show it. If the nails are cyanotic *and the hands are warm,* the cyanosis is central. (Definite central cyanosis is not usually recognized until oxygen saturation is lowered to about 80 percent [13].)

   Peripheral cyanosis is seen only in cool areas such as the nail beds, nose, cheeks, earlobes, and outer surface of the lips.
*2. How can cyanosis be increased in a patient with tetralogy of Fallot if questionable cyanosis is present?
   ANS.: a) By exercising [11]. This increases the right-to-left shunt into the aorta by dilating muscle and skin vessels, thus decreasing peripheral resistance.
   b) By inhaling amyl nitrite or taking a hot bath. This decreases peripheral resistance and favors flow from the right ventricle (RV) into the aorta.
   c) By crying. This increases pulmonary resistance and causes more RV blood to exit from the aorta.
3. How should you test for **clubbing** if it is equivocal or mild?
   ANS.: a) Look for obliteration of the normal angle between the base of the nail and the proximal skin [14].
   b) If you can feel the loose end of the nail root, clubbing is probably present. Your palpating finger must point in the same direction as the patient's finger, that is, you should approach the nail bed from behind and feel the edge of the nail root floating free while you depress the distal portion of the nail with another finger.

Note: No matter how severe the cyanosis, clubbing is rare before 3 months of age.

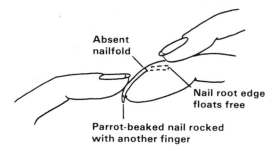

Absent nailfold

Nail root edge floats free

Parrot-beaked nail rocked with another finger

The earliest sign of clubbing is probably the reduction or absence of the groove where the root of the nail slips under the skin. Moist, warm fingertips are often associated signs.

4. What is *differential cyanosis*? What is its significance?

   ANS.: If the hands are pink and the feet are blue, pulmonary hypertension is present with a right–to–left shunt through a PDA.

   Note: Clubbing usually accompanies central cyanosis.

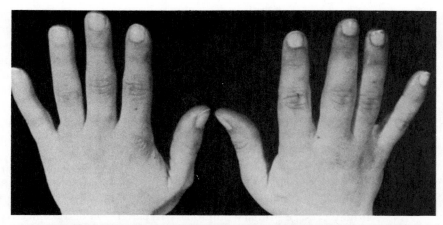

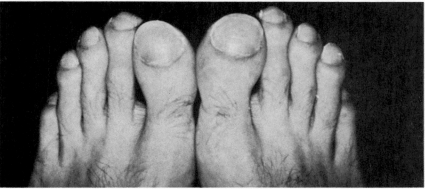

The feet of this 23-year-old man with a reversed shunt through a patent ductus were cyanotic and clubbed, while his hands were normal.

*5. What is suggested by differential cyanosis and clubbing in which the cyanosis and clubbing of the fingers are greater than those of the toes?

ANS.: This situation suggests complete transposition of the great vessels, with either a preductal coarctation or complete interruption of the aortic arch. Slightly less cyanosis of the left arm compared with the right favors coarctation rather than complete aortic interruption.

6. What causes cyanotic cheeks?

ANS.: The "malar flush" used to be considered a mitral facies. However, it can be seen in anyone with very low cardiac output and high pulmonary vascular resistance, high venous pressure, and loss of weight due to chronic heart failure (cardiac cachexia).

*7. What should you suspect if the fingertips are red?

ANS.: This picture is known as *tuft erythema* and may signify intermittent right-to-left shunts due to pulmonary hypertension and a balanced shunt, usually through an ASD.

8. What are the skin signs secondary to the small emboli of **infective endocarditis**?

ANS.: Clubbing, splinter hemorrhages in the nails (not specific for emboli), Osler's nodes (painful, tender, reddish brown raised areas 3–15 mm in diameter, occasionally with a whitish center, on the finger pads, palms, or soles), and Janeway lesions (painless circular or oval pink to tan macules about 5 mm in diameter on the palms and soles that do not blanch with pressure).

Note: a) Most splinter hemorrhages are not embolic; they move with the nail as it grows. Therefore, they are found in the nail substance and usually extend to the distal nail edge. Repeated jarring of the hand is especially likely to cause splinters. They occur in about 20 percent of hospitalized patients, especially in the right hand [5]. The splinter hemorrhages of infective endocarditis are subungual and usually do not extend to the distal nail edge.

b) Osler's nodes are confined to subacute bacterial endocarditis, but Janeway lesions are seen in both subacute and acute forms of endocarditis.

c) Livid reticularis-like mottling of the palmar or plantar aspects of the digits may occur in acute bacterial endocarditis [18].

9. What is the cardiac significance of **Raynaud's phenomenon**?

ANS.: It may presage primary pulmonary hypertension or a connective tissue disease such as scleroderma (cardiac findings include myocardial fibrosis or **cor pulmonale**), disseminated lupus erythematosus (mitral valve vegetations or acute pericarditis, as in Libman-Sacks syndrome), or polyarteritis (coronary artery obstruction and hypertension).

10. What cardiac lesion is suggested by brownish, muddy pigmentation of the skin and signs of hepatic failure, such as loss of axillary and pubic hair?

ANS.: Hemochromatosis with a cardiomyopathy due to intracellular iron deposits in the heart muscle, with secondary interstitial fibrosis.

*11. With which cardiac condition is jaundice most likely to be associated?

ANS.: a) Pulmonary infarction with reabsorption of pigment from broken-down red cells.

b) High venous pressure due to severe TR, secondary to pulmonary hypertension.

*12. What cardiac lesion is associated with multiple lentigines (i.e., multiple pigmented spots that, unlike freckles, begin at about age 6 and do not increase in number with sunlight)?

ANS.: Mild PS or hypertrophic subaortic stenosis [4, 21].

13. With which cardiac conditions may you see facial flushing?

ANS.: *a) Malignant carcinoid heart disease. The serotonin released from the carcinoid tissue in liver metastases can cause a blotchy, cyanotic tinge, which is often associated with abdominal colic and bronchospasm. The cardiac lesions associated with this condition are fused tricuspid or pulmonary valves.

b) If facial flushing occurs in the postsyncopal state, it suggests a **Stokes-Adams** attack. The high carbon dioxide levels and reactive hyperemia resulting from the arrest cause marked vasodilation when circulation resumes.

14. What is livido reticularis? What is its significance?

ANS.: This term indicates a marbling reticulation or fishnet type of mottling of the lower trunk, buttocks, and extremities, which is exaggerated by cold or emotional upsets; occasionally it occurs only when the patient is cold or upset. It occurs in about 20 percent of patients with lupus, periarteritis nodosa, or cryoglobulinemia. If it has occurred recently in a man over age 50, it suggests cholesterol embolization from an abdominal aortic aneurysm [10].

Edema

1. How should you demonstrate peripheral edema even if it is slight?

ANS.: Press on the skin over a bony area for 10 seconds with at least three fingers spread slightly apart, and feel (do not look) for valleys between hills after release. If "slow edema" is present, it will remain pitted for more than 1 minute; this is most likely (but not necessarily) congestive edema. If, however, the pitting disappears in less than 40 seconds ("fast edema"), the cause is almost certainly a low albumin level [6].

2. What should you look for to rule out cardiac disease quickly as a cause of peripheral edema?

ANS.: A normal jugular venous pressure is incompatible with a cardiac cause of edema unless diuretics have been given. Diuretics may lower venous pressure before the edema has had a chance to subside.

Note: a) Only presacral edema may be present if the patient has been in bed for some time.

b) Peripheral edema is a common complaint in normal subjects, especially in women during the premenstrual period or if they wear tight undergarments. It is expected in any obese person due to obstructed lymphatic drainage.

c) At least 10 pounds (4 kg) of body fluid must collect before pitting edema occurs [7].

d) Face and hand edema tends to rule out a cardiac cause.

EXTREMITIES

*1. What cardiac lesion is suggested by short stature and cubitus valgus (medial deviation of the extended forearm)?

ANS.: **Turner's syndrome,** with coarctation as a common abnormality.

> *Note:* When web neck, cubitus valgus, short stature, and hypogonadism are found in males, the condition is called Ullrich-Noonan's syndrome; pulmonary stenosis is the common cardiac abnormality associated with it.

*2. Which abnormalities of the extremities are found with ASDs?

ANS.: a) The thumb may have an extra phalanx ("fingerized thumb"), and it may lie in the same plane as the fingers, so that it is difficult to oppose thumb and fingers [1].

b) There may be distal radial and ulnar deformities, causing difficulty in supination and pronation.

> *Note:* If (a) and (b) are both present, this is the Holt-Oram syndrome, and the ASD is usually of the secundum type [7]. Pectus deformities of the sternum also occur [1A].

3. What hand and wrist signs suggest Marfan's syndrome with its possible cardiac abnormalities of aortic regurgitation or prolapsed mitral valve syndrome?

ANS.: a) Fingers: Slender and long ("spider" fingers, or arachnodactyly).

b) Thumb sign: When a fist is made over a clenched thumb, the thumb should not extend beyond the ulnar side of the hand. (False-positives of this sign occur in 1 percent of white children and 3 percent of black children.)

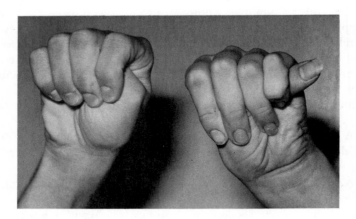

At left is a normal subject, who is unable to protrude his thumb beyond his clenched fingers, as can the patient with Marfan's syndrome at right, who can do this because of a long thumb and lax joints.

c) Wrist sign: When the wrist is encircled by the thumb and little finger (with light pressure), the little finger will overlap at least 1 cm in 80 percent of patients with Marfan's syndrome [22].

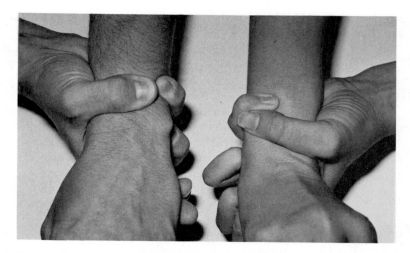

The normal patient at left cannot overlap his thumb and little finger around his wrist because, unlike the patient with Marfan's syndrome at right, his fingers are not long relative to his wrist.

*Note: A forme fruste (incomplete form) of Marfan's syndrome with kyphoscoliosis, pectus carinatum (pigeon breast), and long extremities may occur in homocystinuria, in which there may be thrombosis of intermediate-sized arteries, causing myocardial infarction.

*4. What is the only hand deformity ever correlated with rheumatic heart disease?
 ANS.: Ulnar deviation of the fourth or fifth fingers and flexion at the metacarpophalangeal joints. (This is Jaccoud's arthritis and is very rare.) The fingers can be moved freely into correct alignment [24].

*5. What cardiac lesions are expected in an infant if the fingers are clenched, with the index finger crossing over the third finger?
 ANS.: This is characteristic of trisomy 16-18, in which a ventricular septal defect (VSD) or PDA is common. Also associated is double-outlet RV.
 Note: The facies are abnormal (small mouth and jaw).

6. What is the commonest cardiac lesion associated with rheumatoid arthritic changes in the extremities?
 ANS.: Pericarditis and even occasional constriction.

7. What skeletal deformities suggest that an ejection murmur is due to an ASD?
 ANS.: a) Any skeletal deformity in Marfan's syndrome (see p. 30) suggests not only pulmonary artery or aortic dilatation but also an ASD.
   b) A prominent left precordium suggests not only that the RV was dilated during childhood but also that it was working against a high pressure. This deformity suggests that the ejection murmur is due to an ASD with hyperkinetic pulmonary hypertension.
   c) A thumb deformity such as a fingerlike thumb (three phalanges) or an extra-short thumb, combined with an ASD, is called Holt-Oram syndrome [39]. An ulnar-radial deformity that prevents good forearm supination or pronation may be present with this syndrome.

*8. Which cardiac lesions are expected with the Ellis-van Creveld syndrome (chondroectodermal dysplasia, an extra finger and often an extra toe, hypoplastic fingernails, and dwarfism)?

ANS.: About two-thirds of patients have an ASD, usually of the ostium primum type, or VSD and often a complete endocardial cushion defect or a single atrium.

Note: a) The upper lip of these patients is "tied" down to the alveolar ridge by multiple frenula. It is common among inbreeding communities such as the Amish.

b) The trisomy 13-15 syndrome also involves polydactyly. These patients tend to have a VSD, PDA, and dextrocardia with mental retardation, deafness, and cleft palate.

c) Trisomy 18 patients also have polydactyly; few of these patients survive more than a few months. Rocker bottom feet occur in about 25 percent.

*9. Which congenital syndromes involving heart and vascular abnormalities are also characterized by bradydactyly (short fingers)?

ANS.: Turner's syndrome, Down's syndrome, Ellis-van Creveld syndrome, and mucopolysaccharidoses.

HEAD AND NECK

*1. Which cardiac abnormalities are suggested by webbing?

ANS.: a) Turner's syndrome with coarctation.

b) **Noonan's syndrome** or Ullrich's syndrome with PS and, more rarely, hypertrophic cardiomyopathies [2, 16, 17, 20].

*2. Describe the facies of patients with supravalvular aortic stenosis of the nonfamilial type.

ANS.: a) Broad, high forehead and puffy cheeks.

b) Hypertelorism, strabismus, and sometimes epicanthal folds.

c) Low ears.

d) Upturned nose and long filtrum.

e) Long upper lip and a wide mouth, with pouting, "cupid's bow" lips.

f) Hypoplasia of the mandible, with pointed chin and many dental abnormalities such as small teeth [2].

Note: These patients tend to have deep, somewhat metallic voices, are active, and have a happy outlook [15]. Some are mentally retarded.

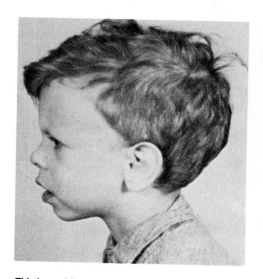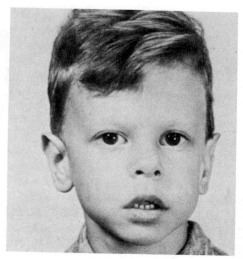

This boy with severe supravalvular aortic stenosis does not have all its facial characteristics; e.g., there is no hypertelorism or strabismus.

*3. What is the facies of some patients with severe pulmonary valve stenosis?

ANS.: Highly colored moon facies, as in Cushing's syndrome. This facies is found in about a third of patients with severe pulmonary stenosis. **Hypertelorism** is often found in pulmonary stenosis with ASD.

*4. What is the velocardiofacial syndrome?

ANS.: These patients have a long face, deep overbite, cleft soft palate (*velum* means palate), and broad nasal bridge, with VSD, tetralogy of Fallot, prolapse of aortic cusp, and right-sided aortic arch, as well as learning disabilities [23].

5. What is de Musset's sign (also called Musset's sign)?

ANS.: Head-nodding movements secondary to the ballistic force of severe AR.

Note: The sign was named after a patient, Alfred de Musset, a French poet whose nodding movements were described by his brother in a biography.

6. What is the facies of myxedema? What cardiac abnormalities are expected?

ANS.: Puffy lids and loss of the outer third of the eyebrows, scanty, dry hair and coarse, dry skin, expressionless face, and an enlarged tongue.

Note: These patients have cardiomyopathies due to increased interstitial fluid and mucoid infiltration. They also have pericardial effusions.

7. What is meant by an earlobe crease, and what is its significance?

ANS.: This is an oblique crease in the earlobe. Ninety percent of patients over age 50 with significant triple vessel coronary disease have a deep one. A unilateral ear crease was found in one study to be associated with an intermediate degree of coronary obstruction [12]. There is no relationship to blood lipids, increased blood pressure, smoking, or obesity in occidentals. However, in the Japanese it is associated more with obesity than with coronary disease [9]. Almost 50 percent of patients with diabetic retinopathy have a diagonal earlobe crease.

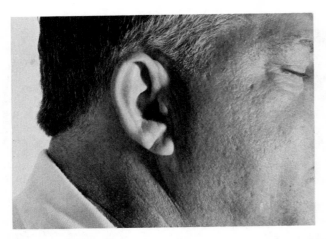

This 47-year-old man had this deep ear crease bilaterally. Although he had no significant coronary disease, his cholesterol-to-HDL ratio was 8 to 1, and he had sinus node dysfunction. He was about 50 pounds overweight.

CHEST AND RESPIRATION

1. What cardiac abnormalities are suggested by a **pectus excavatum**?
    ANS.: a) This may occur in **Marfan's syndrome,** with aortic or pulmonary artery aneurysms or myxomatous degeneration of the mitral or aortic valve with regurgitation. An ASD should also be suspected. (Pectus carinatum, or pigeon breast, may also occur with Marfan's syndrome.)
    b) It may be part of the straight back syndrome (see pp. 290–292).
    *c) It may occur in **Noonan's syndrome,** with pulmonary stenosis or occasionally with PDA.
*2. What should you suspect if only the left anterior chest area bulges?
    ANS.: An ASD with hyperkinetic pulmonary hypertension.
        Note: The RV never enlarges to the right—i.e., the right border of the heart on chest radiographs is never due to the RV, no matter how large it becomes, and RV enlargement never bulges the right anterior chest.
3. What should **Cheyne-Stokes** respiration suggest in a cardiac patient?
    ANS.: Very low output at rest.
4. What is the significance of a short breath-holding time?
    ANS.: It signifies either
        a) Chronic hyperventilation, or
        b) Poor psychophysical control of the breathing apparatus. The normal subject (with legs dangling) can hold his breath for 30 seconds with a little encouragement. Inability to hold it for at least 20 sec is abnormal and can explain dyspnea on exertion.
        Note: Chronic hyperventilation may be due either to a severe pulmonary problem, which should be obvious, or to emotional factors, in which case it could account for nondescript episodes of chest pain, faintness, and syncope.
5. What is a shield chest, and what does it suggest?

ANS.: It is a broad chest with a greater angle than usual between the manubrium and the body of the sternum, as well as widely separated nipples. In a female with neck webbing, wide carrying angle, and short stature (under 5 feet in height) it suggests Turner's syndrome and concomitant coarctation. In a male it is called Noonan's or Ullrich's syndrome and is commonly associated with pulmonary stenosis.

REFERENCES

1. Andresen, A. R., Christiansen, J. S., and Jensen, J. K. *New Eng. J. Med.* 294:1182, 1976.
1A. Antia, A. U. Familial skeletal cardiovascular syndrome (Holt-Oram) in a polygamous African family. *Br. Heart J.* 32:241, 1970.
2. Beuren, A. J., et al. The syndrome of supravalvular aortic stenosis, peripheral pulmonary stenosis, mental retardation and similar facial appearance. *Am. J. Cardiol.* 13:471, 1964.
3. Davies, H., Williams, J., and Wood, P. Lung stiffness in states of abnormal pulmonary blood flow and pressure. *Br. Heart J.* 24:129, 1962.
4. Gorlin, R. J., Anderson, R. C., and Blaw, M. Multiple lentigines syndrome. *Am. J. Dis. Child.* 117:652, 1969.
5. Heath, D., and Williams, D. R. Nail haemorrhages. *Br. Heart J.* 40:1300, 1978.
6. Henry, J. A., and Altmann, P. Assessment of hypoproteinaemic oedema: A simple physical sign. *Br. Med. J.* 1:890, 1978.
7. Holt, M., and Oran, S. Familial heart disease with skeletal malformations. *Br. Heart J.* 22:236, 1960.
8. Kaptein, E. M. Unilateral corneal arcus without carotid artery stenosis. *J.A.M.A.* 238:303, 1977.
9. Kaukola, S., et al. Ear-lobe crease and coronary atherosclerosis. *Lancet* 22/29:1377, 1979.
10. Kazmier, F. J., et al. Livedo reticularis and digital infarcts: A syndrome due to cholesterol emboli arising from atheromatous abdominal aortic aneurysms. *Cardio. Comp.* 1:56, 1966.
11. King, S. P., and Franch, R. H. Production of increased right-to-left shunting by rapid heart rates in patients with tetralogy of Fallot. *Circulation* 44:265, 1971.
12. Lichstein, E., et al. Diagonal ear-lobe crease and coronary artery sclerosis. *Ann. Int. Med.* 85:337, 1976.
13. Lin, Y. T., Yeh, L., and Oka, Y. Pathophysiology of general cyanosis. *New York State J. Med.* 9:1393, 1977.
14. Mellins, R. B., and Fishman, A. P. Digital casts for the study of clubbing of the fingers. *Circulation* 33:143, 1966.
15. Myers, A. R., and Willis, P. W., III. Clinical spectrum of supravalvular aortic stenosis. *Arch. Intern. Med.* 118:553, 1966.
16. Noonan, J. A. Hypertelorism with Turner phenotype. *Am. J. Dis. Child.* 116:373, 1968.
17. Phornphutkul, C., Rosenthal, A., and Nadas, A. S. Cardiomyopathy in Noonan's syndrome. *Br. Heart J.* 35:99, 1973.
17A. Proudfit, W. L. Skin signs of infective endocarditis. *Am. Heart J.* 106:1451, 1983.
18. Scheie, H. G. Evaluation of ophthalmoscopic changes of hypertension and arteriolar sclerosis. *A.M.A. Arch. Ophthalmology* 49:117, 1953.
19. Schrire, V., Beck, W., and Chesler, E. The heart and the eye. *Am. Heart J.* 85:122, 1973.
20. Siggers, D. C., and Polani, P. E. Congenital heart disease in male and female subjects with somatic features of Turner's syndrome and normal sex chromosomes (Ullrich's and related syndromes). *Br. Heart J.* 34:41, 1972.
21. Sommerville, J., and Bonham-Carter, R. E. The heart in lentiginosis. *Br. Heart J.* 34:58, 1972.
22. Walker, B. A., and Murdoch, J. L. The wrist sign. *Arch. Intern. Med.* 126:276, 1970.
23. Young, D., Shprintzen, R. J., and Goldberg, R. B. Cardiac malformations in the velocardiofacial syndrome. *Am. J. Cardiol.* 46:643, 1980.
24. Zvaifler, N. J. Chronic postrheumatic fever (Jaccoud's) arthritis. *N. Engl. J. Med.* 267:10, 1962.

3. *Peripheral Pulses and Pressures*

METHOD OF PALPATING THE ARM PULSES

1. Why is it best to palpate both the brachial and the radial pulses of one arm at the same time?

   ANS.: a) It speeds up the physical examination of the pulses.

   b) It reminds you to palpate the brachials, where you can more easily appreciate rates of rise, the bisferiens (double peaked) pulse, pulse volume, and the hardened vessels of medial sclerosis.

   c) It allows you to estimate the systolic blood pressure without a blood pressure cuff. (See p. 53.)

      Note: If a radial pulse is missing, it is probably due to arterial occlusive disease, as in thoracic outlet syndromes, or to a brachial cutdown used in the Sones technique for cardiac catheterization. You should feel for unilateral absence of the ulnar pulse. An ulnar pulse is not normally absent unilaterally, although it may be bilaterally absent as a normal variant [37].

2. How should you hold the arm for easy simultaneous palpation of the brachial and radial arteries?

   ANS.: Since the brachial artery is a medial vessel, it should be approached medially. The radial artery is a lateral vessel and should therefore be approached laterally.

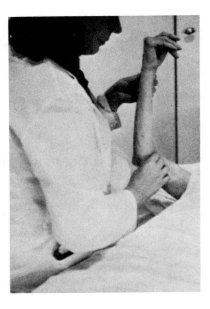

Simultaneous palpation of the radials and brachials speeds up the process and reminds you to palpate the brachials, where you can more easily appreciate rates of rise, the bisferiens pulse, pulse volume, and the hardened vessels of medial sclerosis.

---

*Material marked with an asterisk is for reference and for advanced students in cardiology.

3. When should you compress the brachial artery with the fingers, and when should you use a thumb?

ANS.: If the brachial vessel has a good volume, the thumb is preferable because

    a) The brachial may roll under the fingers; the thumb is better able to fix it.

    b) If more than one finger is used, a pulse wave may be felt to pass from the proximal to the distal finger, producing a false impression of a shoulder or even a double peak effect on the pulse. The fingers, however, are actually more sensitive than the thumb and thus are better for small pulse pressures or volumes.

4. Where on the arm should you feel for the brachial artery?

ANS.: In a younger patient, it may be hidden just under the muscle belly or tendon of the biceps. In older patients, tortuosity of the brachials tends to bring these vessels out medially, away from the biceps.

    Note: Some degree of elbow flexion is often helpful, because extension hides the brachial pulsations in some patients.

5. What are the questions you must answer as you palpate a peripheral pulse?

ANS.: a) What is the rate of rise (i.e., is it slow, normal, or fast)?

    b) What is the contour of the rise (i.e., is there a shoulder on the upstroke or a midsystolic dip, shudder, or thrill)?

    c) What is the pulse volume or pressure (i.e., is it small, normal, or large)?

    d) How hard is the vessel (i.e., does it roll too easily under the fingers)?

    e) What is the blood pressure?

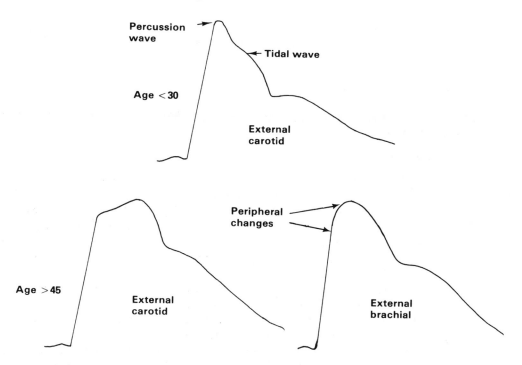

The normal percussion wave (first peak) is felt as a sharp tap. In the older age groups an anacrotic shoulder occurs, resulting in a late tidal wave which is felt as a further outward motion after the initial tap. More peripherally, the shoulder to a high tidal wave disappears.

*6. Why does the tidal wave increase with aging relative to the percussion wave so that eventually the percussion wave becomes an anacrotic shoulder on the way to the peak of the tidal wave?

   ANS.: The percussion wave is associated with flow rates and occurs during the peak velocity of flow; the tidal wave is controlled more by pressure and occurs at peak aortic pressures [90]. With aging, the velocity of the ejection may decrease, thus lowering the percussion wave. If the peripheral resistance rises, the tidal wave becomes higher relative to the percussion wave [66]. It becomes relatively low after the administration of amyl nitrite, which lowers peripheral resistance, and relatively high after administration of a vasopressor agent or with the decreased aortic distensibility of advancing age [34].

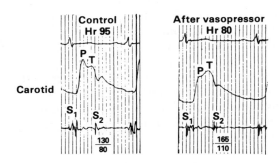

After an artificial rise in blood pressure, the tidal wave (T) becomes higher than the percussion wave (P), just as in older age groups and in hypertension.

RATES OF RISE

Normal Rates of Rise

1. What does the rise of a normal arterial pulse feel like to the finger?
   ANS.: A sharp tap with either light or heavy finger pressure.

2. When and how do you feel a change of slope in the arterial pulse in normal subjects?
   ANS.: In subjects over age 45 the straight upward rise often ends in a change of slope to a late peak known as the tidal wave. The change of slope is called the anacrotic shoulder and is easily appreciated only at the carotid. It is often necessary to vary your finger pressure on the carotid to bring out the anacrotic shoulder. When the correct pressure is applied, you will feel a sharp tap, followed by a more slowly rising nudge or push.

3. What happens to the anacrotic shoulder as you palpate peripherally (i.e., as you compare the brachial and radial pulses with the carotid pulse)?
   ANS.: As the pulse travels peripherally, the percussion wave upstroke becomes steeper and taller, so that the anacrotic shoulder tends to be attenuated and may disappear altogether [35, 84].
   Note: Although the carotid pulse low in the neck may have an anacrotic shoulder, this shoulder may disappear just a few centimeters higher in the neck. The cause for this disappearance is unknown. One analogy

that is used to explain it is that the increased resistance to the pulse wave as it moves peripherally makes it act like a wave coming into shore, that is, the crest of the wave becomes increasingly tall and steep because of the increased resistance due to the upward slope of the shore.

4. What have you ruled out by feeling a normal rate of rise and normal pulse pressure in a carotid pulse?

ANS.: There is not likely to be important fixed-orifice obstruction either at the aortic valve, just distal to the valve, or just below the valve (i.e., there is no significant valvular, supravalvular, or **discrete subvalvular aortic stenosis** (AS). There is also no moderate to severe aortic regurgitation (AR) because such significant AR would have an increased pulse pressure. However, mild obstruction or regurgitation cannot be ruled out by feeling normal peripheral pulses.

Note: An elderly subject with an aorta hardened by atherosclerosis may have a normal rate of rise in the peripheral pulses despite significant valvular AS. A rigid aorta apparently cannot expand slowly.

Slow Rates of Rise

1. How can you recognize a slow rate of rise by palpation?

ANS.: A caressing lift or a gentle push will be felt. There is no tapping sensation, only a push or nudge.

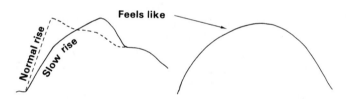

The normal rise is a tap; the slow rise is a caress.

Note: A slowly rising carotid may occasionally consist of a tap followed by a nudge or push. This merely represents a shoulder on the upstroke and requires practice to recognize. If you can elicit a tap, then check to see if the pulse continues to rise after it. Without these tests a moderately slow rise will be missed and called normal. This is the commonest error [99].

2. What conditions can produce a slowly rising pulse besides a fixed aortic outflow obstruction?

ANS.: Arterial stenosis proximal to the site of palpation.

3. List the names given to the slowly rising pulse of AS.

ANS.: a) Anacrotic pulse.
b) Pulsus parvus.
c) Plateau pulse.

4. What is meant by an anacrotic pulse?

ANS.: Anacrotic is derived from the Greek ana-, meaning "up," and krotos, meaning "beat." The literal translation as "upbeat pulse" has no meaning. By

Boldface type indicates that the term is explained in the Glossary.

usage, however, the term has come to mean any slowly rising pulse. Since the literal meaning is so different from the usage meaning, the term is best avoided.

Note: a) The terms *anacrotic shoulder* and *anacrotic notch* are useful terms to retain because they refer to a shoulder or notch on the upstroke.

   *b) It has been suggested that the lower the anacrotic shoulder in the carotid pulse, the higher the gradient across the aortic valve. However, a low anacrotic notch apparently may require a good stroke volume and pulse pressure [91].

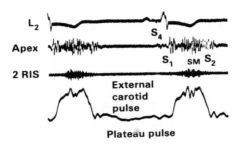

If an almost normal tap is followed by a sustained thrill, this is the plateau pulse of AS. In the above figure L$_2$ = lead 2, and 2 RIS means that the microphone was in the second right interspace.

   c) *Carotid shudder* is a term that was introduced to describe the very short vibration effect that occurs when a patient with combined AS and regurgitation has a double systolic outward movement. It is now known as a bisferiens pulse [27].

   d) A bisferiens pulse can occur in about one-third of patients with severe aortic regurgitation.

6. What happens to the height of an anacrotic shoulder in a patient with AS as you palpate more and more peripherally?

ANS.: The anacrotic shoulder tends to move higher and may even disappear if the AS is mild or moderate.

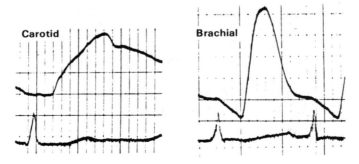

Carotid and brachial pulse contours in a patient with mild AS. By the time the pulse wave reached the brachials, it had become normal.

Note: If the AS is significant or the ventricular contraction weak, an anacrotic shoulder will not disappear at the periphery.

7. What does a slow rise of the carotid pulse (absent percussion wave) tell you about
the degree of aortic valve **gradient?**

ANS.: In the presence of a fairly normal myocardium, the gradient is probably over
50 mm Hg.

Note: a) If the patient has a **cardiomyopathy,** then even in mild AS there
may be a slowly rising pulse that may be transmitted as such even
to the periphery. If, however, the aorta is very rigid owing to
atherosclerosis, as in elderly patients, or if the patient is hypertensive, the percussion wave is exaggerated, and no anacrotic pulse is
felt [22]. A noncompliant aorta due to atherosclerosis often cannot
expand slowly [22]. In this situation only an ejection time will tell
you whether AS or a cardiomyopathy is the cause of the failure (see
pp. 416, 417).

b) If a hypertensive patient with AS has a normal rate of rise, lowering the blood pressure can bring out the anacrotic shoulder.

8. When will the right carotids and brachials have a normal rate of rise and the left
carotids and brachials a slow rise? Why?

ANS.: This situation occurs in supravalvular AS, in which there is streaming of the
jet along the ascending aortic toward the innominate artery.

Note: The pulses will also be stronger and the blood pressure higher on the
right than on the left, usually by about 20 mm Hg [36].

Fast Rates of Rise with Normal Pulse Pressures

1. In which conditions are there very rapid rates of rise but normal pulse pressures?

ANS.: a) When a large volume in the left ventricle (LV) is being ejected but
through two orifices (i.e., mitral regurgitation (MR) or **ventricular septal
defect** (VSD).

b) When there is enhanced systolic ejection due to delayed obstruction to
outflow, as in **hypertrophic subaortic stenosis** (HSS).

Note: A pulse with a rapid rate of rise but a normal volume is also known
as a "brisk" pulse.

2. Why is there an increased volume in the LV in MR?

ANS.: During diastole the ventricle receives two sources of blood from the left
atrium: the blood it would normally receive from the pulmonary veins, and
the blood regurgitated backward into the left atrium during the previous
ventricular systole.

Note: The same reasoning explains the large volume found in the LV in
VSDs, that is, the LV must eventually receive the blood it shunted
into the right ventricle (RV) and pulmonary artery as well as the
normal amounts that entered the RV from the systemic circulation.

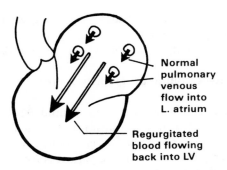

Normal
pulmonary
venous
flow into
L. atrium

Regurgitated
blood flowing
back into LV

This depicts the extra diastolic flow through the mitral valve that takes place when MR occurs during the previous ventricular systole. In MR, the normal pulmonary venous return to the LV is added to the returning regurgitant flow to increase the volume in the LV beyond normal. Thus, in MR, the left atrium is volume-overloaded during ventricular systole and the LV is volume-overloaded during ventricular diastole.

3. Why does the ejection of a large volume from the LV produce a rapid rate of rise in the peripheral arteries if there are two outlets for systole, as in MR or VSD?

   ANS.: The period of ejection into the aorta (ejection time) is not longer than normal in MR or VSD, that is, the LV does not take longer than normal to eject its forward stroke volume of about 60 ml into the aorta. Because the LV is actually moving a greater volume in a normal or even reduced ejection time, it must be moving both the forward and regurgitant streams at a very rapid rate. The LV accomplishes this rapid ejection through the stretched myocardium at the end of diastole, creating a **Starling effect.**

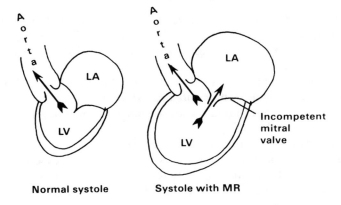

Normal systole   Systole with MR

Note that the arrows representing ejection into the aorta are equal, i.e., the forward stroke volume in MR is not reduced unless the MR is very severe or there is cardiac damage.

4. Why is there a rapid rate of rise in HSS?

   ANS.: In HSS there is no obstruction until the outflow tract contracts, approximating the septum to the mitral valve. (See the figure on p. 298.) When the LV contracts, the **inflow tract** contracts first and the outflow tract contracts last. In HSS early systole is so rapid that as much as 80 percent of ejection has already occurred during the first third of systole.

Note: Doppler flow studies have often shown a systolic M-shaped pattern with two peaks, one in early systole and one in late systole with a midsystolic interruption of flow.

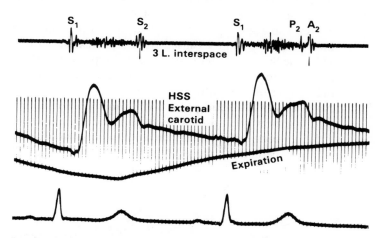

This is a phonocardiogram and pulse tracing from a 34-year-old woman with HSS. The outflow gradient was 70 mm Hg. Some mitral regurgitation was present. There was an S_3 on auscultation and a large LV on x-ray. Note the rapid rate of rise to a high percussion wave and the midsystolic dip that produce the "pointed-finger" carotid pulse contour.

* 5. How can a pulse pressure following a premature ventricular contraction (PVC) help to diagnose HSS?

   ANS.: In HSS the pulse pressure of the post-PVC beat is often the same or smaller than that of the normal beats. This is known as the Brockenbrough effect, and it occurs in only about a third of patients with HSS.

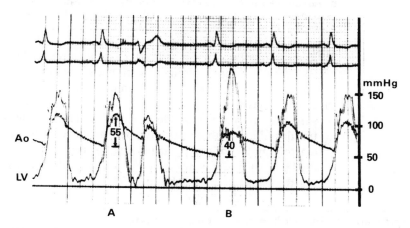

The Brockenbrough effect is seen in the postextrasystolic beat B, because the pulse pressure decreased to 40 mm Hg from 55 mm Hg during normal sinus rhythm A.

In normal subjects or in those with AS due to fixed obstruction, a PVC produces a greater volume and pulse pressure in the postextrasystolic beat due to the combined results of the long diastole, which produces both a

Starling effect and a decrease in afterload, and the inotropic effect of the premature depolarization (the **postextrasystolic potentiation** effect).

In HSS, on the other hand, the drop in aortic pressure that occurs by the end of a long diastole causes a loss of distending force for the LV outflow tract (mitral valve and septum) and produces more obstruction. Furthermore, the increased contractility caused by the postextrasystolic potentiation as well as by the Starling effect may cause the hypertrophied hyperdynamic septum to clamp down more tightly against the anterior mitral leaflet, thus producing further obstruction.

Note: a) On a carotid pulse tracing in a patient with HSS, the post-PVC beat will show a decrease in tidal wave even if the overall pulse pressure is actually increased as a result of an occasionally increased percussion wave [29].

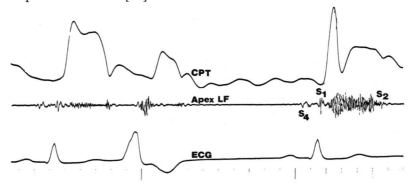

This is a carotid pulse tracing (CPT) and low-frequency (LF) phonocardiogram in a patient with mild HSS. Only after the PVC has produced its Starling and postextrasystolic potentiation effect is there a "pointed finger" carotid pulse contour characteristic of HSS. Note also the marked prolongation of the ejection time in the post-PVC beat. The Brockenbrough effect is difficult to demonstrate with an external carotid pulse unit because these transducers are slightly sensitive to rates of rise, so that the faster the rate of rise, the higher the deflection.

b) Even if the Brockenbrough effect is negative in HSS, the post-PVC beat will have a longer ejection time, whereas in valvular AS there will be a shorter ejection time.

c) In constrictive pericarditis there is also no change in systolic pressure after a long diastole due to a PVC. This is true because ventricular filling with constrictive pericarditis occurs rapidly in early diastole and is abruptly halted by the rigid, unyielding pericardium. Such filling is not time-dependent and cannot increase during the pause of a long diastole [52].

Rapid Rates of Rise with Increased Pulse Pressure

1. What conditions should be considered if there is a rapid rate of rise and a *large* pulse volume (the bounding pulse)?

   ANS.:   The most rapidly rising bounding pulses are found in AR, **persistent ductus arteriosus** (PDA), coarctation, thyrotoxicosis, pregnancy, and severe anemia. AR is by far the commonest cause of a bounding pulse.

*More rarely, a large arteriovenous fistula or a single great vessel arising from the heart (e.g., a persistent truncus or the large aorta in pulmonary atresia) may also cause a large pulse volume and rapid rise.

Note: A PDA is actually a kind of arteriovenous fistula.

2. Why should there be a rapid rate of rise and a large pulse pressure in AR?

ANS.: When the ventricle expands in diastole in AR, it receives not only the regurgitated blood that is leaking back from the aorta but also the normal volume of blood coming from the lungs by way of the pulmonary veins and left atrium through the mitral valve. Therefore, the LV receives a blood volume equal to the normal stroke volume plus the regurgitant volume. This volume from two sources stretches the LV at end-diastole to produce a Starling effect, which propels the increased volume into the aorta at a high velocity.

The increased systolic pressure is due to the increased volume ejected. But the increase in pulse pressure is also partly due to the low diastolic pressure usually found in patients with AR. (See p. 52 for an explanation of the low diastolic pressure in AR.)

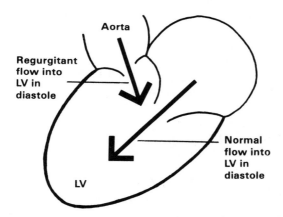

This illustration represents ventricular diastole in a patient with aortic regurgitation. The reason for the large volume in diastole in AR is obvious, since the LV fills from two sources. As long as the LV is healthy, it will eject the usual 60–75% of its increased end-diastolic volume, i.e., its ejection fraction will remain normal. Thus, the aorta will receive a large stroke volume with each systole.

*3. How can you exaggerate the rapid rate of rise of AR?

ANS.: By raising the patient's arm high or by having him stand up [40, 41]. (In subjects *without* AR, standing produces a decrease in the rate of rise.)

Note: In patients with AR, the increased rate of rise of the pulse on standing does not mean that more AR occurs on standing. The expected increase in peripheral resistance on standing should increase the amount of AR, but this effect is attentuated by the decreased venous return, resulting in no significant change in the quantity of AR [40]. However, AR is increased relative to the stroke volume.

Note: Another reason for the increased rate of rise of the brachial pulse on standing is related to the fact that the supine AR patient has more peripheral vasodilatation than normal. The low diastolic pressure seen in AR is mainly due to peripheral vasodilatation caused by a decrease in sympathetic tone. Therefore, the lower than normal sympathetic tone in the supine position changes to an exaggerated increase in sympathetic tone on standing because of the need for enough peripheral vasoconstriction to maintain mean pressure. The increased level of catecholamines or sympathetic outflow causes a more rapid rate of rise of the peripheral pulses [40].

4. What are some of the names given to the pulse in AR other than bounding pulse?

ANS.: *a) **Corrigan's pulse** [21].

*b) **Water-hammer pulse.**

*c) Collapsing pulse.

Note: Because the term *Corrigan's pulse* refers only to a visibly bounding pulse and not to what you feel, the term *water-hammer pulse* requires that you remember the name of an obsolete toy (see p. 443), and the term *collapsing pulse* omits the rate of rise, it may be best to call this a *bounding pulse*, or simply to describe it as a rapidly rising or slapping pulse with a large volume.

5. Why is there a large volume in the LV in PDA, creating a rapid rise and large pulse pressure?

ANS.: The LV receives both the blood shunted from the aorta to the pulmonary artery and the normal volume of pulmonary venous blood.

*6. When may severe AR not produce a large-volume pulse pressure?

ANS.: In sudden, severe AR, the stroke volume may be low or normal or only slightly increased because

a) The high diastolic pressure in the LV may close the mitral valve in mid-diastole, which limits filling from the left atrium, and

b) The LV resists dilatation when it is suddenly presented with a regurgitant volume, probably because the pericardium resists acute stretching.

Note: The pulse pressure is larger than normal in almost all patients with sudden, severe AR, but the systolic pressure is not usually higher than normal. The diastolic pressure tends to be reduced to between 40 and 60 mm Hg, and this is what increases the pulse pressure. In chronic AR, the systolic pressure increases because of the larger forward stroke volume.

7. What traditionally characteristic signs of severe AR can be picked up by auscultation of the femoral arteries?

ANS.: a) Traube's "pistol-shot femorals." This is the loud sound heard when the stethoscope is placed over the rapidly rising large-volume pulsations of the femoral artery.

Note: Venous pistol-shot sounds have been described as the loud systolic sounds heard over a femoral vein in the presence of severe tricuspid regurgitation [49].

b) Duroziez's double murmur. This is

1) The systolic murmur of excessive forward flow produced by placing the stethoscope chest piece on the femoral artery and gradually compressing the artery proximal to the stethoscope with your finger, plus

2) The diastolic murmur produced by gradually compressing the artery distal to the stethoscope. This murmur is due to backflow as the blood

in all the large arteries flows backward toward the aorta in diastole [11].

*Note: a) A double sound over the groin can be heard when a strong atrial contraction occurs. The first sound is from the femoral vein and the second is from the femoral artery [3].

b) These signs are of more historical than practical interest, because usually no more information is gained than that acquired from palpating the pulses and taking the blood pressure.

PULSUS BISFERIENS

1. What is meant by a bisferiens pulse?

   ANS.: *Bis* means "twice," and *feriens* means "beating," i.e., it is a twice-beating pulse. Actually, it is a double-peaked pulse, the two peaks occurring during systole so that there is a midsystolic dip.

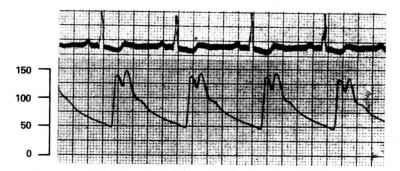

This bisferiens pulse was found in a brachial intra-arterial pressure tracing from a patient with AR. The midsystolic dip that produces this bisferiens pulse is due to the rapid ejection of the excessive volume in the LV.

2. What causes the bisferiens pulse in patients with an increased pulse volume, as in severe AR?

   ANS.: Because it is associated with a rapid ejection of blood through the aortic valve early in systole, one theory proposes that at the peak of flow there is a **Bernoulli effect** on the walls of the ascending aorta, causing a sudden fall in pressure on the inner aspect of the aortic walls. This theory is supported by the correspondence of the dip in pressure with the time of the peak flow rate through the valve.

3. What causes the most marked bisferiens pulse? Why?

ANS.: A combination of moderate AS and severe AR [116]. Moderate AS causes an extra high-velocity jet to be shot out, and this is exaggerated by an increased volume of flow due to the severe AR during the previous diastole. In 1945, *carotid shudder* was suggested as a term for this double-pulse movement [27].

Note: a) A bisferiens pulse will not be present if myocardial contractility is depressed [50].

b) About one-third of patients with severe AR have a carotid thrill instead of a bisferiens pulse [2].

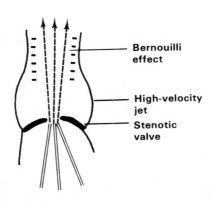

Bernouilli effect

High-velocity jet

Stenotic valve

AS + AR

The fall in lateral-wall pressure during peak velocity requires a high velocity of ejection. This implies the presence of a relatively healthy myocardium.

4. Can normal subjects have a bisferiens pulse?

ANS.: Yes, if the term *bisferiens* is used to refer to a very slight double peak at the height of systole. It may merely signify a hyperkinetic circulatory state. This slight bisferiens often feels like a short thrill at the peak of the carotid pulse. If it is subtle, it will be picked up only with just the right amount of external pressure on the artery.

* Note: A bisferiens pulse can be produced by an intra-aortic tracing only if it is marked.

*5. What kind of pure AS can produce a bisferiens pulse?

ANS.: Hypertrophic subaortic stenosis, because in this condition there is initially no obstruction to outflow. When obstruction occurs in midsystole as the mitral valve approximates the hypertrophied septum, there is a sudden dip in the pulse as the flow virtually ceases: this is often followed by a secondary rise as the LV overcomes the obstruction.

Note: a) The cessation of flow in midsystole can be shown by Doppler techniques.

b) The bisferiens pulse in HSS is often difficult to feel and is a relatively rare palpatory phenomenon. The midsystolic retraction seen in the external carotid tracing of some patients with the prolapsed valve syndrome is also usually difficult to palpate [6].

*THE DICROTIC NOTCH AND INCISURA

*1. What is the difference between a dicrotic notch and an incisura?

ANS.: The dicrotic notch is the post-tidal wave dip that occurs on a carotid pulse tracing. The same thing in an aortic pressure tracing is called the incisura.

*2. What controls the depth of the dicrotic notch?

ANS.: The distensibility and recoil ability of the aortic valve [93]. The absence of the incisura in severe calcific aortic stenosis is due to thickening and calcification of the aortic leaflets because little or no stretch or recoil can occur. In severe AR, the failure of the valve to close completely results in inability of the valve to distend downward into the LV.

Note: a) In children with congenital AS, the leaflets are fused but may retain their distensibility and permit enough recoil to produce a good dicrotic notch.

b) With increasing age, the level of the dicrotic notch becomes higher (i.e., it moves closer to the peak of the tidal wave).

*3. How can the dicrotic notch suggest significant AS in adults?

ANS.: Only about 2 percent of patients with a gradient over 50 have a distinct dicrotic notch [23].

*THE PALPABLE DICROTIC WAVE

*1. What is the dicrotic wave?

ANS.: This is the small wave that follows the dicrotic notch in an external carotid pressure tracing.

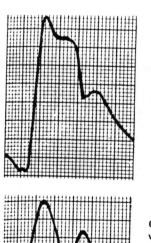

Normal carotid pulse

Carotid with large dicrotic wave

Short ejection time

At first glance, a large dicrotic wave gives the appearance of a bisferiens pulse because of the short ejection time seen in all patients with severe heart failure; the large dicrotic wave is usually seen only in such patients.

*2. When does a dicrotic wave become palpable?

ANS.: When there is a very low output, a soft, elastic aorta, and a high peripheral resistance. The commonest causes of a palpable dicrotic wave are

a) Severe congestive failure, usually secondary to a dilated cardiomyopathy.

b) **Tamponade** [72].

c) The low output state following open heart surgery, especially after aortic valve replacement for AR [5].

Note: a) A low stroke volume is important for the production of a palpable dicrotic wave; therefore it is more likely to appear or to become accentuated after a sudden short diastole, after the weaker beats of a pulsus alternans, in the straining phase of a Valsalva maneuver or the inspiratory phase of respiration, or when there is a pulse rate of over 90 beats per minute.

b) Soft, elastic blood vessels seem to be necessary to make a dicrotic wave palpable, as shown by the rarity of the palpable dicrotic wave when blood pressure is over 140 mm Hg and in subjects over 40 years old [72].

c) Occlusive pressure distal to the site of palpation will tend to bring out the dicrotic wave during inspiration.

d) A dicrotic pulse after open heart surgery for AR correlates with continued LV dilatation by echocardiography and decreased left ventricular function [75].

*3. How do you diagnose or recognize an excessive dicrotic wave from a carotid tracing?

ANS.: a) The dicrotic notch is abnormally low (i.e., 10 percent or less of the total pulse pressure [28]).

b) About 50 percent or more of the pulse pressure occurs from the dicrotic notch to the peak of the dicrotic wave [28].

PALPATION OF THE PERIPHERAL LEG PULSES

1. What can you learn about the heart from palpating the popliteal arteries?

ANS.: Vascular disease of the lower extremities is highly correlated with the presence of coronary disease.

Note: Obstructive disease of the carotids with an arterial murmur in the neck is also highly correlated with coronary atherosclerosis.

2. What is the most important aid in palpating the popliteal pulses?

ANS.: You must not try to feel a popliteal blood vessel, but instead must concentrate on trying to feel an area of transmitted pulsation. You may only feel this as a faint, diffuse pulsatile mass in a small segment of popliteal space. It does not feel like a carotid or brachial artery.

3. How do you examine for faint popliteal pulses with the patient supine?

ANS.: a) Place the fingers of both hands in the popliteal space with the palms of your hands in complete contact with the patient's skin including the anterolateral aspect of the knee. (Air over one part of the palm with skin over another part may prevent the detection of a faint pulsatile kinesthetic sensation in one area.)

b) Relax the muscles around the popliteal area by bouncing the knee up and down a few times.

c) Squeeze with the entire hand (i.e., with the thumbs as well as the fingers), so that the sensation is equal all through the hand. Usually firm pressure is necessary to feel the movements due to popliteal pulsations.

d) Slight dorsiflexion of the foot to stretch the popliteal artery may help to bring out the pulsation.

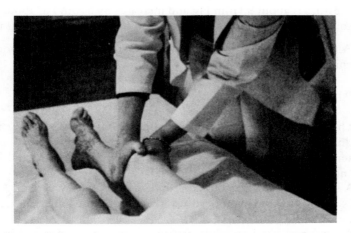

It will not be necessary to place the patient in the prone position if you remember that the key to popliteal palpation is to feel for an area of transmitted pulsation.

4. How can you sometimes bring out a faint posterior tibial or dorsalis pedis pulse?

ANS.: Maximum dorsiflexion can be used. Use two hands and dorsiflex the foot to various degrees with one hand as you palpate with the other [1]. A tendon passes diagonally over the dorsalis pedis, and the extensor retinaculum of the ankle crosses perpendicularly over it. Plantar flexion may tighten these overlying structures and obliterate the pulse. Dorsiflexion separates them from the artery beneath them.

Note: There are many normal variations of foot pulses. The dorsalis pedis may not be palpable in the usual line between the great toe and the index toe, or it may be absent in as many as 10 percent of normal subjects [51]. Normal adult subjects may have a palpable posterior tibial or dorsalis pedis only on one side. For this reason it is more important to document the foot pulses as a baseline for future follow-up in case peripheral vascular problems develop.

BLOOD PRESSURE

1. How do the heart and blood vessels control arterial systolic and diastolic pressure levels?

ANS.: Systolic blood pressure (the highest pressure reached by the arteries) is controlled by the stroke volume of the heart and the stiffness of the arterial vessels that receive the stroke volume. Diastolic blood pressure (the lowest pressure found in the aorta and its branches after maximal run-off into the periphery) is controlled primarily by peripheral resistance.

2. What is normal systolic and diastolic blood pressure?

ANS.: In the adult, the upper limit of normal blood pressure should probably be considered to be about 140/90 mm Hg.

  * In infants and children, you may use the rule that by age 1 year the systolic pressure is about 90 mm Hg and increases by 5 mm Hg about every 3 years, so that by age 13 or 14 it has reached the adult level of 120 mm Hg.

  A rough rule of thumb, then, would be that the systolic blood pressure in a child would be roughly:

$$90 + \frac{(\text{the age} \times 5)}{3}$$

  The diastolic pressure tends to be about 60 ± 10 mm Hg in infants and children of all ages.

3. What arterial abnormality can cause a rise in systolic pressure and leave diastolic pressure normal?

ANS.: A stiff aorta secondary to atherosclerosis in elderly patients.

4. Why does severe AS usually not cause a lower blood pressure than normal despite a low output?

ANS.: As the stroke volume falls, peripheral resistance rises and keeps the blood pressure normal. In very severe AS, however, a decrease in systolic blood pressure may occur as the patient progresses toward cardiac failure.

  Note: The highest blood pressure reported in severe valvular AS was 280/140 mm Hg [116].

5. How does AR affect blood pressure?

ANS.: The increased stroke volume causes a higher systolic pressure than normal, while the decreased peripheral resistance causes a lower diastolic pressure than normal. However, in young subjects with soft blood vessels, even severe AR may not raise the systolic blood pressure to more than about 140 mm Hg. In older patients with stiff vessels, even moderate AR may raise the systolic pressure to as high as 180 mm Hg. In hypertensive patients, the increased peripheral resistance can produce a normal or even high diastolic pressure despite severe AR.

  Note: The low diastolic blood pressure in AR is due mostly to the low peripheral resistance, which is presumably a reflex response to the large pulse pressure on the carotid and aortic baroceptors.

BLOOD PRESSURE DIFFERENCES IN THE ARMS

1. What should you suspect if the blood pressure is higher in one arm than in the other?

ANS.: a) Arterial obstructive disease may be present, either atherosclerotic or embolic, or it may be due to a thoracic outlet syndrome such as a cervical rib.

  b) It may be an artifact due to the lack of simultaneous recording.

c) If it is higher on the right, it may be due to supravalvular AS, which directs its jet preferentially up the innominate artery. The average difference is about 20 mm Hg [36]. A difference in carotid pulsation, as well as the presence of a murmur of AS, gives additional information. (See p. 32 for the facies of supravalvular AS.)

2. In what percentage of patients is there a difference of 10 mm or more in *systolic* blood pressure between the arms if the pressure in both arms is taken (a) separately or (b) simultaneously, if hypertensive patients are included?

ANS.: If the blood pressure is taken separately, 25 percent of patients will have at least a 10-mm difference in systolic blood pressure. If it is taken simultaneously, only 5 percent will have such a difference [45].

Note: When taken simultaneously only in normotensive patients, the maximum blood pressure difference between the arms was found in one study to be 20 mm Hg systolic and 5 mm Hg diastolic [107].

Note: If the history suggests vertebral-basilar insufficiency and the blood pressure is lower in one arm than the other, a **subclavian steal** should be suspected [102]. (See Checklist, p. 15.)

*BLOOD PRESSURE BY PALPATION ALONE

*1. How can you take a systolic blood pressure by palpation alone, that is, without a blood pressure cuff or stethoscope?

ANS.: While simultaneously palpating the brachial and radial arteries, apply slight, moderate, and marked pressure on the brachial in an attempt to obliterate pulse transmission to the radial. If only slight pressure on the brachial is required to obliterate the radial pulse, the systolic pressure is probably 120 mm Hg or less. If moderate pressure is needed, the pressure is probably between 120 and 160 mm Hg. If marked pressure is required, the blood pressure is probably over 160 mm Hg.

Note: If too little pressure is applied to the radial, the pulse will appear to be falsely obliterated. The radial should be palpated with enough pressure to give a maximum pulse pressure. If you do not apply pressure squarely on the the brachial but instead push the artery to one side, no amount of pressure on the brachial will obliterate the radial pulse. Comparing the pulse in both arms helps to prevent a false reading.

If the pulse pressure in the radials is too small, you will obliterate the radial pulse sensation too easily and may get a false impression of a normal or low blood pressure.

*2. How can you take a blood pressure reading by cuff (sphygmomanometer) and palpation alone (i.e., without auscultation)?

ANS.: With the thumb on the brachial just under the distal edge of the cuff, you can easily palpate the systolic pressure as the cuff is deflated and the pulse returns. As the cuff is further deflated toward diastole, the brachial pulse becomes increasingly more slapping and hyperdynamic, until it suddenly changes to a more normal rate of rise. This point of change correlates well with the diastolic pressure at about the time of muffling [26, 79].

Note: a) The diastolic point is difficult to appreciate at the radial pulse.

b) It is useful to obtain the diastolic pressure by palpation alone in subjects in shock and in those without a sharp disappearance or muffling point, as occurs in AR, when the Korotkoff sounds may be heard down to zero [26].

KOROTKOFF SOUNDS

1. What is meant by Korotkoff sounds?

   ANS.: These are sounds produced by the pulsations of the artery under a partially constricting blood pressure cuff (described by the Russian physician N. S. Korotkoff in 1905).

   * *Note:* a) Arterial-wall oscillations have been shown to be the major components of the sounds [103].

   b) Five phases of Korotkoff sounds are conventionally recognized: Phase 1, onset of tapping sounds; Phase 2, at a pressure of about 10 to 15 mm lower than phase 1, a murmur may be heard after the tap; Phase 3, reappearance of only the tapping sound; Phase 4, muffling; Phase 5, disappearance of sounds.

2. Does one hear the heart sounds at the brachial area?

   ANS.: Not usually. If they are very loud, they may be transmitted by bone conduction to that area (e.g., after vigorous exercise, and also prosthetic aortic valve sounds). Korotkoff sounds are *not* transmitted heart sounds.

3. What can make the Korotkoff sounds difficult to hear?

   ANS.: a) A slow rate of rise in the pulse wave, as in AS.

   b) Poor blood flow to the limbs.

   c) A small pulse pressure.

4. How can inaudible blood pressure sounds in a limb be made audible, or soft ones made louder?

   ANS.: a) Have the subject open and close his fist about 10 times, either before or during cuff inflation. If the popliteal or foot blood pressure is being taken, have him flex and extend the ankle. This increases flow and dilates the forearm or leg blood vessels. Thus it may increase the gradient of the blood volume and pressure between the proximal and distal cuff blood vessels.

   Note: This degree of mild exercising of the hand or foot does not alter the blood pressure reading.

   b) Elevate the arm before you inflate the cuff. This empties the arteries beyond the cuff, thus increasing the gradient between the arteries proximal and distal to the cuff [8].

   c) Inflate the cuff quickly. This minimizes the quantity of venous blood trapped in the forearm during the low occlusion pressures that are acting as a venous tourniquet during inflation before arterial occlusion pressure is reached. This decreases the tissue pressure distal to the cuff, thus increasing the flow gradient for the arterial blood passing under the cuff.

   * *Note:* A patient recording his own blood pressure will often get a slightly higher blood pressure reading than another person taking it a few minutes later or before. This result probably occurs because the patient may squeeze the sphygmomamometer bulb to inflate the cuff with the same hand as the arm with the cuff on it. This will make the Korotkoff sounds louder, resulting in a truer systolic blood pressure than if another person took the blood pressure [13].

5. Which is the true diastolic pressure, the point of muffling or the disappearance of the Korotkoff sounds?

ANS.: Comparative studies have shown that muffling occurs at a point about 10 mm Hg higher than the diastolic pressure obtained by direct intra-arterial needle [33]. The point of disappearance of the Korotkoff sounds is probably more accurate when compared with the intra-arterial manometer reading in the brachial artery beyond the cuff [62]. In hyperkinetic states such as AR, however, the disappearance point is often very low and also far from the muffling point. In AR, therefore, muffling is probably closer to the true intra-arterial diastolic pressure. In any condition in which the disappearance point is more than 10 mm Hg lower than the muffling point, muffling is probably the more accurate blood pressure reading. Recording both the muffling and the disappearance points aids in communication. Thus, a blood pressure might read 140/70–40.

6. What are the other advantages of taking the disappearance point rather than the muffling point as the diastolic pressure?

ANS.: a) It is easier to agree on where the disappearance point is than where muffling is. The muffling point has often been controversial because some people take a sudden change from loud tapping to quieter tapping, and others take full muffling as the diastolic point.

b) Because the disappearance point will give a slightly lower diastolic pressure, you are less likely to overtreat on the basis of a questionable blood pressure elevation.

c) Repeatedly clenching the fists can eliminate the muffling phase altogether, suggesting its unreliability [87].

*Note: The idea that muffling denotes diastolic blood pressure was introduced by Erlanger in 1921, in an experiment in which blood from the heart was pumped into an exposed segment of artery enclosed within an air compression chamber. As the pressure in the chamber was reduced, the Korotkoff sounds muffled just as the artery first became full and round throughout the pulse cycle. Low-frequency muffled sounds (fourth phase of Korotkoff sounds) continued for a further short period of decompression [33].

7. Is the systolic blood pressure higher by palpation or by auscultation?

ANS.: The blood pressure obtained by auscultation is higher because the Korotkoff sounds are heard with the slightest pulse movement at the edge of the cuff (at least 5–10 mm Hg higher than by palpation).

8. Why should you record blood pressure to the nearest 5 or 0 mm Hg despite the fact that manometer dials are graduated in increments of 2?

ANS.: Recording a blood pressure as 132 instead of 130 mm Hg gives a false sense of accuracy. It is unscientific because the significance of the last figure is not to the nearest 2 mm Hg (i.e., blood pressure is not accurate to the nearest 2 mm Hg) because:

   a) The National Bureau of Standards has set a figure of $\pm$ 3 mm Hg as the limit of tolerance for sphygmomanometers.
   b) The blood pressure changes by at least 2 mm spontaneously from moment to moment and may vary by as much as 30 mm Hg systolic and 20 mm Hg diastolic when continuous recordings are made during 24 hours [57].
   c) The Korotkoff sounds will occur at different levels of cuff deflation if different observers have differences in hearing acuity, deflate or inflate the cuff at different rates, have different concepts of the diastolic end-point, or place the stethoscope at different sites.
   Note: Blood pressure recorded with the patient in a recliner chair has been shown to be as much as 25 mm Hg lower in systolic and 20 mm Hg in diastolic levels than when the patient is dangling on an examination table. Sitting on a hard chair gave intermediate blood pressure readings [109].

9. What are the advantages or "bonuses" for being scientific?
   ANS.: a) It is easier to remember three numbers than six numbers between each 10 mm Hg. For example, between 120 and 130 there are only three numbers—120, 125, and 130—if you record the blood pressure to the nearest 5 or 0, but if you record the pressure to the nearest 2 there are six possibilities to remember, namely, 120, 122, 124, 126, 128, and 130.
   b) It is faster to estimate to the nearest 5 or 0 because it takes unnecessary time to try to be sure that you are exactly on a division of 2 when the Korotkoff sounds first appear or when they disappear because of the slight fluctuations in blood pressure that occur from moment to moment.

10. In taking blood pressure, where should you place the stethoscope chest piece in relation to the cuff?
   ANS.: As close to the cuff edge as possible, preferably partly under the edge of the cuff. The farther the stethoscope is from the cuff edge, the softer will be the Korotkoff sounds. A diaphragm placed completely under the center of the cuff produces the loudest Korotkoff sounds. Even if no Korotkoff sounds at all are heard at the edge of the cuff (as in patients in shock), they can be heard if the diaphragm can be placed deep under the cuff [118].

11. Should a bell or a diaphragm be used for Korotkoff sounds?
   ANS.: Because soft Korotkoff sounds consist mostly of low and medium **frequencies,** it seems logical to use a bell. But a diaphragm is preferable because it is difficult to get a good air seal on a rounded arm with a large-diameter bell, the edge of the diaphragm can be slipped under the cuff edge, and most diaphragms are not very efficient in attenuating low and medium frequencies.
   Note: When the sounds are soft, as when a patient is in shock, the bell may be preferred because the higher frequencies tend to disappear, and only very low-frequency components of the Korotkoff sounds may remain [67, 113].

*DOPPLER METHOD OF TAKING A BLOOD PRESSURE

1. How does a Doppler instrument detect blood flow?

    ANS.: A Doppler instrument probe generates high-frequency sound and also receives sound waves reflected back to the probe from moving particles. In accordance with the Doppler principle, motion in the path of the sound beam will alter the frequency of the reflected sound. When the instrument placed over a blood vessel receives reflected sound that differs in frequency from the transmitted sound, an audible signal is produced that is due mainly to the motion of the blood through the vessel.

*2. When is it especially useful to take blood pressure by a Doppler probe rather than by stethoscope?

    ANS.: a) In infants [48].

    b) In legs, especially when there is arterial occlusive disease, coarctation, or a low output state [17].

    c) In shock states [12].

    d) During cardiopulmonary resuscitation, to test for effectiveness of blood flow.

    Note: a) The blood pressure obtained by a Doppler probe can be accepted as nearly the same as that obtained by a stethoscope [106].

    b) Only a systolic BP can be obtained by Doppler.

SOURCES OF ERROR IN TAKING BLOOD PRESSURE

1. What is meant by an accurate zero recording for an aneroid (rotating needle type) manometer?

    ANS.: The zero recording is accurate if the indicator needle is within the zero circle on the dial before inflating the cuff. The manometer is more likely to be accurate if an accurate zero recording is present, but it still must be periodically checked against a mercury manometer.

    Note: About 15 percent of hospital aneroid manometers were found to be wrong by about 10 mm Hg when tested against a mercury manometer [78]. There appears to be no place for an aneroid manometer in office practice, where bulk is not a significant obstacle to using the more accurate and stable mercury manometer.

2. What precautions must be taken concerning the level of the brachial artery in recording a sitting or standing blood pressure in the arm?

    ANS.: The brachial artery must be near heart level. If it is much below heart level, gravity will add its pressure (equal to the hydrostatic column in the artery below heart level) to the brachial artery pressure.

    *Note: It takes about 90 seconds of holding an arm unsupported, before the diastolic pressure increases by about 5 mm Hg due to isometric contraction effort [96].

3. What is the advantage of decreasing the inflation pressure slowly when one is first beginning to deflate the cuff?

    ANS.: Spasm of the artery occurs on initial compression. Also, the patient may be anxious and apprehensive on feeling the discomfort of the pressure, causing the blood pressure to be too high. Slow initial deflation will allow spasm and anxiety to disappear by the time the blood flow occurs under the cuff.

> *Note:* Deflation of a mercury manometer cuff at the slow rate of about 5 mm Hg per heartbeat or per second is recommended, both to prevent missing the first Korotkoff sounds and to prevent negative pressure from forming above the mercury column. It will also enable you to detect a slight degree of pulsus alternans (see p. 60) and pulsus bisferiens (see p. 47).

4. What errors occur if the rubber part of the cuff balloons beyond its covering, or if the cuff is so loose that central ballooning occurs?

ANS.: Both will require excessive cuff pressure to compress the artery, and the readings will be falsely high [38, 74, 75A].

5. How does the blood pressure obtained with an average cuff on a fat arm compare with intra-arterial pressure?

ANS.: Because the cuff is too small, most often the pressure is too high, sometimes by as much as 100 mm Hg [7].

6. How can you overcome the small-cuff problem in a fat arm if there is no large cuff available?

ANS.: a) Place the cuff on the forearm and either auscultate or use a Doppler probe over the radial artery.

*b) Use the formula 32 − (1.05 × arm circumference in cm). If the number is positive, add it to the recorded blood pressure. If the number is negative, subtract it [68].

7. How can you determine accurately if the cuff is the correct width for the limb?

ANS.: For most adult arms it must be at least 20 percent wider than the diameter of the arm (multiply the diameter of the limb by 1.2). The cuff width according to the above formula should be at least 40 percent of the arm circumference.

> One study showed that as long as the width of the cuff is at least 12 cm, and the length of the bladder encompasses at least one-half the circumference of the arm, the reading will be reliable even for a fat arm when compared with intra-arterial pressure. This requires that the rubber bladder be placed over the brachial artery. Larger or longer cuffs were found to be no more accurate for the fat arm [14].

> *Note:* a) Several studies have shown that the ideal pneumatic bag bladder pressure is transmitted with the least delay to the underlying artery when the rubber bag completely circles the arm. Some studies have shown that there are no falsely low readings when unusually wide cuffs are used in the adult, and that the width may even be more than half the arm circumference. In the thin arm of a child, however, you should expect at least a 5 percent underestimation of the blood pressure if too large a cuff is used [38, 103]. Using the 12-cm cuff and an average adult it has been shown that a cuff width of 40 percent of the circumference of the arm will give the most accurate blood pressure. If it is 50 percent of the arm circumference, the underestimation will be 5 percent. If it is 30 percent of the arm circumference, the overestimation will be about 5 to 10 percent [38].

> *b) Maximum accuracy in pediatric age groups requires cuffs of several sizes. From birth to age 1, a cuff that is 2.5 cm in width should

be available. For ages 1 to 4, a 5–cm cuff is usually needed. For ages 4 to 8, a 9–cm cuff may be needed to achieve a width that is almost half the circumference of the arm.

*8. What is the effect of calcified brachial arteries ("pipestem" brachials) on blood pressure taken by cuff?

   ANS.: Medial sclerosis of the brachial arteries (Monckeberg's arteriosclerosis), may be severe enough to strongly resist compression by a blood pressure cuff. This could give a falsely high systolic pressure of over 300 mm Hg despite an intra-arterial needle blood pressure of only 130 mm Hg [98].

   Note: Studies that use femoral or radial intra-arterial pressures to prove that hard brachial arteries, as in elderly patients, produce a falsely elevated blood pressure by cuff may themselves produce falsely low intra-arterial pressures because of the effect of standing waves [98].

THE AUSCULTATORY GAP

1. Why is it often taught that we should start taking a blood pressure by feeling for the radial pulse and inflating the cuff until the radial pulse disappears?

   ANS.: This is said to be necessary in order to avoid the auscultatory gap.

2. Why should we discourage first feeling the radial pulse disappear to get the correct systolic blood pressure?

   ANS.: Because

   a) The auscultatory gap is eliminated if the Korotkoff sounds are elicited properly.

   b) It takes extra time to feel for a radial pulse and to note its disappearance in patients with low volume pulses.

3. What is meant by an auscultatory gap?

   ANS.: It is the silence caused by disappearance of the Korotkoff sounds after their first appearance. The gap ends when the Korotkoff sounds reappear at a lower cuff pressure level but before the diastolic blood pressure level is reached.

   *Note: The auscultatory gap has been said to occur only when there is venous distention in the arm. This is merely another way of saying that Korotkoff sounds may be faint when the tissue pressure is high distal to the cuff [81, 85].

4. What proof is there that the auscultatory gap is dependent on decreased blood flow to the extremities?

   ANS.: a) It can be induced in some elderly subjects with coronary disease by using a tourniquet above the cuff to decrease the flow to the arm [85].

   b) It can be eliminated by exercising the hand (repeatedly clenching and extending the fingers) for about 10 seconds before taking the blood pressure [87], by inflating the cuff rapidly, or by elevating the arm during cuff inflation.

*5. What kind of pulse contour is necessary before a reduced blood flow can produce an auscultatory gap?

   ANS.: An anacrotic shoulder, as in subjects with AS or in elderly subjects with sclerotic aortas or hypertension.

PULSUS ALTERNANS

1. What is meant by pulsus alternans?
   ANS.: This is an alternating fluctuation in pulse pressure (i.e., in every other beat, the blood pressure is lower).

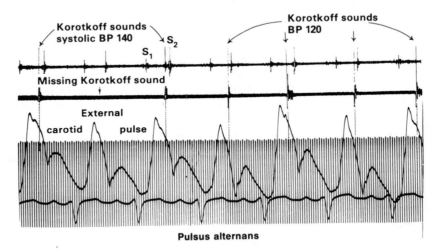

Pulsus alternans

The heart sounds are shown in the top line. The next line is taken with a microphone over the brachial artery distal to a blood pressure cuff. Note the doubling of the number of Korotkoff sounds when the cuff has been deflated from 140 to 120 mm Hg.

2. What is the significance of pulsus alternans?
   ANS.: a) It is usually associated with myocardial damage of the type that is either
      1) Severe enough to cause gross failure, or
      2) Mild but associated with LVH, as in hypertension or AS.
   b) It may be secondary to tachycardias even in a normal heart [58].
      *Note: An alternating pulmonary artery pulse has been seen in the presence of atrial fibrillation [39].
3. What can start a short run of pulsus alternans in a patient who either has been or is in heart failure?
   ANS.: a) A sudden increase in venous return, as with a deep inspiration or after a PVC in the postextrasystolic cycle [59, 60].
   b) A decrease in venous return due to onset of tachycardia or to sitting up. (Testing for pulsus alternans in the sitting position may provoke alternans when it is absent in the supine position.)
   c) Exercise [89].
      *Note: a) There is no significance to the disappearance of pulsus alternans at rest in a patient who has been or is in heart failure, because pulsus alternans may disappear with either improvement or worsening of the failure [89].
      b) If nitrates do not increase cardiac output in patients with heart failure, the decreased preload may cause the onset of pulsus alternans [18].
      c) Pulsus alternans is often first apparent only after vigorous diuresis with resultant decrease in venous return [55].

4. How much difference in pulse pressure is detectable by finger palpation?

   ANS.: Usually, at least a 20-mm Hg difference must be present between beats [58]. Because in pulsus alternans there is usually less than a 10-mm Hg difference between the beats, a blood pressure cuff is usually required to detect it.

5. What is the cause of pulsus alternans?

   ANS.: Three theories are widely held.

   *a) It is due to an atrial-carotid reflex started by a sudden strong or weak beat.

   *b) It is due to a sudden critical change in diastolic filling period [101].

   c) It is due to an alternation in the number of cardiac fibers contributing to each systole.

   *Note: a) The atrial-carotid reflex explanation for pulsus alternans is based on the concept that a sudden strong beat (as in a post-PVC beat) reflexly weakens atrial contraction by way of the carotid sinus, resulting in decreased LV contraction and a small carotid pulse, which in turn reflexly stimulate the carotid sinus to excite the atrium to a stronger contraction. The mechanism for alternation is thereby set up [92].

   b) Pulsus alternans has been reported in the pulmonary circulation and is associated with pulmonary embolism, primary pulmonary hypertension, and acute myocardial infarction [15, 31, 94].

   c) When an S_4 is present, it is louder before the weak beats [59].

6. Is electrical alternans (alternating differences in QRS configuration) associated with pulsus alternans?

   ANS.: Pulsus alternans occurs in only about 10 percent of patients with electrical alternans. (Electrical alternans is most frequently associated with large pericardial effusions.)

SUMMARY OF HOW TO TAKE ARM BLOOD PRESSURE BY LISTENING FOR KOROTKOFF SOUNDS

1. Ask the patient to extend his arm with the palm upward. This clarifies the position of the brachial artery.

2. Be sure that the center of the cuff bladder is over the brachial artery, and if you are using an aneroid manometer, make sure that the indicator needle is in the zero area on the dial before inflating the cuff. (A mercury manometer should be used in the office to avoid having to check and calibrate your aneroid manometer repeatedly.)

3. Place the diaphragm of your stethoscope partly under the cuff directly over the brachial artery.

4. Raise the cuff pressure to a reasonable level, such as 140 mm Hg, with the arm at heart level and listen for Korotkoff sounds. If they are present at 140 mm Hg, pump the cuff up another 20 mm Hg. Repeat the listening and pumping until no Korotkoff sounds are heard. (This avoids applying excessive and painful pressure and shortens the time taken to reach systolic pressure.)

5. If the Korotkoff sounds are very soft, eliminate any auscultatory gap by having the patient open and close his hand about ten times, raising the arm up at 45 degrees or higher before inflating the cuff and pumping up the bladder quickly.

6. Deflate the cuff at a rate of about 5 mm Hg per heartbeat or per second until the first Korotkoff sounds are heard. This is the systolic blood pressure, and it should be read to the nearest 5 or 0 mm Hg.
7. Listen for pulsus alternans. This requires slow cuff deflation when the first Korotkoff sound is detected.
8. Deflate the cuff further until muffling is heard. Then deflate further until the Korotkoff sounds disappear. If the difference in pressure between the muffling point and the disappearance point is less than 10 mm Hg, report the disappearance point as the diastolic pressure. If, however, the difference is greater than 10 mm Hg, report both numbers (to the nearest 5 or 0 mm Hg).
9. If the arm is so fat that the cuff width or bladder length is less than 40 percent of arm circumference, use a thigh cuff. If no thigh cuff is available, use an arm cuff above the radial artery.

BLOOD PRESSURE AND PULSES IN THE LEGS

Normal Pressures

1. How does the blood pressure in the legs compare with that in the arms?
   ANS.: It depends on the cuff size used, which leg artery is occluded, and on whether the pressure is measured by an intra-arterial needle, by Korotkoff sounds, or by Doppler techniques. With a proper size cuff over the thigh, the popliteal systolic pressure in adults should be either the same or as much as 20 mm higher than in the arms. In children the pressure in the popliteal artery is usually about 10 mm Hg higher than the pressure in the arms [75]. If the systolic pressure in the legs is lower than that in the arms, occlusive disease anywhere beyond the origin of the subclavian arteries should be suspected [16, 30, 117].
   Note: a) By Doppler methods, with the cuff placed above the malleolus, the blood pressure in the foot vessels is normally only slightly higher than that in the brachials [117].
      *b) If an intra-arterial manometer in the femoral artery is used, the systolic and diastolic pressure in the legs is usually the same as that in the arms [9, 76, 77].
2. What happens to the popliteal blood pressure if the thigh cuff is too short?
   ANS.: If there is not enough length to overlap the edges so that you can double the thickness of the edges, the edges of the bladder will bulge at the sides when the cuff is inflated, so that less of the cuff will be in contact with the skin. This will require more pressure to compress the artery, and the blood pressure will appear too high.
     *Note: The blood pressure reading can tell you that the cuff is too small for the thigh because with a proper size cuff, even though the systolic pressure may normally be higher in the leg, the diastolic pressure tends to remain the same as in the arm. Thus, if the diastolic pressure is higher in the leg than in the arm, the cuff is probably too small.
3. Where is the most reliable place to auscultate for blood pressure in the legs?
   ANS.: Over the popliteal artery, with a large cuff on the thigh.

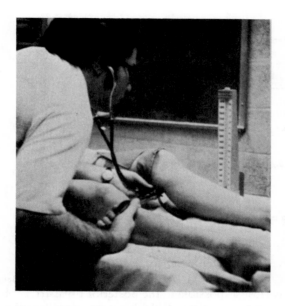

The usual commercial leg cuff, such as that shown here, must be rolled diagonally around the thigh to keep the edges snug against the skin. The systolic blood pressure in the legs should not be over 20 mm Hg higher than in the arms and should not be lower.

* *Note:* a) In severe AS, the slow rate of rise may make it impossible to hear Korotkoff sounds in the popliteals because the audibility of the sounds depends partly on the rate of rise.

        b) Compressing the thigh with a blood pressure cuff can cause enough discomfort to cause a false elevation of pressure. When accurate comparison with the brachials is necessary, as in patients with suspected coarctation or aortic regurgitation, the arm and thigh measurements should be done by two persons simultaneously.

4. How can you fit a cylindrical cuff to the usual conical thigh?

    ANS.: It is impossible to make an exact fit. Therefore, you must use a spiral occlusion cuff, an extra-large cuff, or an extra-thick cuff.

      * *Note:* With a sickle-shaped leg cuff you can achieve an exact fit. A second-best method is to use either an extra-large cuff, so that the edges can be well doubled, or an extra-thick canvaslike material that cannot bulge easily.

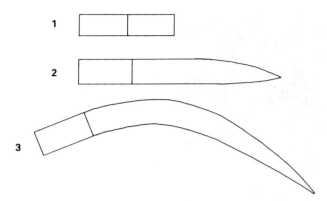

1. Arm cuff. 2. Commercial leg cuff. 3. Curved leg cuff to fit conical thigh and long enough for obese patient.

5. How is a blood pressure taken in the lower legs?

   ANS.: Place an ordinary arm cuff over the lower part of the calf, just above the malleolus (i.e., as close as possible to the posterior tibial artery) but without including the protuberance of the malleolus. Use a small (pediatric) bell to auscultate the posterior tibial artery. If no Korotkoff sounds are audible, auscultate or palpate the dorsalis pedis instead. If no Korotkoff sounds are present over any foot artery, the Doppler method of taking a blood pressure can be used (see p. 57).

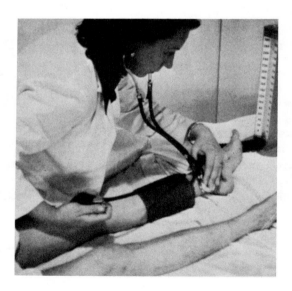

A convenient method of taking a leg pressure if you do not have a thigh cuff. A pediatric bell should be used to achieve an easy air seal behind the medial malleolus.

6. What are the advantages of using the foot for taking blood pressure in a lower limb?

   ANS.: a) No special size or shape of cuff is necessary.

b) It is more comfortable for the patient. About 1 in 3 patients will complain of pains with the thigh cuff.

7. What are the disadvantages of using the foot rather than the thigh for taking a blood pressure?

ANS.: a) No Korotkoff sounds can be elicited in about 10 percent of patients over the posterior tibial or dorsalis pedis.

b) Marked peripheral constriction, as in a cold room, may cause the blood pressure to be as much as 50 mm Hg lower in the foot than in the arm.

8. How is blood pressure taken in an infant?

ANS.: a) By the flush method: The limb is raised until it is blanched (some bind the forearm with a bandage to empty it of blood first). Then the cuff is inflated. The first distal flush as the cuff is deflated is read as the mean pressure.

b) By Doppler ultrasound and a cuff about 2.5 cm wide (see p. 57 for a description of Doppler sounds).

LEG BLOOD PRESSURE IN AORTIC REGURGITATION

1. How does AR affect the blood pressure in the legs in comparison with that in the arms? What is this sign of AR called?

ANS.: AR exaggerates the tendency for the leg systolic pressure to be higher than that in the arms. If the difference in greater than normal, it is known as a Hill's sign [47].

Note: It is easy to remember because blood pressure increases, i.e., goes "uphill" in AR as the examiner goes down the body.

2. Why is the cuff systolic pressure in AR higher in the legs than in the arms?

ANS.: One theory is that the increased forward initial flinging of blood through the aortic valve causes a percussion wave that builds up as it moves peripherally against resistance, just as an ocean wave often becomes higher and higher as it approaches shore. Another theory is that reflected waves from the periphery summate with forward waves. These summated waves are known as standing waves.

*Note: Intra-arterial pressure measurements have not always shown this difference in blood pressure [77]. It is not due to too small a cuff for the leg, because a higher pressure in the leg in AR can be elicited with a large sickle-shaped cuff on the thigh or an ordinary arm cuff above the malleolus. It is more likely that standing waves cause pressures that are always higher in some parts of the arterial system than in others so that the femoral arteries may always have a lower systolic pressure than the popliteals, even in patients with AR. In a dog, if a catheter is withdrawn from the arch of the aorta to the lower extremities, the iliac pressure will be seen to be 20 mm Hg higher than that in the proximal part of the aorta, and the femoral artery pressure is then seen to be lower than that in the iliacs. Therefore, if it is femoral arterial catheter pressures that are always compared with brachial pressures, then no Hill's sign will be found.

3. Can Hill's sign be used to grade the severity of AR?

ANS.: Yes, roughly. In mild AR the difference is up to 20 mm Hg (i.e., the difference is in the normal range). In moderate AR the difference is 20 to 40 mm Hg; in severe AR the difference is over 60 mm Hg. A difference of between 40 and 60 mm Hg may represent either moderate or severe AR [32].

4. What produces a falsely low Hill's sign (i.e., less difference is found between the arms and the legs than would be expected from the severity of the AR)?

ANS.: a) Congestive heart failure, presumably because of the poor stroke volume. A positive Hill's sign may depend, at least in part, on a strong myocardial contraction.

b) Significant AS.

   Note: Mild AS will not eliminate the normal brachial-popliteal gradient usually found by the Korotkoff sounds method.

THE LEG PULSES AND BLOOD PRESSURE IN COARCTATION OF THE AORTA

1. When should you suspect coarctation of the aorta?

ANS.: In any patient with hypertension.

2. What are the characteristics of the pulses proximal to and beyond an aortic coarctation?

ANS.: The proximal pulses, that is, the carotid and brachial pulses, are large, bounding, fast-rising pulses. The parts of the body beyond the coarctation (i.e., usually beyond the left subclavian artery) receive blood through enlarged collaterals that do not transmit the percussion wave well. Therefore, not only do the lower extremity pulses have a low pulse pressure, but also their rate of rise is slow and they have a late peak, that is, the pulse wave is almost purely a tidal wave.

   Note: In infants and children with coarctation the diastolic pressure in the brachials is normal despite a higher than normal systolic pressure.

3. If the onsets of the femoral and radial pulses are almost simultaneous, what causes the sensation of the delayed peak in the femorals?

ANS.: Because of the decreased initial flow rate through the femorals, their percussion wave is so low that only the tidal wave is felt in the femorals. In the radials, the usual percussion wave is easily felt because there is no obstruction to flow, and the velocity of flow and pulse pressure are increased due to their position proximal to the coarctation.

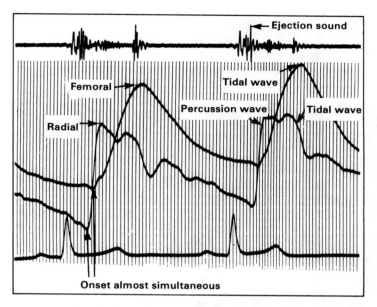

Intra-arterial pressure tracings in a patient with coarctation of the aorta show that the onsets of the femoral and radial pulses remain almost simultaneous. In coarctation, a delay in the femoral is felt on palpating both arteries simultaneously because the percussion wave distal to an obstruction is obliterated by an anacrotic shoulder, which is imperceptible. Thus only the later tidal wave is felt in the femoral artery, whereas the earlier percussion wave is felt in the unobstructed radial artery.

4. What may make it difficult to compare pulse peaks in the femoral and radial arteries?
ANS.: They have different pulse pressures, and the finger on the radial may be too far from the finger on the femoral.
5. How can you overcome the difficulties in comparing the femoral and radial pulses?
ANS.: a) Place the patient's wrist over the femoral artery, so that your fingers on the radial and femoral are on top of one another.
b) Vary the compression force until both pulse pressures feel equal.
c) Use the lightest possible pressure, so that you can allow comparison of peaks.

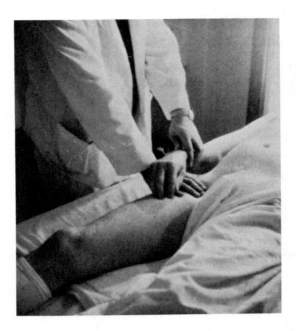

By placing the patient's wrist over his femoral artery as you palpate both, you can best perceive the obvious delay of the femoral pulse peak over that of the arm. In using the radials rather than the brachials to
test for differences between the arm and leg, you take advantage of the increased rapidity of pulse rise as
you palpate more peripherally down the arm.

6. When may the femoral pulse be easily palpable in coarctation?
   ANS.: It is especially important to test for femoral pulse peak delay in suspected
   coarctation when coexistent AR is present (as may occur with a bicuspid
   valve). This test is needed because with AR all peripheral pulses become
   more bounding, so that the femoral pulses may be well enough preserved to
   have normal volume despite coarctation.
   Note: a) As many as 50 percent of patients with coarctation may have a
   bicuspid aortic valve, which is commonly regurgitant.
       b) Even if the AR is severe, the diastolic pressure in the arms may be
   normal, despite coarctation [16].
      * c) Kinking of the aortic arch without any pressure gradient across the
   kinked segment (pseudocoarctation) can also delay the femoral
   pulse peak when compared with the radials [112]. Experimental
   progressive constriction of the aorta in animals will produce a
   delayed femoral peak when the aorta is constricted to 40 percent of
   its cross-sectional area, whereas a significant gradient will not develop until the aorta is narrowed to 30 percent of its original area
   [112].
      * d) Supravalvular AS [61] can also cause a radial-femoral lag. Only a
   delay between the *right* radial and the femoral will occur. (The left
   radial may also be delayed.)
      * e) The blood pressure may not be elevated in the arms in coarctation
   in patients in whom there is

1) Significant AS plus PDA [56].
2) Severe MR [114].
* f) You must always palpate the abdomen of a patient with suspected
coarctation. If a strong aortic pulsation in the epigastrium suddenly
disappears lower down, an abdominal aortic coarctation should be
suspected [80].

PULSUS PARADOXUS

What is meant by pulsus paradoxus?
ANS.: It is a marked fall, that is, a fall of 8 mm Hg or more, in systolic blood
pressure on inspiration, usually due to **tamponade.** An inspiratory fall of less
than 8 mm is physiological.

Normal Effect of Respiration on Blood Pressure

1. Does the systolic blood pressure normally increase or decrease with inspiration?
Why?
ANS.: It decreases because
a) Lung capacity increases with inspiration and the pulmonary vascular bed
expands; therefore, less blood moves from the lung into the left heart.
b) Intrathoracic pressure decreases with inspiration. Because the aorta is an
intrathoracic organ, its pressure will also drop.
2. If the systolic pressure normally decreases with inspiration, what is paradoxical
about a pulsus paradoxus?
ANS.: Nothing. It is simply an exaggeration of a normal phenomenon.
3. Why did the term *paradoxus* come into use?
ANS.: A. Kussmaul, in the late 1800s, originally described a marked drop in, or
even loss of, blood pressure on inspiration in patients with constrictive
pericarditis [53]. He decided to call it a "pulsus paradoxus" because he
noticed that the apex beat did not change in any way, despite the loss of
radial pulse with inspiration. Kussmaul also thought it was paradoxical that
although the peripheral pulse seems at first to be irregular, it actually comes
and goes regularly [110].
4. What might be a more descriptive term than pulsus paradoxus?
ANS.: A marked inspiratory fall in blood pressure.
5. How much systolic pressure is normally lost during (a) normal, (b) deep, and (c)
very deep inspiration?
ANS.: a) 2 to 6 mm Hg.
b) Up to 10 mm Hg.
c) Up to 15 mm Hg.

How to Elicit a Pathological Inspiratory Fall in Blood Pressure

1. With what depth of respiration is the test done?
ANS.: Not more than a moderate depth of respiration. If the patient is breathing
too shallowly, tell him to breathe "just a little more deeply, but not too

deeply," only enough for you to see the chest movements easily while watching the manometer out of the corner of your eye.

> *Note:* If respirations are rapid or irregular, raise your arm for inspiration and lower it for expiration, and ask the patient to follow the movements of your hand.

2. On moderate inspiration and expiration, what is a positive paradoxus (i.e., how much blood pressure fall on inspiration is definitely abnormal)?

ANS.: A fall of 10 mm Hg or more is generally agreed on in the literature. With practice, however, experience shows that an inspiratory fall of about 6 mm Hg is the upper limit of normal. Some of the probable reasons for believing that between 8 and 10 mm Hg could be normal are errors such as the following:

  a) The subject is asked to breathe too deeply or even to hold his breath on inspiration and expiration.

  b) The physician may fail to realize that as he is lowering the cuff pressure slowly below the level of the first Korotkoff sound on expiration, the blood pressure itself is often falling. Therefore, after the physician hears the Korotkoff sounds both on inspiration and expiration for the first time, he fails to reinflate the cuff to see if the systolic pressure has actually dropped while he was performing the test. One need not reinflate the cuff from the zero point but merely from the point where the sounds were heard on both inspiration and expiration.

  c) A fall of 5 mm Hg could be a significant loss of systolic pressure and actually mean **tamponade** if the pulse pressure were markedly reduced, for example, to 20 mm Hg (e.g., if the blood pressure were 110/90, a 5-mm Hg decrease with inspiration could occur with tamponade [4]).

> *Note:* If you always test for pulsus paradoxus while taking a patient's blood pressure for the first time, you will get enough practice to make your results more reliable. Also, this way you will automatically pick up pulsus alternans or pulsus bisferiens.

The Mechanism of Inspiratory Fall in Tamponade or Constriction

1. Why is there a more marked drop in stroke volume on inspiration in tamponade than in normals?

ANS.: Because much less blood enters the left atrium on inspiration than in normal subjects.

2. Why does much less blood enter the left atrium on inspiration in tamponade?

ANS.: Because on inspiration the left ventricular and left atrial pressure does not drop so far as does the intrathoracic pressure. Thus, the pressure in the left atrium may exceed the pressure in the pulmonary veins and blood may even flow backward into the lungs on inspiration.

3. Why does left atrial and left ventricular pressure not drop proportionately to intrathoracic pressure in the presence of tamponade?

ANS.: The following is one plausible explanation: Tamponade almost always affects both sides of the heart. With inspiration the filling pressure and volume of the right ventricle are increased. The pericardium is stretched, and its intrapericardial pressure is increased. This increased intrapericardial pressure is transmitted to the left atrium (which is covered with pericardium), and its pressure is raised during inspiration [25]. Septal bowing into the LV on inspiration also contributes to the decrease of LV volume on inspiration.

Causes of False-Positive and False-Negative Tests for Inspiratory Fall in Blood Pressure

1. Why do some asthmatic patients seem to have a marked inspiratory fall in blood pressure?

    ANS.: If expiration raises the intrathoracic pressure too high as a result of broncho-spasm (similar to a Valsalva maneuver), inspiration will, by contrast, seem to lower the systolic pressure excessively. Actually, it is an expiratory rise in blood presure, not an inspiratory fall. There are, however, patients with emphysema who also have some *inspiratory* obstruction that causes an exaggerated inspiratory fall of intrathoracic pressure as well (similar to a **Müller maneuver**).

    It is surprising how severe chronic emphysema can be with only a slight expiratory rise in blood pressure.

    Note:*a) The pulse of tamponade may differ from the pulse of a patient with bronchospasm and a marked expiratory rise in blood pressure because in bronchospasm the pulse pressure often remains the same on inspiration and expiration because cardiac output is only slightly affected by the phasic changes in intrathoracic pressure. In tamponade, on the other hand, the pulse pressure (as well as the systolic pressure) decreases on inspiration because the cardiac output drops markedly on inspiration. Consequently, although the tamponade pulsus paradoxus may occasionally be palpable, the pulsus paradoxus due to bronchospasm alone rarely is.

    *b) The diastolic pressure in tamponade changes very little, whereas in bronchospasm it varies as much as does systolic pressure. An occasional patient with bronchospasm will have an exaggerated decrease in stroke volume on inspiration; this is thought to be due to the bulging of the ventricular septum into the LV caused by the Müller maneuver.

    *c) The degree of pulsus paradoxus correlates with the severity of the asthmatic attack. A drop of up to 20 mm Hg of blood pressure on inspiration is found in moderate degrees of asthma. A fall of more than 20 mm Hg is a sign of a severe attack [108].

2. Which patients have the greatest inspiratory fall in systolic pressure, those with constriction or those with tamponade?

    ANS.: Only with tamponade are inspiratory drops of 20 mm Hg or more found during quiet breathing [54, 82].

    In chronic constrictive pericarditis, a pulsus paradoxus is actually uncommon unless it is subacute, with some fluid still present (effusive-constrictive).

    *Note: In the effusive-constrictive type of pericarditis, a tense effusion adds pressure to a constricting visceral pericardium, which still causes constriction even after complete pericardiocentesis. While the relatively small effusion is present, there is likely to be a marked pulsus paradoxus, just as in pure tamponade [43].

*3. Why may congestive heart failure by itself sometimes cause a falsely exaggerated inspiratory fall in blood pressure?

ANS.: It is always associated with marked cardiomegaly when it does occur. It may be partly due to a cardiomegaly so great that it stretches even the normal pericardium to its maximum, causing inspiration to create such pressure on the outer cardiac walls that it makes the pericardium behave like a noncompliant restrictive band.

*4. What conditions that are neither cardiac nor bronchospastic can cause a marked inspiratory fall in blood pressure? Why?

ANS.: a) Extreme obesity, which possibly causes excessive compression of the inferior vena cava at the thoracic inlet on inspiration.

b) Pregnancy, presumably because the large uterus obstructs the free forward flow of blood in the inferior vena cava during expiration. (Blood flows forward in the abdomen mainly during expiration, when intra-abdominal pressure is lowest.)

c) Compression, on inspiration, of one subclavian artery by a fibrous band or anterior scalenus muscle in thoracic outlet syndromes may account for the occasional unilateral paradoxus effect [20, 104].

d) Acute pulmonary embolism, usually with a cardiomyopathy [19, 69].

e) Shock [24].

*Note: Shock can cause a marked inspiratory fall in blood pressure only if it is associated with hypovolemia. This occurs presumably because the depletion of the venous reservoir will cause less blood than normal to be ejected into the lungs on inspiration. Because the pulmonary reservoir is underfilled and has a low mean pressure, an excess amount of pulmonary blood is withheld from the LV on inspiration, thus markedly decreasing the left ventricular output and blood pressure.

*5. What is the cause of the marked inspiratory fall in blood pressure seen in some patients with a large acute pulmonary embolism?

ANS.: Since it is associated with a decrease in pulse pressure during inspiration, there are several possibilities:

a) An acutely dilated RV on inspiration may encroach on the LV in diastole and reduce the LV stroke volume, as in a reversed **Bernheim effect.**

b) The lungs are so empty that there may be excessive pooling in the lungs on inspiration.

*6. When will there be no significant inspiratory fall in blood pressure despite marked tamponade?

ANS.: a) If AR is present, the LV can fill from the aorta during inspiration. Therefore, if dissection of the aortic root causes both AR and tamponade, do not expect a pulsus paradoxus.

b) In patients with a large ASD the normal increase in systemic venous return on inspiration is balanced by a decrease in left-to-right shunt, so that the right ventricular volume changes very little during inspiration [115].

Note: When venous return to the right atrium is held constant in experimental tamponade, pulsus paradoxus cannot be elicited [95].

c) In patients with isolated right heart tamponade (usually patients with chronic renal failure) [82].

Note: Hypertrophic subaortic stenosis has been reported to cause a reversed pulsus paradoxus [65]. The reason for this is unknown.

CAPILLARY PULSATION

1. How do you elicit capillary pulsation (Quincke's sign)?

ANS.: Compress the skin of the face or hands with a glass slide, or exert slight pressure on the nail beds and watch for intermittent flushing. You can also transilluminate the nail bed with a flashlight against the pad of the patient's finger while shading the finger with your other hand.

2. What is the mechanism of capillary pulsation? What noncardiac conditions can cause it?

ANS.: The mechanism is the transmission of the arterial pulse through dilated capillaries to the subpapillary venous plexus. It is found in any condition that causes capillary dilatation, such as hot weather, a hot bath, fever, anemia, pregnancy, or hyperthyroidism.

3. Which cardiac conditions cause capillary pulsation?

ANS.: Any cardiac condition that causes a large pulse pressure, such as AR, systolic hypertension, or marked bradycardia, as in complete atrioventricular block.

Note: When severe, all the preceding cardiac conditions can cause such marked capillary pulsation that it can be seen merely by inspecting the palms, cheeks, or forehead, without compressing the skin [64].

HOW TO TELL CARDIAC FUNCTION BY BLOOD PRESSURE RESPONSE TO A VALSALVA MANEUVER

The Normal Valsalva Hemodynamics

1. What happens to the blood pressure immediately on performing a Valsalva strain and why?

ANS.: During the strain, the blood pressure rises by an amount equal to the increase in intrathoracic pressure because the aorta, like all structures in the thorax, must reflect changes in intrathoracic pressure.

2. What happens to the blood pressure, pulse pressure, and heart rate while the strain is maintained for 10 seconds?

ANS.: The blood pressure and pulse pressure decrease, and the heart rate increases. This occurs because the increased intrathoracic pressure obstructs venous return and therefore progressively decreases stroke volume and cardiac output. The reflex increase in sympathetic outflow due to the decreased stroke volume and blood pressure causes tachycardia.

*Note: The LV volume decreases by about 50 percent during the strain phase.

3. What happens to the blood pressure, pulse rate, and heart rate on release of the strain?

ANS.: For a few beats the blood pressure falls further due to decreased flow into the

LV because there are a few seconds of decreased flow from relatively empty pulmonary vessels. Then the blood pressure overshoots to above control levels, and the pulse pressure increases because the increased sympathetic outflow caused by the Valsalva maneuver persists for at least 5 to 10 seconds after the release of the strain. The temporary increase in venous return to the heart of blood that had been dammed up by the increased intrathoracic pressure then causes an increase in LV stroke volume. The increased stroke volume, together with the increased peripheral resistance due to the persistent excess sympathetic outflow, causes an increase or "overshoot" in blood pressure. The increased pressure on the carotid sinus, in turn, causes a reflex bradycardia.

  * *Note:* In mitral stenosis, the left atrial pressure overshoots more in the post-strain period than when there is a normal valve. This should prove useful in bringing out a mitral stenosis murmur [10].

The Valsalva Effect in Patients with Depressed Myocardial Function

1. What is the blood pressure response to a Valsalva strain if the ejection fraction is normal, i.e., 60 ± 10% by angiography or 50 ± 10% by radionuclide methods?

   ANS.: If the cuff pressure is held at 25 mm Hg above systolic pressure during the strain, a few Korotkoff sounds heard at the beginning of the strain reflect the increased intrathoracic pressure. Then the Korotkoff sounds will disappear as the blood pressure falls, due to the decreased venous return. Post-Valsalva, the Korotkoff sounds will reappear due to an overshoot of at least 25 mm Hg if the ejection fraction is normal. If no overshoot is obtained, hold the cuff pressure at 15 mm Hg above the control pressure. If there is an overshoot to 15 mm Hg, the ejection fraction may be low normal or it may be slightly reduced.

2. What kind of blood pressure response to the Valsalva occurs with a markedly reduced ejection fraction?

   ANS.: During the entire strain, the blood pressure stays up, and after the Valsalva maneuver there is no overshoot or bradycardia. This is known as a "square wave" response. This is partly due to the excess lung blood volume in the congested lungs, which continues to empty into the LV during the entire 10 seconds of strain.

3. How does the square wave response relate to ejection fraction and end-diastolic pressure in the LV?

   ANS.: It has been found that the ejection fraction is about 30 ± 10 percent by angiography (20 ± 10% by radionuclide methods). The end-diastolic pressure in the LV is likely to be very high (i.e., as much as 40 mm Hg [19]).

4. What happens to the blood pressure response to the Valsalva if the ejection fraction is reduced to 50 ± 10 percent by angiography, or 40 ± 10 percent by nuclear methods, and has a normal ejection fraction only with the help of a high end-diastolic pressure?

   ANS.: The blood pressure and pulse pressure decrease during the strain, but there is no post-strain overshoot [119]. This is presumably due to the excess sympathetic tone to which hearts with reduced ejection fractions are subject. Therefore, the strain does not stimulate enough further sympathetic drive to produce an overshoot after release of the strain.

Note: The end–diastolic pressure in the LV with this kind of response is also high (i.e., as much as 35 mm Hg).

5. What can produce a falsely abnormal absence of overshoot despite a normal heart?

ANS.: 1) Any cause of autonomic imbalance. Some rarely considered ones are:

a) Any cause of orthostatic hypotension.

b) Administration of beta blockers.

c) Parkinsonism.

2) Other conditions in a normal heart that have been found to be associated with an absent overshoot. These are:

a) Prerenal azotemia.

b) Decreased blood volume.

c) Hypokalemia.

d) A moderate or large ASD [46].

Note: A large ASD may even produce a square wave response [44, 71].

6. How can you help the patient to perform a Valsalva if he cannot comprehend or cooperate enough to carry out the maneuver?

ANS.: a) Press on the abdomen with one hand and ask the patient to push your hand away with his abdomen [42]. If this does not work, then

b) Have the patient blow up an aneroid manometer to 40 mm Hg through a rubber tube connection. (Use of a 20-gauge needle inserted into the rubber tube will ensure that continuous expiration through an open glottis is moving the manometer needle and prevents the needle from moving if only intraoral pressure is raised.)

REFERENCES

1. Abramson, D. I. Some simple clinical tests for the study of the arterial circulation in the extremities. *Am. J. Cardiol.* 3:597, 1959.
2. Alpert, J. S., Vieweg, W. V. R., and Hagan, A. D. Incidence and morphology of carotid shudders in aortic valve disease. *Am. Heart J.* 92:435, 1976.
3. Alzamora-Castro, V., and Battilana, G. The double femoral sound. *Am. J. Cardiol.* 5:764, 1960.
4. Antman, E. M., Cargill, V., and Grossman, W. Low-pressure cardiac tamponade. *Ann. Intern. Med.* 91:403, 1979.
5. Barner, H. B., Willman, V. L., and Kaiser, G. C. Dicrotic pulse after open heart operation. *Circulation* 42:993, 1970.
6. Benchimol, A., Harris, C. L., and Desser, K. B. Graphic techniques in cardiology. Midsystolic carotid pulse wave retraction in subjects with prolapsed mitral valve leaflets. *Chest* 62:614, 1972.
7. Berliner, K., et al. Blood pressure measurements in obese persons. *Am. J. Cardiol.* 8:10, 1961.
8. Berry, M. R. The mechanism and prevention of impairment of auscultatory sounds during determination of blood pressure of standing patients. *Staff Meet. Mayo Clin.* 15:699, 1940.
9. Bertrand, C. A. Arm and leg blood pressures. *J.A.M.A.* 227:942, 1974.
10. Bjork, V. O., and Malmstrom, G. Simultaneous left and right atrial pressure curves during Valsalva's experiment. *Am. Heart J.* 50:742, 1955.
11. Braunwald, E., and Morrow, A. G. A method for the detection and estimation of aortic regurgitant flow in man. *Circulation* 17:505, 1958.
11A. Brooker, J. Z., Alderman, E. L., and Harrison D. C. Alterations in left ventricular volumes induced by Valsalva manoeuvre. *Br. Heart J.* 36:713, 1974.

12. Buggs, H., et al. Comparison of systolic arterial blood pressure by transcutaneous Doppler probe and conventional methods in hypotensive patients. *Anesth. Analg.* 52:776, 1973.
13. Burch, G. E. Of recording your own blood pressure. *Am. Heart J.* 89:813, 1975.
14. Burch, G. E., and Shewey, L. Sphygmomanometric cuff size and blood pressure recordings. *J.A.M.A.* 225:1215, 1973.
15. Calick, A., and Berger, S. Pulmonary arterial pulsus alternans associated with pulmonary embolism. *Chest* 64:663, 1973.
16. Campbell, M., and Baylis, J. H. The course and prognosis of coarctation of the aorta. *Br. Heart J.* 18:475, 1956.
17. Carter, S. A. Clinical measurement of systolic pressures in limbs with arterial occlusive disease. *J.A.M.A.* 207, 1869, 1969.
18. Chandraratna, P. A. N., Langevin, E., and Langevin, J. Pulsus alternans induced by glyceryl trinitrate paste in a patient with alcoholic cardiomyopathy. *Br. Heart J.* 41:354, 1979.
19. Cohen, S. I., et al. Pulsus paradoxus and Kussmaul's sign in acute pulmonary embolism. *Am. J. Cardiol.* 32:271, 1973.
20. Cohn, J. N., Tristani, F. E., and Pinkerson, A. L. Mechanism of parodoxical pulse in clinical shock. *J. Clin. Invest.* 46:1744, 1967.
21. Constant, J. Arterial and venous pulsations in cardiovascular diagnosis. *J. Cardiovasc. Med.* 5:973, 1980.
22. Corrigan, D. J. Permanent patency of the mouth of the aortic valves. *Edinb. Med. Surg. J.* 37:225, 1832.
23. Cousins, A. L., Eddleman, E. E., Jr., and Reeves, T. J. Prediction of aortic valvular area and gradient by noninvasive techniques. *Am. Heart J.* 95:308, 1978.
24. Curtiss, E. I., Lindsey, R. L., Jr., and Reddy, P. S. Diagnostic criteria for pulsus paradoxus and abnormal inspiratory decrease of ejection time in cardiac tamponade. *Pericardial Disease.* New York: Raven Press, 1982, p. 201.
25. Dornhorst, A. C., Howard, P., and Leathart, G. L. Pulsus paradoxus. *Lancet* 1:746, 1952.
26. Enselberg, C. D. Measurement of diastolic blood pressure by palpation. *N. Engl. J. Med.* 265:272, 1961.
27. Evans, W., and Lewes, D. The carotid shudder. *Br. Heart J.* 7:171, 1945.
28. Ewy, G. A., Rios, J. A., and Marcus, F. I. The dicrotic arterial pulse. *Circulation* 39:655, 1969.
29. Falicov, R. E., and Wang, T. Analysis of post-extrasystolic beats in the diagnosis of idiopathic hypertrophic subaortic stenosis. *Am. J. Cardiol.* 33:931, 1974.
30. Felix, R., Jr., et al. Ultrasound measurement of arm and leg blood pressures. *J.A.M.A.* 226:1096, 1973.
31. Ferrer, M. E., et al. Cardiocirculatory studies in pulsus alternans of the systemic and pulmonary circulations. *Circulation* 14:163, 1956.
32. Frank, M. J., et al. The clinical evaluation of aortic regurgitation. *Arch. Intern. Med.* 116:357, 1965.
33. Freis, E. D. Auscultatory indication of diastolic blood pressure. *Cardiol. Digest* 3:13, 1968.
34. Freis, E. D., et al. Changes in the carotid pulse which occur with age and hypertension. *Am. Heart J.* 71:757, 1966.
35. Freis, E. D., and Kyle, M. C. Computer analysis of carotid and brachial pulse waves. *Am. J. Cardiol.* 22:691, 1968.
35A. Freis, E. D., and Sappington, R. F., Jr. Dynamic reactions produced by deflating a blood pressure cuff. *Circulation* 38:1085, 1968.
36. French, J. W., and Guntheroth, W. G. Explanation of asymmetric upper extremity blood pressures in supravalvular aortic stenosis. *Circulation* 40:31, 1970.
37. Friedman, S. A. Prevalence of palpable wrist pulses. *Br. Heart J.* 32:316, 1970.
38. Geddes, L. A., and Whistler, S. J. The error in indirect blood pressure measurement with the incorrect size cuff. *Am. Heart J.* 96:4, 1978.
39. Gould, L. Pulmonary artery alternation with atrial fibrillation. *J.A.M.A.* 207:1515, 1969.
40. Gould, L., and Lyon, A. F. Postural changes in the brachial artery first derivative in the normal and pathologic state. *Dis. Chest* 53:476, 1968.
41. Gould, L., and Shariff, M. Comparisons of the left ventricular, aortic, and brachial artery first derivative. *Vasc. Surg.* 3:34, 1969.
42. Hamby, R. I. Accurate Valsalva maneuver made actually easy. *Am. Heart J.* 82:838, 1971.
43. Hancock, E. W. Subacute effusive-constrictive pericarditis. *Circulation* 43:183, 1971.

44. Hancock, E. W., et al. Valsalva's maneuver in atrial septal defect. *Am. Heart J.* 65:50, 1963.
45. Harrison, E. G., Jr., Roth, G. M., and Hines, E. A., Jr. Bilateral indirect and direct arterial pressures. *Circulation* 22:419, 1960.
46. Henrich, W. L. Autonomic insufficiency. *Arch. Intern. Med.* 142:339, 1982.
47. Hill, L., and Rowlands, R. A. Systolic blood pressure: (1) in change of posture, (2) in cases of aortic regurgitation. *Heart* 3:219, 1911–1912.
48. Hockberg, H. M., and Saltzman, M. D. Accuracy of an ultrasound blood pressure instrument in neonates, infants, and children. *Ther. Res.* 13:482, 1971.
49. Hultgren, H. N. Venous pistol shot sounds. *Am. J. Cardiol.* 10:667, 1962.
50. Ikram, H., Nixon, P. G. F., and Fox, J. A. The haemodynamic implications of the bisferiens pulse. *Br. Heart J.* 26:452, 1964.
51. Ison, J. W. Palpation of dorsalis pedis pulse. *J.A.M.A.* 206:2745, 1968.
52. Kaul, U., et al. Characteristic postextrasystolic ventricular pressure response in constrictive pericarditis. *Am. Heart J.* 102:461, 1981.
53. Kussmaul, A. Ueber schweilige Mediastinopericarditis und den paradoxen Pulse. *Klin. Wochenschr.* 10:443, 1873.
54. Lange, R. L. et al. Diagnostic signs in compressive cardiac disorders, constrictive pericarditis, pericardial effusion, and tamponade. *Circulation* 33:763, 1966.
55. Lee, Y-C, and Sutton, F. J. Pulsus alternans in patients with congestive cardiomyopathy. *Circulation* 65:1533, 1982.
56. Little, J. A., et al. Coarctation of the aorta associated with aortic stenosis and a patent ductus arteriosus. *Am. J. Cardiol.* 12:570, 1963.
57. Littler, W. A., et al. The variability of arterial pressure. *Am. Heart J.* 95:180, 1978.
58. Littmann, D. Alternation of the heart. *Circulation* 27:280, 1963.
59. Littmann, D. Cardiac alternation. Alternation of heart sounds and murmurs. *Am. J. Cardiol.* 14:420, 1964.
60. Liu, C. K., and Luisada, A. A. Halving of the pulse due to severe alternans (pulsus bisectus). *Am. Heart J.* 50:927, 1955.
61. Logan, W. F. W. E., et al. Familial supravalvar aortic stenosis. *Br. Heart J.* 27:547, 1965.
62. London, S. R., and London, R. E. Critique of indirect diastolic end-point. *Arch. Intern. Med.* 119:39, 1967.
63. Lopez-Sendon, J., et al. Pulmonary pulsus alternans in acute myocardial infarction. *Am. J. Cardiol.* 42:577, 1978.
64. MacGregor, G. A. Spontaneous capillary pulsations in complete heart block. *Br. Heart J.* 21:225, 1959.
65. Massumi, R. A., et al. Reversed pulsus paradoxus. *N. Engl. J. Med.* 1973.
66. Masuda, Y., et al. Carotid pulse wave contour in normal and diseases: The relation of percussion wave and tidal wave. *J. Cardiography* 6:725, 1976.
67. Maurer, A. H., and Noordergraaf, A. Korotkoff sound filtering for automated three-phase measurement of blood pressure. *Am. Heart J.* 91:584, 1976.
68. Maxwell, M. H., et al. Error in blood-pressure measurement due to incorrect cuff size in obese patients. *Lancet* 2:33, 1982.
69. McDonald, I. G., et al. Acute major pulmonary embolism as a cause of exaggerated respiratory blood pressure variation and pulsus paradoxus. *Br. Heart J.* 34:1137, 1972.
70. McIntosh, H. D. Discordant pulsus alternans. *Circulation* 26:214, 1960.
71. McIlroy, M. B. The clinical uses of oximetry. *Br. Heart J.* 21:293, 1958.
72. Meadows, W. R., Draur, R. A., and Osadjan, C. E. Dicrotism in heart disease. *Am. Heart J.* 82:596, 1971.
73. Mitchell, J. H., Sarnoff, S. J., and Sonnenblick, E. H. The dynamics of pulsus alternans: Alternating end-diastolic fiber length as a causative factor. *J. Clin. Invest.* 42:55, 1963.
74. Nuessle, W. F. The importance of a tight blood pressure cuff. *Am. Heart J.* 52:905, 1956.
75. Orchard, R. C., and Craige, E. Dicrotic pulse after open heart surgery. *Circulation* 62:1107, 1980.
75A. Park, M. D., and Guntheroth, W. G. Direct blood pressure measurements in brachial and femoral arteries in children. *Circulation* 40:231, 1970.
76. Pascarelli, E. F., and Bertrand, C. A. Comparison of blood pressures in the arms and legs. *N. Engl. J. Med.* 270:693, 1964.

77. Pascarelli, E. F., and Bertrand, C. A. Comparison of arm and leg blood-pressures in aortic insufficiency: An appraisal of Hill's sign. *Br. Med. J.* 2:73, 1965.
78. Perlman, L. V., Chiang, B. N., and Keller, J. Accuracy of sphygmomanometers in hospital practice. *Arch. Intern. Med.* 125:1000, 1970.
79. Putt, A. M. A comparison of blood pressure readings by auscultation and palpation. *Nurs. Res.* 15:311, 1966.
80. Pyorala, K., et al. Coarctation of the abdominal aorta, review of twenty-seven cases. *Am. J. Cardiol.* 6:650, 1960.
81. Ragan, C., and Bordley, J. The accuracy of clinical measurements of arterial blood pressure. *Bull. Johns Hopkins Hosp.* 69:504, 1941.
82. Reddy, P. S., et al. Cardiac tamponade: Hemodynamic observations in man. *Circulation* 58:265, 1978.
83. Rittenhouse, E. A., and Strandness, D. E., Jr. Oscillatory flow patterns in patients with aortic valve disease. *Am. J. Cardiol.* 29:568, 1971.
84. Robinson, B. The carotid pulse. II. Relation of external recordings to carotid, aortic, and brachial pulses. *Br. Heart J.* 25:61, 1963.
85. Rodbard, S., and Ciesielski, J. A relation between auscultatory gap and the pulse upstroke. *Am. Heart J.* 58:221, 1959.
86. Rodbard, S., and Ciesielski, J. Duration of arterial sounds. *Am. J. Cardiol.* 8:18, 1961.
87. Rodbard, S., and Margolis, J. The auscultatory gap in arteriosclerotic heart disease. *Circulation* 15:850, 1957.
88. Rose, G. Standardization of observers in blood-pressure measurement. *Lancet* 1:673, 1965.
89. Ryan, J. M., et al. Experiences with pulsus alternans, ventricular alternation and the stage of heart failure. *Circulation* 14:1099, 1956.
90. Sabbah, H. N., et al. Effect of turbulent blood flow on systolic pressure contour in the ventricles and great vessels: Significance related to anacrotic and bisferious pulses. *Am. J. Cardiol.* 45:1139, 1980.
91. Sabbah, H. N., and Stein, P. D. Valve origin of the aortic incisura. *Am. J. Cardiol.* 41:32, 1978.
92. Sarnoff, S. J., et al. Regulation of ventricular contraction by the carotid sinus: its effect on atrial and ventricular dynamics. *Circ. Res.* 8:1123, 1960.
93. Sawayama, T., and Yamamoto, S. Semi-quantitative analysis of carotid arterial wave form— its physiological changes with aging in normal subjects. *Kawasaki Med. J.* 3:1, 1977.
94. Scoblionko, D. P., and Lozner, E. C. Pulsus alternans: A review of current concepts. *Cardiovasc. Rev. Rep.* 2:581, 1981.
95. Shabetai, R., et al. Pulsus paradoxus. *J. Clin. Invest.* 44:1882, 1965.
96. Silverberg, D. S., et al. The unsupported arm—a cause of falsely elevated blood pressure readings. *Br. Med. J.* 2:1331, 1977.
97. Spence, J. D., Sibbald, W. J., and Cape, R. D. Pseudohypertension in the elderly. *Clin. Sci. Molecular Med.* 55:399, 1978.
98. Spence, J. D., Sibbald, W. J., and Cape, R. D. Direct, indirect and mean blood pressures in hypertensive patients. The problem of cuff artefact due to arterial wall stiffness, and a partial solution. *Clin. Invest. Med.* 2:165, 1980.
99. Spodick, D. H., et al. Rate of rise of the carotid pulse. An investigation of observer error in a common clinical measurement. *Am. J. Cardiol.* 49:159, 1982.
100. Spodick, D. H., Khan, A. H., and Quarry, V. M. Systolic and diastolic time intervals in pulsus alternans. *Am. Heart J.* 87:5, 1974.
101. Spodick, D. H., and St. Pierre, J. R. Pulsus alternans: Physiologic study by noninvasive techniques. *Am. Heart J.* 80:766, 1970.
102. Sproul, G. Basilar artery insufficiency secondary to obstruction of left subclavian artery. *Circulation* 28:259, 1963.
103. Steinfeld, L., Alexander, H., and Cohen, M. L. Updating sphygmomanometry. *Am. J. Cardiol.* 33:107, 1974.
104. Swinton, N. W., Jr., et al. Paradoxical pulse. *Arch. Intern. Med.* 124:492, 1969.
105. Taguchi, J. T., and Suwangool, P. "Pipe-stem" brachial arteries. *J.A.M.A.* 228:733, 1974.
106. Tahir, A. H., and Adriani, J. Usefulness of ultrasonic technique of blood pressure determination. *Anesth. Analg.* 52:699, 1973.

107. Toole, J. F. Bilateral simultaneous sphygmomanometry: A new diagnostic test for subclavian steal syndrome. *Circulation* 10:35, 1966.
108. Vaisrub, S. Pulsus paradoxus of the airways. *J.A.M.A.* 232:1041, 1975.
109. Viol, G. W., et al. Seating as a variable in clinical blood pressure measurement. *Am. Heart J.* 98:913, 1979.
110. Wagner, H. R. Paradoxical pulse: 100 years later. *Am. J. Cardiol.* 32:91, 1973.
111. Waltemath, C. L., and Preuss, D. D. Determination of blood pressure in low-flow states by the Doppler technique. *Anesthesiology* 34:77, 1971.
112. Wang, K., Harrington, D., and Gobel, F. L. Delayed systolic peak of the femoral pulse from kinking of the aortic arch. *Am. J. Cardiol.* 33:286, 1974.
113. Warren, S. E., and Vieweg, W. V. R. Artifacts in the indirect measurement of arterial pressure. *Practical Cardiol.* 5:111, 1979.
114. Wigle, E. D., and Auger, P. Coarctation of the aorta associated with severe mitral insufficiency. *Am. J. Cardiol.* 21:190, 1968.
115. Winer, H. E., and Kronzon, I. Absence of paradoxical pulse in patients with cardiac tamponade and atrial septal defect. *Am. J. Cardiol.* 44:378, 1979.
116. Wood, P. Aortic stenosis. *Am. J. Cardiol.* 1:553, 1958. Classic article.
117. Yao, S. T., Hobbs, J. T., and Irvine, W. T. Ankle systolic pressure measurements in arterial disease affecting the lower extremities. *Br. J. Surg.* 56:676, 1969.
118. Zahir, M., and Gould, L. A new method for measurement of blood pressure in clinical shock. *Am. Heart J.* 79:572, 1970.
119. Zema, M. J., et al. Left ventricular dysfunction—bedside Valsalva manoeuvre. *Br. Heart J.* 44:560, 1980.
120. Zema, M. J., Caccavano, M., and Kligfeld, P. Detection of left ventricular dysfunction in ambulatory patients. *Am. J. Med.* 75:241, 1983.

4. Jugular Pressure and Pulsations

VENOUS PRESSURE BY JUGULAR INSPECTION

1. With which chambers of the heart are the jugular veins in continuity in systole and in diastole?

   ANS.: In systole the jugular veins are in continuity only with the right atrium because the tricuspid valve is closed. In diastole, when the tricuspid valve is open, the jugulars are in continuity with both the right atrium and the right ventricle (RV). Therefore, examination of the jugulars may reveal the contour and pressures in the right atrium and the right ventricle without the need for catheterization.

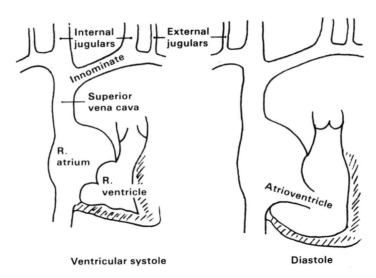

   In diastole, the atrium and ventricle are in continuity and become an "atrioventricle." Note also that the internal jugulars are in a more direct line with the superior vena cava than are the external jugulars.

2. What is the location of the venous valves between the jugulars and the superior vena cava?

   ANS.: In both the external and the internal jugulars. (The external jugular valves can often be demonstrated by occluding the external jugulars with a finger, preventing venous flow from the head.)

   Note: Competent valves between the superior vena cava and the internal jugulars have been demonstrated when the intrathoracic pressure is raised, as in coughing or chest compression [11A]. The valves usually become incompetent in the presence of tricuspid regurgitation (TR). Doppler studies show no retrograde flow even in the presence of high venous pressure unless there is tricuspid regurgitation.

3. Do these valves interfere with the use of the jugulars as a manometer for the measurement of venous pressure (i.e., as reflectors of right atrioventricular events)?

ANS.: No. Apparently elevated internal jugular venous pressures can be transmitted through the venous valves, which presumably are open during both systole (descent of base of ventricle effect) and diastole (opening of tricuspid valve effect).

*Note: If the venous valves of the arms are destroyed by phlebitis, as in chronic heroin users, the normal jugular pulsations will be transmitted to the arm veins [1]. Any vein in the body may transmit jugular pulsations if there is marked elevation of venous pressure or volume of pulsations, as in severe TR. Varicose veins in the leg are especially likely to pulsate in the presence of severe TR because their valves are incompetent.

4. Why is the criterion of "filling from below" a poor method for determining that there is an elevated jugular pressure?

ANS.: All jugulars fill from below up to the level of the right atrial pressure. This may or may not make even normal jugulars visible, depending on the angle of the patient's chest. Therefore, "filling from below" alone has no meaning without noting the vertical height to which the jugular fills from below (i.e., above some stated reference level and at a standardized chest angle).

5. How can you estimate venous pressure by jugular inspection?

ANS.: By using the internal jugular veins as a manometer. The external jugulars are poor manometers [9].

6. Why is the external jugular a poor vein to use as a manometer?

ANS.: External jugulars are often invisible or reflect a falsely low pressure despite high internal jugular pressure. This is because

a) Poor transmission of superior vena cava pulsations to the external jugulars, which are not in a direct line with the superior vena cava (see figure on page 80).

b) The external jugulars may be poorly developed anatomically.

c) Severe venous constriction due to the very high venous tone which may occur in conditions that produce high venous pressure. This is especially likely to occur in shock states.

7. Can you see an internal jugular vein?

ANS.: Only in the presence of severe TR is this vein visible as a discrete structure.

8. If you cannot ordinarily see the internal jugular veins, how can they be used as a manometer?

ANS.: The *pulsations* of the internal jugulars are transmitted to the skin of the neck. The top level of neck pulsations is taken as the venous pressure. Thus, the jugular is used as a "pulsation manometer."

9. Why should the right rather than the left internal jugular veins be used?

ANS.: Normally, the pressure in the right jugulars is either slightly greater than or the same as that in the left jugulars. Upper levels of normal have been established for the right side. In some arteriosclerotic patients the left jugular pressure may be falsely elevated owing to compression of the innominate vein between the sternum anteriorly and large tortuous arteries arising from a high unfolded aortic arch posteriorly [45A]. (An aortic **aneurysm** may also

*Material marked with an asterisk is for reference and for advanced students in cardiology.
Boldface type indicates that the term is explained in the Glossary.

be the cause of innominate vein compression, but this is rare in comparison with arteriosclerotic compression.)

Note: a) Taking a deep breath will decrease manubrial compression against the innominate vein and help to exclude this left jugular artifact [45A]. You can also reduce innominate vein compression by lowering venous pressure through diuresis [12].

b) A persistent left superior vena cava that drains into the coronary sinus will cause a slightly higher pressure in the left jugulars than that in the right, possibly owing to a relatively greater emptying resistance [24]. A persistent left superior vena cava is especially likely in the presence of an atrial septal defect (ASD) [16].

10. How can you detect jugular pulsations that are difficult to perceive?

ANS.: a) Shine a light tangentially from behind the neck to throw a jugular shadow anteriorly, or from in front of the neck to throw the jugular shadow posteriorly.

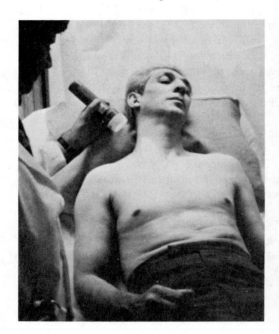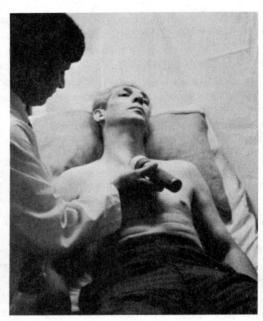

Jugular movements may be very subtle. Any slight movement of the hand holding the light can produce as much artifactual movement as movement from the jugulars themselves. Therefore, you must support your hand on either the pillow behind or the chest in front.

b) Examine the silhouette of the neck for pulsations. This is the most accurate way of finding the top level of pulsations. When you are examining the right side of the neck, you must lean over to the left side of the patient or stand on the left side of the bed temporarily to obtain a good view of the silhouette of the skin overlying the right internal jugular.

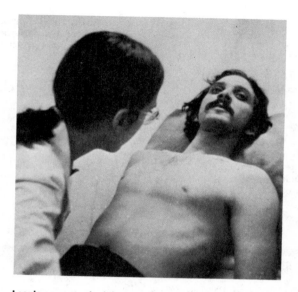

Leaning over to the left side of the patient to view an outline of the neck against the pillow will show you more subtle motion than could be seen even with an oblique light. Therefore, the true upper level of motion is best seen from this viewpoint.

c) Check for slight earlobe movement. If the internal jugular pressure is high, the earlobes often pulsate. Unfortunately, a strong carotid pulse pressure can also cause slight earlobe pulsations.

11. Why is the phrase "distended neck veins," which is so widely used as a sign of high venous pressure, a poor expression?

ANS.: This expression suggests that the observer is probably accustomed to looking mainly at the external jugulars, because the internal jugular veins are rarely visibly distended. A high level of pulsation in the internal jugulars may be associated with invisible (nondistended) external jugulars. When you use the jugulars as a manometer, you should state the height of the top level of internal jugular pulsations in centimeters above a certain reference point with the patient in a certain position. You should be interested in the top level of pulsations, not in distention of the veins.

Note: One of the difficulties in judging the top level of jugular pulsations is that they tend to diminish toward the upper level—that is, the top level of pulsation is very much like a fulcrum of movement. Determining the top level of venous pressure really means looking for the fulcrum of internal jugular movement.

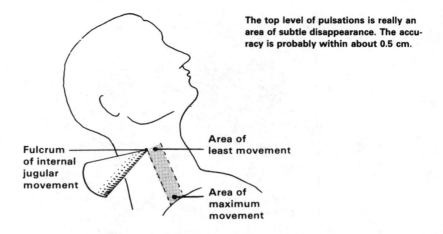

The top level of pulsations is really an area of subtle disappearance. The accuracy is probably within about 0.5 cm.

HOW TO READ THE JUGULAR MANOMETER

1. What reference level may be used as zero? Why?

    ANS.: The **sternal angle,** or angle of Louis. This landmark was once thought to bear a constant relationship to the right atrium when the body is in either the recumbent or the sitting position. Although this is doubtful, an arbitrary zero level is practical, provided normal standards for venous pulsations above this zero level are established.

2. What upper limits of normal have been suggested for jugular pulsations in (a) the supine and (b) the 45-degree position using the sternal angle as the zero reference level?

    ANS.: a) In the supine position, the upper limit is 2 cm.

    b) At 45 degrees, the upper limit is 4.5 cm. (It is easy to remember 4.5 cm at 45 degrees.)

    Note: These upper limits of normal represent a central venous pressure of about 15 cm of water with the patient supine and with zero level at the mid-axillary line.

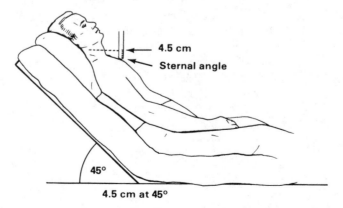

4.5 cm at 45°

Venous pressure can be estimated by observing the upper level of internal jugular pulsations above the sternal angle. If it is over 4.5 cm at 45°, it indicates an elevated right atrial pressure.

If you find a normal or low venous pressure when you suspect a low cardiac output, inquire about the ingestion of diuretics. You may find that a lowered blood volume has normalized the venous pressure.

3. Why does the upper limit of normal for jugular pulsations above the sternal angle rise as the chest is raised?

ANS.: This may be due to

    a) An actual change in the relationship between the right atrium and the sternal angle as the upright position is assumed.

    b) An increase in venous tone as the chest is raised.

4. Why is it important to know what the venous pressure is at 45 degrees?

ANS.: When the patient is supine, the jugular pressure may be normal, but the top level of pulsations may be so high that they are above the level of the angle of the jaw. This occurs because in some supine patients the sternal angle may be even above the horizontal level of the jaw.

    Note: Normal subjects have been shown to have about the same absolute venous pressure in the supine position as in the 45-degree chest position relative to the right atrium.

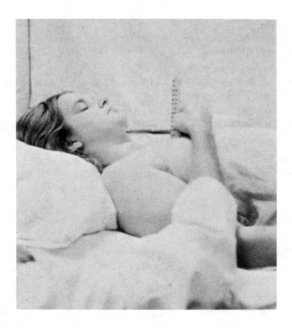

The 2-cm level is above the angle of the jaw in this patient. Therefore, only if her top level of pulsations were lower down at sternal-angle level would the upper level be measurable. At 45 degrees, her top level of jugular pulsations was below jaw level and was measurable.

5. What effect does inspiration have on the absolute height or top level of jugular pulsations in the normal subject?

ANS.: The top level may be lowered because the drop in intrathoracic pressure on inspiration may be reflected in the jugulars. Inspiration may, however, make jugular pulsations easier to see because the right atrium has more vigorous pulsations on inspiration.

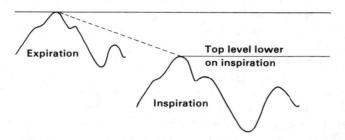

Note the higher absolute level but smaller amplitude of pulsations on expiration. With bronchospasm, jugular pulsations with normal pressures may only be visible above the clavicle during expiration due to the effect of straining, which elevates intrathoracic pressure with each expiration.

THE ABDOMINAL COMPRESSION TEST (HEPATOJUGULAR REFLUX)

1. How can you tell that a venous pressure that is below the upper limit of normal is actually relatively high for a particular person?

    ANS.: Abdominal compression will cause and maintain a rise of at least 1 cm in the top level of pulsations only if the venous pressure is relatively high. The greater the rise with abdominal compression, the higher the venous pressure. This is called the *hepatojugular reflux* [8, 39A] (not reflex).

    Note: The effect of abdominal compression is more important than the absolute jugular pressure in determining whether or not the venous pressure is normal or relatively high.

2. What happens to the top level of jugular pulsations if abdominal compression is applied to a patient without heart failure?

    ANS.: In the normal patient the jugular pulsation level will either remain the same or fall.

3. In the normal subject, what causes the fall in jugular pressure if abdominal compression is maintained?

    ANS.: a) Pressure on the abdomen obstructs femoral venous return almost as effectively as venous tourniquets on the thighs. Thus, less blood reaches the right atrium.

    b) The response of many patients to interference with diaphragmatic descent by abdominal compression is to breathe in a more inspiratory position. This causes a decreased intrathoracic pressure, which is reflected in the jugulars as a decrease in jugular pressure.

    Note: One bonus derived from testing for jugular pressure with abdominal compression is the possible discovery of a low vital capacity. Abdominal compression that causes an increase in dyspnea or the use of accessory muscles of respiration implies that the patient's vital capacity is so reduced that he cannot tolerate any further decrease produced by pushing up on the diaphragm.

4. What is wrong with the historical term *hepatojugular reflux?*

ANS.: This term was first applied in 1885, when it was thought not only that pressure on a large liver was an essential part of the test but also that the procedure was a test only for tricuspid regurgitation [39A]. Actually, the effect can be achieved with a normal-sized liver and with compression on any part of the abdomen, although pressure on the right upper quadrant produces the greatest response [8]. If the right upper quadrant is tender, do not hesitate to compress other areas instead.

The term *hepatojugular reflux* must be retained because it is so widely known that it is useful for indexing and referencing as well as for communication among physicians.

5. Why does abdominal compression cause a sustained rise in pressure in a patient with congestive failure?

ANS.: a) In patients with peripheral venous congestion (high venous pressure and peripheral edema) there is increased venous tone that not only counteracts the thigh tourniquet effect but also decreases the ability of the veins flowing into the superior vena cava to dilate and absorb the displaced visceral blood [53]. This inability to dilate further is accentuated by the increased venous volume caused by salt and water retention [53, 56].

b) The patient with peripheral venous congestion also commonly has a large RV and RA. Right upper quadrant compression transmitted to the RV and RA can interfere with their filling, especially if there is increased tone of those chambers and they are near the limit of their compliance. This may account for the fact that right upper quadrant pressure may cause a decrease in cardiac output despite the apparently higher filling pressure [18].

6. What causes the increased venous tone in congestive heart failure?

ANS.: Inadequate cardiac output eventually causes
    a) Sympathetic outflow along the autonomic nerves.
    b) Increased catecholamines in the blood.
        Note: a) The increased sympathetic outflow and catecholamines are reflected in the sinus tachycardia seen in patients with heart failure.
            b) Their increased venous tone, or tension, has been proved by plethysmography, in which volume and pressure in an encased limb are used to solve for tension by using Laplace's law: pressure is proportional to tension/volume.
            c) Increased venous tone has been found in all patients with so-called **right ventricular failure,** that is, peripheral venous congestion (increased venous pressure and peripheral edema due to inadequate cardiac output) [44]. If diuretics have normalized the absolute height of venous pressure, abdominal compression may still demonstrate the increased tone.

7. What are the common causes of a false rise in the height of jugular pulsations with abdominal compression?

ANS.: a) Inability to tolerate the resistance to downward movement of the diaphragm when pressure on the abdomen raises the diaphragm in patients with severe obstructive pulmonary disease or in any other condition that causes severe loss of vital capacity [33].

b) Increased blood volume [23].

c) Increased sympathetic stimulation due to such causes as nervousness, pain, intravenous catecholamines, or an acute infarct [8].

d) Abdominal compression often exaggerates the amplitude of the jugular pulsations without actually raising the upper levels, and by merely revealing the true upper level of pulsations, which were difficult to perceive before compression, it may give a false impression of a rise in venous pressure.

* Note: An obstruction of the superior vena cava below the azygos vein is a rare cause of a positive abdominal compression effect.

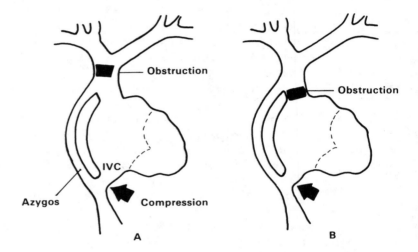

(A) Partial obstruction of the superior vena cava above its junction with the azygos will elevate jugular venous pressure. Abdominal compression will not elevate it further because the displaced abdominal blood can reach the area below the obstruction. (B) Obstruction, partial or complete, below the junction of the azygos with the superior vena cava will also elevate venous pressure, and abdominal compression will prevent the jugular blood from emptying freely into the azygos, thus further elevating the jugular pressure.

8. How should you compress the abdomen in order to prevent false elevations due to sympathetic outflow?

ANS.: a) Compress with warm hands or with a garment or sheet between your hand and the abdomen.

b) Spread the fingers apart, so that there is as little local pressure as possible.

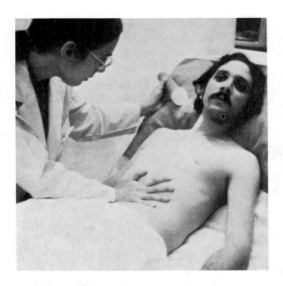

Spreading the fingers allows you to distribute pressure over a large area, so that more pressure can be applied without producing discomfort. Sometimes, only marked abdominal pressure will raise jugular pulsations enough to show that they are abnormal.

    c) Start by pressing gently, and gradually increase the pressure to just below the point of discomfort.

    d) Ask the patient to tell you if you are pressing too hard, and warn him that it spoils the test if you produce discomfort.

*9. What is Kussmaul's sign?

ANS.: Historically, it is the rise in the height of jugular pulsations during inspiration in patients with chronic constrictive pericarditis. However, it is found in only a minority of patients with constrictive pericarditis, and it often occurs with peripheral venous congestion from any cause [28].

    Note: a) Inspiration raises the intraabdominal pressure and can produce an effect like that of abdominal compression [54]. Therefore, in any patient with high venous pressure, inspiration may cause a further pressure increase. Also, any patient with a strong right atrial contraction may have a stronger one on inspiration, because that is when more blood is drawn into the right atrium.

    b) This sign should alert you to the presence of RV infarction in a patient with acute inferior infarction and no signs of left ventricular (LV) failure because it will be present in a majority of such patients [2A].

JUGULAR PULSE CONTOURS

The Normal Jugular Pulse Contours

1. What is the difference between the jugular and right atrial pulse contours?

ANS.: None, for all practical purposes, except when jugular pulse tracings pick up carotid artifacts. Therefore, the right atrial contours will be explained first, because it is right atrial events that produce the jugular contours.

    * *Note:* The delay between right atrial and jugular events during recording of jugular pulsations depends on the recording site used. There is a much more delayed response in the narrow external jugulars than in the larger internal jugulars. Thus, among various investigators, the delay has been found to vary from an insignificant 10 msec (0.01 sec) at the jugular bulb to as much as 100 msec (0.10 sec) at the external jugulars.

2. What is the normal right atrial contour and what are the letters given to the important crests and descents?

    ANS.: The normal right atrial contour consists of the waves A, C, and V, and the descents X, X prime, and Y.

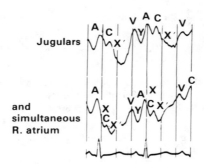

The atrial and jugular waves are very similar. The crests are A, C, and V; the descents are X, X', and Y.

THE A WAVE AND THE X DESCENT

1. What produces the A wave? Relate the right atrial A wave to the electrocardiogram (ECG).

    ANS.: The A wave is produced by right atrial contraction and relaxation.

    * *Note:* The right atrial pressure rise begins about 90 msec after the onset of the P wave. (Left atrial pressure begins to rise about 30 msec later.)

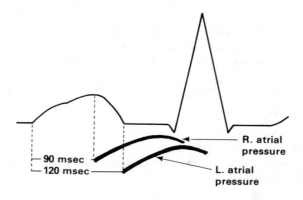

The A wave of the atrium and jugular pulse is produced by right atrial contraction, which in turn is produced by depolarization of the right atrium, as represented by the first third of the P wave. (The last two-thirds of the P wave represents left atrial depolarization.)

2. What is the descent produced by atrial relaxation called?
   ANS.: The X descent. It occurs just before the ventricle contracts.

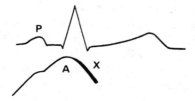

Atrial relaxation produces the drop in pressure known as the X descent.

Note: a) The rises in atrial contours are not named. Only the peaks and descents are given letters.

*b) A review of the literature on jugular contours shows that about half the writers on the subject do not actually name the atrial diastolic descent as a separate entity, and those that do name it call it the X descent [7].

THE C WAVE

1. What produces the rise in pressure that eventually makes the upstroke of the C wave in the right atrial pressure pulse?
   ANS.: Tricuspid valve closure due to RV contraction, which causes the valves to bulge upward into the right atrium, raising its pressure slightly. This occurs at the beginning of **isovolumic contraction**.

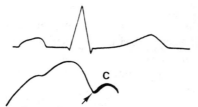

The right atrial C wave is probably due to tricuspid valve bulging, but in the jugulars only the first part of the C wave is due to such bulging. The huge jugular C waves seen in some tracings are certainly not all due to tricuspid valve movement.

Onset of RV contraction and beginning of tricuspid valve upward movement

*2. What produces the ascending part of the C wave in jugular tracings taken with a cone or other pickup device applied to the neck?
   ANS.: This is a fusion of the tricuspid bulging effect plus carotid artifact. It is usually (although not always) due to carotid artifact on the pulse tracing (i.e., when isovolumic contraction finishes and the aortic valve opens, the aortic pressure rises and expands the carotid arteries). The expansion of the carotid pulse is picked up by the pulse unit on the neck despite an attempt, usually unsuccessful, to isolate the jugular pulse. Sometimes a double upward dome is seen at the end of atrial relaxation, the first bulge due to tricuspid closure and the second to carotid artifact [22, 41].

*Note: a) Mackenzie, in 1902, in his book on the pulse, was the first to use the term *C wave* to symbolize the word *carotid*, because he believed that the C wave was always entirely due to carotid artifact [29]. He described an experiment in which pure jugular tracings were taken before and after the jugulars were dissected away from the carotid. The carotid C wave, which had been present before, disappeared after dissection. Mackenzie also described the various amplitudes of C wave that could be obtained merely by varying the pressure or site of the pickup. The theory attributing the C wave in jugular pulse tracings to upward bulging of the tricuspid valve was tested and also found wanting by Wiggers [52], who described right atrial pressure and jugular pulses taken at various levels. When he recorded pulse contours at successively higher levels, from the right atrium to low in the neck, the changes in contour that were due to tricuspid valve closure completely disappeared, and only the carotid artifact C wave remained.

In complete atrioventricular (AV) block, simultaneous jugular and right atrial pulse tracings have shown a persistent C wave in the jugulars following the onset of each ventricular contraction even when the C wave is absent in the atrial tracing [11].

If the carotid arterial component is electronically subtracted from the jugular tracing, the C wave becomes diminutive or disappears [35].

THE X PRIME DESCENT

1. What is meant by the X prime (X′) descent on an atrial or jugular pulse contour?
   ANS.: It is the systolic descent that occurs during ventricular contraction and is usually the major descent during systole. It contributes to the formation of the downslope of the C wave on a jugular or atrial pulse tracing.

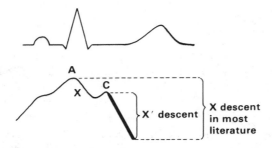

The jugular pulse descent during systole should not be called X, as it is by most authors, because the X descent is due to atrial relaxation, whereas the jugular systolic descent is due mostly to the pulling down of the base of the ventricle during systole. As shown in the pulse wave diagram, the diastolic X descent precedes the visible systolic jugular descent, which is now termed the X′ descent.

2. The following illustration numbers the four possible movements of the right ventricle that cause contraction and eject its blood. In the following diagram, which movements actually make the right ventricle smaller in systole?
   1) Does the free wall move in toward the septum?
   2) Does the septum move laterally toward the free wall of the right ventricle?
   3) Does the apex rise toward the base?
   4) Does the base move down toward the apex?

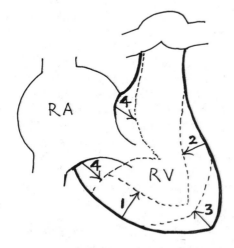

The broken lines represent the four possible inward movements of the RV that could eject its blood.

ANS.: 2) and 3) do not assist in RV contraction during systole. The apex does *not* move toward the base, and the septum does *not* normally move toward the free wall. (Echocardiograms show that the septum normally moves away from the RV free wall during systole.) The only mechanisms for RV contraction are 1) and 4) (i.e., the free wall moves inward and the base descends).

3. How do these RV contraction movements cause the X′ descent?

ANS.: If you watch carefully the next time you see a cineangiogram of a ventricle contracting, you will note that the base of the ventricle (floor of the atrium) descends toward the apex with ventricular contraction. Physiologists have called this the systolic "descent of the base," meaning the descent of the AV ring. Because the atria are firmly attached by their tributary veins to the surrounding structures, when the atrial floor is pulled down, a decline in atrial pressure results, the X′ descent.

* *Note:* a) A tricuspid closure C wave bulge may be expected in a jugular pulse tracing if there is right atrial or right ventricular overload, as in ASDs or congestive heart failure [4].

b) The anatomy of the LV lends itself well to a downward pull on the atrial floor because its syncytium has two prominent columns parallel with the long axis of the ventricle, each inserting into the trigones of the AV ring [17].

c) Since intrapericardial pressure falls during ventricular contraction because the heart shrinks during systole, the decreased intrapericardial pressure is transmitted to the right atrium, and this probably contributes to the X′ descent.

d) Other explanations for the systolic jugular descent do not stand up well against criticism.

1) Atrial relaxation has been said to be partly responsible [39]. Because an X′ descent occurs in patients with atrial fibrillation and even in atrial standstill, it cannot be due to atrial relaxation [20]. If venous return is reduced by limb tourniquets plus tilting, a jugular tracing will show a progressively smaller A wave and a larger C wave until the A wave is eliminated. The systolic descent, although smaller, remains [34].

2) Another explanation given for the systolic descent is that it is caused by the pressure drop in the thorax secondary to the loss of blood from the chest due to LV ejection. This ignores the increase in thoracic blood volume that occurs during simultaneous RV systole. Flowmeters and angiograms have shown that forward flow into the heart occurs chiefly during RV systole, which produces a "suction effect" on vena caval blood as it draws the floor of the atrium down [14, 51].

e) In a thorough review of the nomenclature used by 36 authors who have described jugular contours, it was noted that almost half of these authors left the systolic venous descent unnamed [7]. It was called X by seven authors; it was combined with atrial relaxation under the letter X by an equal number; and it was called X prime (X′) by nine authors [7].

4. What are the advantages of using the term X′ for the systolic jugular descent?
   ANS.: a) It is a compromise with those who have always used an X to represent the descent of the base.

   b) No other name has been given to it by anyone who wanted to distinguish it from the X of atrial diastole ever since it was first used by Mackenzie in 1907, in what was apparently the first attempt to distinguish the atrial diastolic X descent from the systolic descent [30]. Mackenzie showed a tracing with a delay in ventricular contraction due to first-degree AV block (long P-R interval). The systolic jugular descent was so obviously not due to atrial diastole, which showed its descent long before, that he felt obliged to give a different name to the descent during systole, calling it X′. He correctly ascribed it to a drawing down of the floor of the atrium by the RV contraction.

THE V WAVE AND Y DESCENT

1. What causes the ascending limb of the V wave?
   ANS.: During systole the tricuspid valve is closed, and atrial filling from the venae cavae finally overcomes the "descent of the base" when ventricular contraction becomes too weak to cause any more base descent. Therefore, toward the end of systole atrial pressure begins to rise. Because the V wave is a right

atrial filling wave built up during systole, it is crucial to remember that the V wave is mainly a systolic event, resulting entirely from blood pouring into the right atrium while the tricuspid valve is closed. It may help the novice to call the V wave a *V-illing* wave (i.e., right atrial *filling* wave).

  * *Note:* The X' descent ends at a nadir called the X' trough, from which the V wave begins its rise.

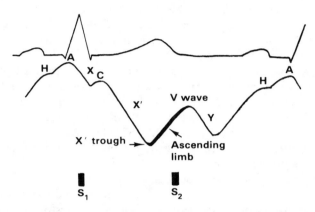

The jugular V wave is built up during systole, and its height will reflect the rate of filling and the elasticity of the right atrium. Between the bottom of the Y descent (Y trough) and beginning of the A wave is the period of relatively slow filling of the "atrioventricle" or diastasis period. The wave built up during diastasis is the H wave. The H wave height also reflects the stiffness of the right atrium.

2. What causes the Y descent, or descending limb, of the V wave?

   ANS.: When ventricular systole ends and the ventricle expands rapidly, the ventricular pressure will quickly fall to below right atrial pressure, which is about 5 mm Hg. At this point the tricuspid valve opens, and there is rapid inflow into the expanding RV. This causes a rapid drop in right atrial pressure because the right atrium empties more rapidly than it can fill. This fall in right atrial pressure is known universally as the *Y descent.*

   Note: * a) The bottom of the descent is known as the *Y trough.*

   b) It is easiest to understand that the right atrium empties faster than it fills if you assume that RV expansion is not a passive process but an active one that can create a suction effect on the right atrium.

   c) The common pressure chamber produced by the opening of the tricuspid valves might be called an "atrioventricle."

3. What is the wave called that is produced by the passive pressure rise in the atrioventricle as it fills in diastole after the Y trough?

   ANS.: The diastasis wave, or H wave [22]. (See figure above.)

   * *Note:* The H wave may be absent in tricuspid stenosis because the Y descent is too slow unless there is a bradycardia.

* 4. When is forward flow through the superior vena cava and right atrium greatest in the normal heart, during ventricular systole or diastole?

   ANS.: Vena caval forward flow is normally greater during ventricular systole than during diastole. This is reflected by the fact that the X' descent is normally deeper than the Y descent [45].

CONTOUR RECOGNITION BY INSPECTION

Normal Jugular Movement

1. Why is it easier to decipher jugular movements by observing the descents, or down-ward-collapsing movements, rather than ascents, or upward movements?

   ANS.: The jugular descents or collapsing movements are usually larger and faster than the ascents because the X′ descent is due to the rapid RV contraction and the Y descent is due to the rapid phase of RV expansion. The eye perceives and times the deeper, faster descents more easily than it does the slower, shallower ascents.

   Note: You will see on page 101 that it is easier to time jugular descents by either auscultation of heart sounds or pulse synchronization, especially when A waves are absent as in atrial fibrillation or flutter.

2. Can you see a C wave by inspection of the normal jugulars?

   ANS.: No. The C wave is not normally visible because it is too small. In jugular tracings it is mostly carotid artifact. The V wave is also often too small to be seen in normal adults.

3. Can you separate the X from the X′ descent by eye?

   ANS.: Not easily, because the C wave that separates them is invisible.

   Note: After much experience a subtle double systolic descent or break in the descent can be seen in some subjects, denoting a separate X and X′ descent.

4. Why is the V wave not always visible in the normal jugular pulse even though it is usually seen on a jugular pulse tracing?

   ANS.: Because the right atrium is a very compliant or distensible chamber, that is, the right atrium is too distensible to allow its pressure to rise very much when the tricuspid valve is closed.

   Note: The left atrium is a thicker chamber and has a much more visible V wave and Y descent. Also, it may receive some contribution from the slightly delayed pulmonary artery pressure pulse.

5. How can the knowledge that the normal jugular is mainly a systolic descent (X + X′) help in recognizing whether or not a jugular contour is normal?

   ANS.: Because the descent of the base, which causes the X′ descent, is a systolic event, it must end at the end of systole, which at the bedside is marked by the second heart sound (S_2). With your stethoscope on the chest, you can time the dominant jugular descent or collapse to see if it appears to fall onto the S_2. If it does, it is an X plus X′, and the wave preceding it must be an A wave. If, on the other hand, the dominant descent does not fall onto the S_2, it must be a Y descent, and the preceding wave must be a V wave.

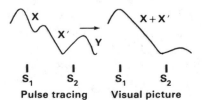

Pulse tracing   Visual picture

Although the X′ trough actually ends *before* the S_2, to the eye and ear it seems to end *at* the S_2; i.e., the jugular descent seems to fall onto the S_2.

Note: a) If there is only a V wave and a Y descent, it may help to time the peaks because the peak of the jugular pulse will coincide with the S_2.

b) If there is no A wave, as in atrial fibrillation or flutter, the wave preceding a systolic descent is the H wave.

c) The X′ actually ends before the S_2, but it appears to end *at* the S_2 because the eye sees movement later than the ear hears sound— that is, a movement that ends just *before* a sound appears to end *at* the sound. (Visual perception has been shown to be delayed by about 60 msec compared with auditory perception.)

Note: With this technique, the type of wave that is present can be inferred from the recognition of descents. If, for example, in sinus rhythm, there is an X′ descent but very little Y descent, a dominant A wave is present. If, on the other hand, there is a large Y and very little X′ descent, the presence of a dominant V wave can be inferred. If we see equal X′ and Y descents, we can infer that the A and V waves are nearly equal in amplitude.

6. What relation should the X′ and Y descents have to the carotid or radial pulse as felt by the finger?

ANS.: The X′ should seem to be immediately initiated by the peak of the carotid or radial pulse.

Note: If you say "C" simultaneously with the tap of the carotid pulse and "down" with the observed X′ jugular descent, the rhythm will be "C-down" as quickly as you can say it. The jugular X′ descent and a peripheral arterial pulse such as the radial will be synchronous. The Y descents should be later so that they seem to occur about the same distance from the carotid or radial pulse as the two heart sounds are from one another. Therefore, if you say "C-down" slowly enough to equal the lub-dup of a first and second heart sound rhythm, you will have it about right.

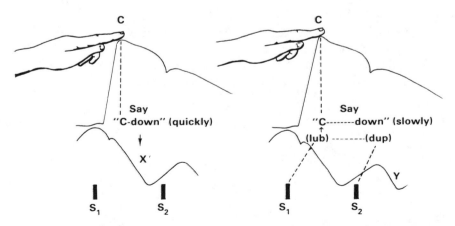

With a quick "C-down," the "down" will time with the X′ descent. With a slow "C — — — down," the "down" will time with the Y descent.

7. Why is it normal for young people to have a Y descent that is moderately easy to see (i.e., a fair V wave)?

ANS.: Because the circulation time is slightly fast in most young people, the atrial filling wave or V wave will be slightly exaggerated. However, the X' descent will still be dominant.

Making Jugular Movements More Visible

1. Which jugulars should you examine for contours, the internal or the external jugulars? Why?

ANS.: Because they have the freest communication with the right atrium, the internals are best. Occasionally, however, the external jugulars show the only easily analyzable movement, and then they must be used for contour analysis.

2. In what position do you place the patient to examine for jugular contours?

ANS.: In the supine position, because in this position more blood returns to the right atrium. Further, when the chest is raised, the jugulars may disappear below the clavicles.

3. How can you exaggerate jugular movement that is too small to be easily timed?

ANS.: Try to increase the venous return by the following maneuvers:

a) Elevate the subject's legs.

b) Have the subject take deeper breaths. Deep inspiration can draw more blood into the right atrium, making movements of larger amplitude.

Note: Holding the breath is sometimes necessary when the use of accessory muscles of respiration interferes with jugular visibility. This, however, often produces a slight Valsalva maneuver, which may eliminate all venous movement.

DIFFERENTIATING THE JUGULAR FROM THE CAROTID PULSE

1. How does sitting up affect the jugular and carotids?

ANS.: The more upright the chest, the lower the jugular pulsations are in relation to the clavicle, because the right atrium becomes lower in relation to the clavicle in the upright position. The carotid, on the other hand, appears higher in the neck as the chest becomes more upright.

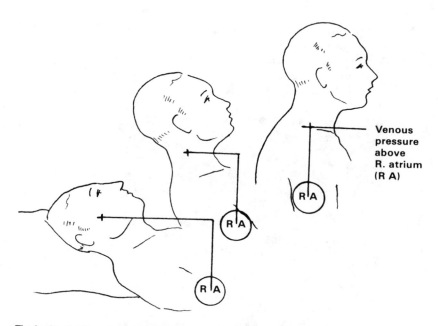

Venous
pressure
above
R. atrium
(R A)

The horizontal line represents the top level of jugular pulsations. Note that jugular pulsations fall relative to the clavicle with a subject in the upright position. Visible carotid pulsations remain the same distance superior to the clavicle in all chest positions.

2. How can you tell a jugular from a carotid by palpation?

ANS.: Normal jugulars are not palpable. If venous pressure is high, you may occasionally feel a very compressible gentle undulation. The carotids produce a strong, almost incompressible impulse.

3. How does abdominal compression differ in its effect on jugular and carotid pulsations?

ANS.: In normal subjects sudden abdominal compression momentarily displaces some blood into the RV, which therefore has a greater output for a few beats. This produces a greater descent of the base effect and therefore a more marked X' descent; because of the momentary increase of venous return, the V wave may also become higher for a few beats. In patients with congestive failure, the jugulars may be more visible for as long as abdominal compression is maintained. Abdominal compression has no effect on carotid pulsations.

4. What is the effect of inspiration on jugular and carotid pulsations?

ANS.: It increases the amplitude of jugular pulsations but has little visible effect on carotid pulsations.

5. Why will inspiration increase the amplitude of jugular pulsations?

ANS.: Inspiration decreases intrathoracic pressure, which in turn acts as an expanding bellows or suction pump to bring more blood into the RV during systole. The greater RV contraction in response to this increased volume causes a greater "descent of the base" (the X' descent). A greater filling wave (V wave) and Y descent are also produced.

6. How can pencil or finger pressure on the neck reveal whether one is dealing with jugular or carotid pulsations?

ANS.: Moderate pressure on the neck below the level of pulsations will obliterate jugular but not carotid pulsations.

Note: When jugular pressure is high, obliteration of its pulsation may occur only with compression that is applied at least one-third or even one-half of the way up the neck.

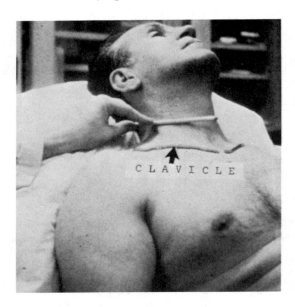

A very strong jugular pulsation with a high venous pressure will not be eliminated by pressure just above the clavicle, probably because the sternomastoid tendons prevent adequate pressure against the vein.

Summary of Differences Between Jugular and Carotid Pulsations

1. The carotid pulse has only one descent, or collapse; the jugular often has two, the X' and the Y.
2. The carotid descent is slow, whereas the jugular X' descent is rapid. If the fastest and greatest movement is a collapse, or descent, it is a jugular pulse.
3. A pencil pressed firmly just above the clavicle will obliterate all but the highest pressure jugular pulsations but will not affect carotid pulsations.
4. Inspiration may exaggerate jugular pulsations (although it may lower their vertical level) but will, if anything, diminish carotid pulsations.
5. Sitting up will make the carotids appear higher in the neck, but the jugulars will appear lower in the neck.
6. The carotid, if visible, is always easily palpable with firm pressure. The normal jugular is rarely palpable, except as a slight fluttering sensation with light pressure. The jugular is relatively easily compressible.
7. The X' descent appears to end at the S_2, whereas the carotid descent appears to begin with the S_2.
8. Sudden abdominal compression makes the jugulars momentarily more visible but has no effect on the carotids.

Summary of How to Recognize Normal Jugulars

1. With the patient supine, palpate the carotid or radial pulse. If the jugular descent occurs either a fraction of a second after the carotid pulse or simultaneously with the radial pulse, a dominant X′ descent is present.
2. Listen to the heart sounds and time the descents. If the nadir (bottom) of the descent falls onto the S_2, the dominant descent is an X′.
3. If you are still uncertain because of an irregular rhythm, you can confirm your impression by looking at the peaks of the jugular outward movements. If the dominant peak is simultaneous with the S_1, there is a dominant A wave, which is one of the characteristics of a normal contour.

ABNORMAL JUGULAR CONTOURS

Abnormalities of the A Wave

1. What can cause a stronger than normal atrial contraction, thereby producing an exaggerated or giant A wave?
   ANS.: a) Obstruction to outflow from the atrium, as in tricuspid stenosis (TS) or right **atrial myxoma** [38].
   b) A poorly compliant (stiffer) RV, as in pulmonary stenosis (PS) or pulmonary hypertension.
2. Why does a RV systolic (pressure) overload, as in PS or pulmonary hypertension, cause a stronger right atrial contraction?
   ANS.: When the RV has a **pressure load** to overcome, it becomes thicker and less compliant than normal. Because in diastole the atrium and ventricle are in continuity, the pressure in this "atrioventricle" rises very rapidly as it fills with blood. The stretch of the atrium produces a **Starling effect** and a powerful atrial contraction, which stretches the ventricle before it contracts. This in turn produces a Starling effect on the ventricle that can result in a ventricular contraction that is more powerful than usual.
   Note: a) There may seem to be only an A wave in the jugular pulse in severe PS because RV systole may be so prolonged that the V wave is also prolonged. (Remember that the V wave is built up during ventricular systole when the AV valves are closed.) If there is a slight tachycardia or a first-degree AV block, the atrium is ready to contract at the time of the V wave peak and the AV valve opens. Therefore, the giant A wave may begin to rise almost as soon as the late peak of the V wave is reached.
   b) In the presence of pulmonary hypertension the peak of the A wave comes earlier. One study has shown that if the patient has chronic obstructive pulmonary disease (COPD) and the ratio of P to peak of A over the P-R interval is less than 1, the mean pulmonary artery pressure is above 22 mm Hg [49].
   c) A giant A wave can produce a presystolic sound if you auscultate over the jugulars [10].
3. What else besides a strong atrial contraction increases the amplitude of the A wave?

ANS.: An atrial contraction during ventricular systole. If the atrium contracts when the tricuspid valve is closed, it will transmit its pressure backward to form a large A wave called a cannon wave. Cannon waves may occur either in the presence of **atrioventricular dissociation** or when there is an early P wave (e.g., as with a premature atrial depolarization or junctional pacemaker).

Note: a) A strong right atrial contraction that produces a larger A wave than normal but not a cannon wave is known as a giant A wave.

b) Cannon waves are usually very difficult to see unless the atrial contraction is very strong, as when there is loss of **compliance** (increased stiffness) of the RV as in pulmonary hypertension. Because they are easily recorded they probably were given the name cannon waves from the appearance of the recordings rather than from the appearance of the slight variations in jugular pulsation amplitude seen in the neck.

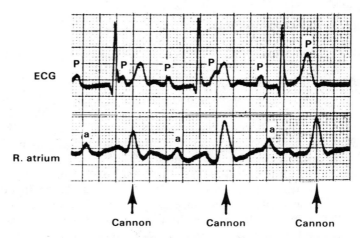

Note that in this patient with complete atrioventricular block, every other P wave happens to fall on a T wave, i.e., it occurs during ventricular systole when the tricuspid valve is closed. Thus, there is a cannon A wave with every other P wave.

*4. How can the jugular A wave suggest **hypertrophic subaortic stenosis** in a patient with an aortic ejection murmur?

ANS.: If the jugulars show a giant A wave, RV outflow obstruction due to an excessively thick septum is suggested.

Abnormalities of the X′ Descent

1. What can cause a smaller than normal or even absent X′ descent?

ANS.: a) A poor RV contraction, as in heart failure, or absence of an atrial presystolic Starling effect stretch, as in atrial fibrillation, atrial flutter, or right atrial standstill [20].

b) Tricuspid regurgitation (TR). The X′ descent is encroached on in proportion to the degree of regurgitation.

*c) Loss of pericardium, for instance, if the surgeon fails to close the pericardium after open heart surgery or if there is congenital absence of the pericardium.

d) Build up of the V wave earlier than usual, as with loss of capacitance of the right atrium (e.g., when filled by tumor [right atrial myxoma]) or with loss of compliance of the right atrium due to hypertrophy (e.g., as in TS or stiffening by sutures in the right atrium after open heart surgery).

*2. What condition besides increased volume in the RV (as in ASD) can produce an increased descent of the base and X' descent?

ANS.: a) Increased pressure in the RV, as in pulmonary hypertension or PS.

  b) **Pericardial tamponade.**

Abnormalities of the V Wave

1. What can cause a higher than normal jugular V wave or relatively deep Y descent?

ANS.: a) Rapid or excessive right atrial filling while the tricuspid valve is closed, as in ASD.

  b) Tricuspid regurgitation, if one calls the regurgitant wave a V wave.

   Note: A poor descent of the base of the RV, as in the presence of a poor stroke volume, does not produce an absolutely higher V wave but a relatively higher V wave than normal due to the shallow X' descent.

  c) A high venous pressure or right atrial and ventricular diastolic pressure in mid and late diastole, as in congestive heart failure or severe pulmonary hypertension.

  d) Loss of compliance of the right atrium, as in constrictive pericarditis or after heart surgery in which sutures are placed in the right atrium [21, 31, 42]. A severe pectus excavatum may also restrict right atrial filling and cause a poor X' descent and a relatively high V wave [13].

   Note: a) If the X' is smaller than the Y descent after heart surgery, the myocardium has probably been damaged by the surgery or was depressed before surgery. It is also possible that if the pericardium is not closed after surgery, interpericardial pressure changes during systole will be blunted and will decrease the X' descent.

    b) A calcified pericardium without constriction of the ventricles may constrict only the atria and produce a relatively high V wave.

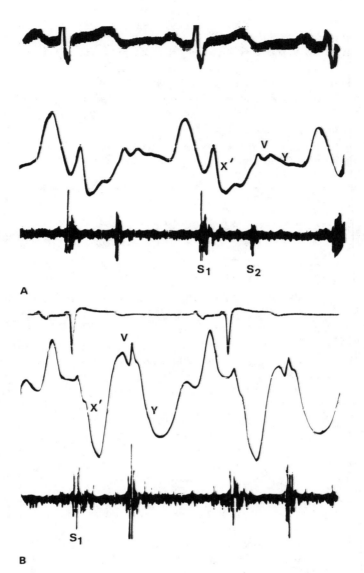

(A) The preoperative jugular tracing with a dominant X + X′ descent. (By inspection the C wave was not visible.) **(B)** The jugular tracing after bypass surgery. Note the dominant Y descent.

  e) Loss of capacitance of the right atrium, as in right atrial myxoma.
 *f) Severe MR [45] produces a large right atrial V wave possibly by displacing the atrial septum into the right atrium during ventricular systole.
 *g) A pleuropericardial defect [55].
2. What can cause rapid atrial filling, thus producing a relatively high V wave?
 ANS.: a) Rapid **circulation times,** such as those occurring in exercise, anemia, anxiety states, and hyperthyroidism.
  b) Filling of the right atrium from extra sources as in ASD, **anomalous pulmonary venous drainage** into the right atrium, or TR.
  Note: *a) A patent foramen ovale may be stretched by severe MR or a

large left-to-right shunt such as patent ductus arteriosus or VSD, thus producing an atrial left-to-right shunt that can enlarge the right atrial V wave [36].

b) In ASD, the overloaded right atrium contracts strongly owing to the Starling effect, producing a prominent A wave and X descent. The large volume ejected by the RV causes a deep X′ descent. The large V wave, as well as the deep X plus X′, produces a characteristic jugular pulse with both deep X plus X′ and deep Y descents (i.e., a prominent A wave and a relatively high V wave). (See figure on page 381.)

3. Why will double filling of the right atrium by TR not produce deep X′ and Y descents as it does with ASDs?

ANS.: In TR the tendency to increase the descent of the base is counteracted by the regurgitant stream. Therefore, with increasing amounts of TR, the X′ descent becomes more and more shallow and the Y descent increasingly deep.

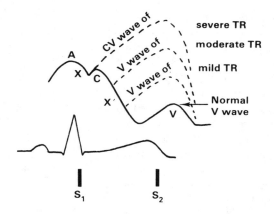

As the degree of TR increases, the X′ descent is increasingly encroached upon. With severe TR, no X′ descent is seen, and the jugular pulse wave is said to be "ventricularized."

*4. On inspection of the jugulars alone severe TR is often confused with which lesion? Why?

ANS.: Severe AR. The large single regurgitant CV wave resembles the large carotid pulse wave of severe AR.

*5. Why will a poor descent of the base, such as occurs with a poor RV contraction, cause a high V wave?

ANS.: Both the X′ descent and the V wave are produced during systole (i.e., while the triscuspid valve is closed). The V wave can appear only when atrial filling can overcome the fall in pressure produced by the descent of the base. A poor descent of the base will be overcome much earlier by atrial filling from the venae cavae, resulting in a larger V wave.

*6. Why is it logical to call the atrial wave caused by TR a V wave, even though it is the result of a different mechanism than the usual V wave?

ANS.: Other sources besides the usual venae cavae blood often contribute to the V wave; for example, in ASDs, blood from the left atrium is added to it, and an anomalous pulmonary vein draining into the right atrium can also contribute to it. Regurgitant flow from the RV contributing to the V wave in

TR should not force us to use a different term for this large wave. However, if the entire X' is replaced, the systolic wave may justifiably be called a CV wave.

*7. How does the V wave in patients with congestive (dilated) cardiomyopathy differ from normal on a pulse tracing?

ANS.: The horizontal distance from the V peak to the Y trough (V–Y time) becomes shorter, due to decreased distensibility of the RV (i.e., a slight restrictive effect) causing the Y trough to begin at a higher pressure and therefore earlier.

Note: In hypertrophic cardiomyopathies the V–Y time is prolonged, reflecting the poor compliance of the ventricles and their slow expansion in diastole.

The Jugulars in Pericardial Tamponade and Constrictive Pericarditis

*1. Why may the X' descent in tamponade be very deep?

ANS.: Unlike constriction, in which diastolic flow is not restricted until the end of early diastole, in tamponade diastolic flow is restricted throughout diastole, including the period of early rapid expansion of the ventricle. Therefore, in tamponade forward flow depends almost entirely on the descent of the base. It is not surprising that in the absence of diastolic forward flow the entire forward flow occurs during ventricular systole and a dominant X' descent is always present. Cardiac output can be maintained only by tachycardia or more complete systolic emptying, or both.

Note: In constrictive pericarditis systole is also often restricted, as shown by the below normal or low normal cardiac output and stroke volume at rest [2, 37, 50].

*2. How can a jugular contour help differentiate constrictive pericarditis, effusive-constrictive pericarditis, and tamponade?

ANS.: In constrictive pericarditis the Y descent is dominant. In effusive-constrictive pericarditis the X' is either dominant or equal to the Y descent even in atrial fibrillation. In tamponade there is almost always a dominant X' descent and occasionally no Y at all [27].

Note: When the X' descent is dominant, an S₃ or pericardial knock (p. 139) is usually absent [20].

*3. When should you suspect that a deep X' descent is due to the presence of tamponade or effusive-constrictive pericarditis?

ANS.: If the venous pressure is high, a deep X' is rarely seen unless there is tamponade or effusive-constrictive pericarditis, especially if the patient is in atrial fibrillation.

Note: In severe chronic MR and AR (and perhaps in other conditions causing LV dilatation) a **Bernheim effect** that may have the same effect as effusive-constrictive pericarditis may occur [43, 45]. This may produce a deep X' descent (as well as a Y) in the presence of a high venous pressure [3].

*4. How can a jugular tracing help suggest constrictive pericarditis?

ANS.: It will reflect the right atrial pressure curve, which usually shows a dominant V wave and a steep Y descent with a rapid rise to a diastolic plateau type of H wave [19]. The diastolic part of this curve reflects RV pressure events known as the "square root sign," or the early diastolic dip and plateau, which are commonly seen at cardiac catheterization in constrictive pericarditis. One theory attributes the early diastolic dip to work performed during contraction on the fibrotic or calcific pericardium that is fixed to the ventricular wall—(i.e., it is deformed in the manner of a loaded spring) [5]. The sudden release of the loaded spring in diastole causes the ventricular wall to recoil excessively, resulting in a rapid fall in ventricular pressure (which is reflected in the rapid jugular Y descent). The limited expansion due to the encasement causes the ventricular pressure to rise steeply after the early dip. The same mechanism does not well explain the dip and plateau in the right atrial pressure tracing in some patients with RV infarction or myocardial infiltrate causing a restrictive cardiomyopathy, as in amyloid disease [47].

Note: a) If in the presence of a high venous pressure the Y descent is either equal to or greater than the X' descent and the patient has neither constrictive pericarditis nor recent heart surgery, then pulmonary hypertension should be considered even without significant TR.

b) In the presence of constriction due to pericardial fibrosis without calcification the jugular findings are similar to those of tamponade in that there is a dominant X' descent, but they are unlike tamponade in that the Y descent is slightly exaggerated [25].

*5. How can we explain the small V wave in tamponade and the large V wave in constrictive pericarditis?

ANS.: Because fluid does not have as much effect on atrial compliance as does the stiff encasement of the atrium with fibrous tissue and calcium, as in constrictive pericarditis, tamponade does not build up as large a V wave.

Abnormalities of the H Wave

*1. When does a steeply rising H wave occur?

ANS.: When there is a restriction of RV expansion, as in constrictive pericarditis and restrictive cardiomyopathy, occurring, for instance, in amyloidosis [47].

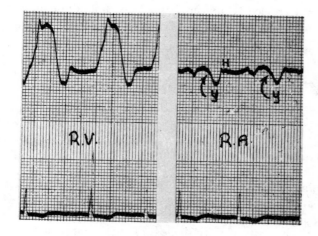

Right ventricular (RV) and right atrial (RA) pressures from a patient with constrictive pericarditis and atrial fibrillation. Note the square root sign in the RV pressure curve reflected in the RA curves (i.e., a Y descent that terminates in a rapid rise to an H plateau). Note that despite atrial fibrillation, a small X' descent is present.

Note: a) Right ventricular infarction has the same effect as a restrictive cardiomyopathy [26]. The jugulars show the "square root sign" seen in the right atrial and RV pressure curves [6, 32].

b) An H wave may be absent in tricuspid stenosis because the Y descent is too slow, unless there is a bradycardia.

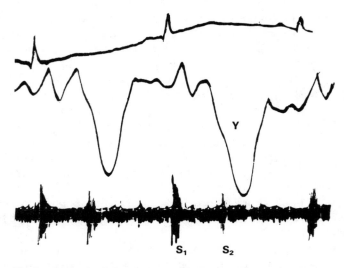

This jugular tracing is from a 60-year-old woman one month after an inferior myocardial infarction that was diagnosed as extending to the RV. Note the "square root sign," i.e., the dominant Y descent rises steeply to a plateau-type H wave.

THE JUGULAR PULSE IN ARRHYTHMIAS

1. How does atrial fibrillation affect the jugular pulse contour?
   ANS.: a) No A wave is present.

   b) There is a decreased X′ descent, usually with a dominant Y descent.

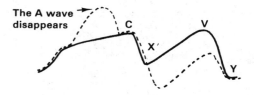

The dominant descent in atrial fibrillation is almost always the Y descent, i.e., it has the superficial appearance of the pulse wave of TR.

2. Why is there a diminished X′ descent in the presence of atrial fibrillation?
   ANS.: The absent atrial "kick" at the end of diastole causes a poor RV contraction because the RV is not stretched at the end of diastole and therefore loses some of its Starling effect. With the loss of atrial contraction, the otherwise normal heart may decrease its stroke work by about 10 percent, but the heart with RV overload may decrease its stroke work by as much as 30 percent.

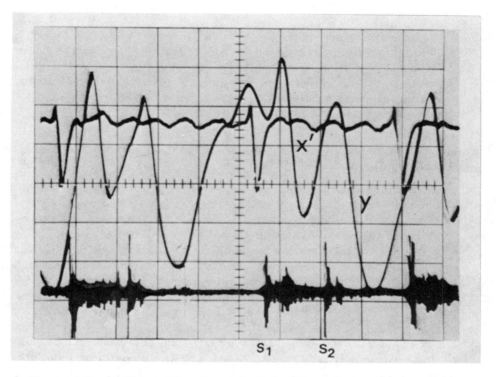

The wave before the X′ cannot be an A wave since it is not due to atrial contraction. It is really a prolonged H wave. Note the good X′ descent, despite the dominant Y descent, in this patient with moderate rheumatic MR.

3. What other reasons are there for a poor X′ descent in atrial fibrillation if there is also a high venous pressure?

ANS.: a) A high venous pressure due to heart failure implies poor RV contraction and therefore a poor descent of the base. The poor RV contraction also causes a smaller decrease in intrapericardial pressure, which in turn produces a smaller fall in right atrial pressure during systole.

b) The right atrium in a patient in heart failure is under increased tension both from excess sympathetic stimulation and from the high pressure in the atrioventricle when the AV valve is open. Thus, the atrium is less compliant than normal and there will be a steeper rise of pressure as it receives its blood from the venae cavae to build up a V wave during ventricular systole.

Note: a) Some TR tends to occur in the presence of atrial fibrillation and high venous pressures, which tend to obliterate the X′ descent further.

b) If only a systolic wave (CV wave) and Y descent are present, forward flow into the right atrium will occur only in diastole [45].

4. What is the name of the wave that precedes the descent of the base or X′ descent in a patient with no atrial contraction (as in atrial fibrillation)?

ANS.: An H wave. (The tradition of not naming the diastolic wave in atrial fibrillation supports further the concept of naming descents rather than waves because most physicians are not accustomed to describing H waves on jugular inspection.)

* 5. How are jugular pulsations affected by atrial flutter?

    ANS.: Multiple small A waves may result, one for each F wave, with higher ones occurring during systole when the AV valves are closed. These are difficult to see unless the venous pressure is elevated. (Even coarse atrial fibrillation has produced irregular small A waves in jugular tracings.)

*HOW TO RECORD A JUGULAR PULSE

* 1. Where must one place a pulse pickup on the neck for best recording of an internal jugular pulsation?

    ANS.: Over the right jugular bulb [2]. This is located just above the clavicle, between the two origins of the sternocleidomastoid muscle.

    It is often helpful to remove the pillow from beneath the patient's head, raise his chin slightly, and push it to the left in order to expose the right jugular bulb area as well as to relax the muscle overlying the jugular bulb.

* 2. Which is preferable, a photoelectric cell method of recording the silhouette of a jugular as it interrupts a light source, a cone that picks up volume changes, or a pressure-sensitive device that is placed on the jugulars?

    ANS.: The photoelectric cell method exaggerates carotid artifacts and also causes marked time delays. Thus, either a cone or a pressure-sensitive transducer is preferable.

*SPECIAL INFORMATION FROM JUGULAR TRACINGS

* 1. What is meant by the P_2 to V peak interval, and what hemodynamic event does this represent?

    ANS.: The distance between the pulmonary component of the S_2 and the peak of the V wave of a simultaneously recorded jugular pulse tracing represents the isovolumic relaxation time of the RV.

* 2. What controls the P_2 to V peak interval?

    ANS.: a) Heart rate. Bradycardia makes it longer.

    b) Rapidity of intrinsic ventricular expansion time. In uncomplicated ASD the rate of expansion is inordinately rapid.

    c) Height of the pulmonary artery pressure and right atrial V wave pressure. Pulmonary hypertension prolongs isovolumic expansion time, thereby prolonging the P_2 to V peak interval, provided the venous pressure is normal and the height of the V wave is not thereby increased.

    Note: The P_2 to V peak interval is well correlated with mean pulmonary artery pressure in isolated VSDs, in which the regression equation for mean PA pressure is $812 \times (P_2$ to V$) - 37$, with a standard error of 12 mm. Roughly, a P_2 to V peak interval of 80 msec (0.08 sec) separates normal from elevated PA pressure [15]. It is probable that the kind of pulse unit necessary to make use of these figures is one that utilizes volume displacement by a funnel or cup. The P_2 to

V peak interval in ASD or in PS correlates poorly with PA pressure.

REFERENCES

1. Ali, N. Pulsations of arm veins in the absence of tricuspid insufficiency. *Chest* 63:41, 1973.
2. Armstrong, T. G., Lewis, B. S., and Gotsman, M. S. Systolic time intervals in constrictive pericarditis and severe primary myocardial disease. *Am. Heart J.* 85:6, 1973.
2A. Baigrie, R. S., et al. The spectrum of right ventricular involvement in inferior wall myocardial infarction: A clinical, hemodynamic and noninvasive study. *J. Am. Coll. Cardiol.* 16:1396, 1983.
3. Bernheim, P. Right ventricular stenosis, accompanied by deformation of the septum in eccentric hypertrophy of the left ventricle and consequent venistasis. *J. Practitioners* 29:721, 1915.
4. Bonner, A. J., Jr., and Tavel, M. E. The relationship of the jugular "C" wave to changing diastolic intervals. *Am. Heart J.* 84:441, 1972.
5. Burch, G. E., and Giles, T. D. Theoretic consideration of the post-systolic "dip" of constrictive pericarditis. *Am. Heart J.* 86:569, 1973.
6. Coma-Canella, I., and Lopez-Sendon, J. Ventricular compliance in ischemic right ventricular dysfunction. *Am. J. Cardiol.* 45:555, 1980.
7. Constant, J. The X prime descent in jugular contour: nomenclature and recognition. *Am. Heart J.* 88:372, 1974.
8. Constant, J. Arterial and venous pulsations in cardiovascular diagnosis. *J. Cardiovasc. Med.* 5:973, 1980.
9. Davison, R., and Cannon, R. Estimation of central venous pressure by examination of jugular veins. *Am. Heart J.* 87:279, 1974.
10. Dock, W. Loud presystolic sounds over the jugular veins associated with high venous pressure. *Am. J. Med.* 20:853, 1956.
11. Feder, W., and Cherry, R. External jugular phlebogram as reflecting venous and right atrial hemodynamics. *Am. J. Cardiol.* 12:383, 1963.
11A. Fisher, J., et al. Determinants and clinical significance of jugular venous valve competence. *Circulation* 65:188, 1982.
12. Fred, H. L., Wukash, D. C., and Petrany, Z. Transient compression of the left innominate vein. *Circulation* 29:758, 1964.
13. Fukuda, N., et al. Phono- mechano- and echocardiographic studies of patients with funnel chest, especially on the changes of the jugular phlebogram and interventricular septal motion. *J. Cardiography* 11:161, 1981.
14. Gabe, I. T., et al. Measurement of instantaneous blood flow velocity and pressure in conscious man with a catheter-tip velocity probe. *Circulation* 40:603, 1969.
15. Gamboa, R., et al. External measurement of the isovolumic relaxation phase as an indicator of pulmonary artery pressure in ventricular septal defects. *Am. J. Cardiol.* 16:665, 1965.
16. Gensini, G. G., et al. Persistent left superior vena cava. *Am. J. Cardiol.* 4:677, 1959.
17. Grant, R. P. Notes on the muscular architecture of the left ventricle. *Circulation* 32:301, 1965.
18. Hamosh, P., and Cohn, J. N. Mechanism of the hepatojugular reflux test. *Am. J. Cardiol.* 25:100, 1970.
19. Hansen, A. T., Eskildsen, P., and Gotzsche, P. Pressure curves from right auricle and the right ventricle in chronic constrictive pericarditis. *Circulation* 3:881, 1951.
20. Harley, A. Persistent right atrial standstill. *Br. Heart J.* 38:646, 1976.
21. Hartman, H. The jugular venous tracing. *Am. Heart J.* 59:698, 1960.
22. Hirschfelder, A. D. Some variations in the form of the venous pulse. *Johns Hopkins Hosp. Bull.* 195–196:265, 1907.
23. Hitzig, W. M. On the mechanism of inspiratory filling of the cervical veins and pulsus paradoxus in venous hypertension. *J. Mt. Sinai Hosp.* 8:625, 1941.
24. Horwitz, S. et al. Clinical diagnosis of persistent left superior vena cava by observation of jugular pulses. *Am. Heart J.* 86:759, 1973.

25. Ikram, H., Banim, S. O., and Makey, A. R. Clinical features of non–tuberculous constrictive pericarditis. *Thorax* 29:204, 1974.
26. Jensen, D. P., Goolsby, J. P., Jr., and Oliva, P. B. Hemodynamic pattern resembling pericardial constriction after acute inferior myocardial infarction with right ventricular infarction. *Am. J. Cardiol.* 42:858, 1978.
27. Kesteloot, H., and Denef, B. Value of reference tracings in diagnosis and assessment of constrictive epi– and pericarditis. *Br. Heart J.* 32:675, 1970.
28. Lange, R. L., et al. Diagnostic signs in compressive cardiac disorders: Constrictive pericarditis, pericardial effusion and tamponade. *Circulation* 33:763, 1966.
29. Mackenzie, J. *The Study of the Pulse.* London: Pentland, 1902.
30. Mackenzie, J. The interpretation of the pulsations in the jugular veins. *Am. J. Med. Sci.* 134:12, 1907.
31. Matsuhisa, M., et al. Postoperative changes of jugular pulse tracing. *J. Cardiography* 6:403, 1976.
32. Matsuhisa, M., et al. Right ventricular infarction: Graphic studies of three cases. *J. Cardiography* 9:375, 1979.
33. Matthews, M. D., and Hampson, J. Hepatojugular reflux. *Lancet* 1:873, 1958.
34. McKay, I. F. S. An experimental analysis of the jugular pulse in man. *J. Physiol.* 106:113, 1947.
35. McKay, I. F. S., and Walker, R. L. True venous pulse wave. *Nature* 205:1220, 1965.
36. Nagel, M. R., Ronan, J. A., Jr., and Roberts, W. C. Left–to–right shunt at atrial level after rupture of papillary muscle from acute myocardial infarction. *Am. Heart J.* 86:112, 1973.
37. Nakhjavan, F. K., and Goldbert, H. Hemodynamic effects of catecholamine stimulation in constrictive pericarditis. *Circulation* 52:487, 1970.
38. Nasser, W. K., et al. Atrial myxoma. *Am. Heart J.* 83:810, 1972.
39. Nixon, P. G. F., and Polis, O. The left atrial X descent. *Br. Heart J.* 24:173, 1962.
39A. Pasteur, W. Note on a new physical sign of triscupid regurgitation. *Lancet* 2:524, 1885.
40. Rapaport, E., Weisbart, M. H., and Levine, M. The splanchnic blood volume in congestive heart failure. *Circulation* 18:581, 1958.
41. Rich, L. L., and Tavel, M. E. The origin of the jugular C wave. *N. Engl. J. Med.* 284:1309, 1971.
42. Roguin, N., Amikam, S., and Riss, E. Prolapsing right atrial myxoma. Clinical and haemodynamic considerations. *Br. Heart J.* 39:577, 1977.
43. Russek, H. I., and Zohman, B. L. The syndrome of Bernheim. *Am. Heart J.* 30:427, 1945.
44. Sharpey–Schafer, E. P. Venous tone. *Br. Med. J.* 2:1589, 1961.
45. Sivaciyan, V., and Ranganathan, N. Transcutaneous Doppler jugular venous flow velocity recording: Clinical and hemodynamic correlates. *Circulation* 57:930, 1978.
45A. Sleight, P. Unilateral elevation of the internal jugular pulse. *Br. Heart J.* 24:726, 1962.
46. Spring, D. A., et al. Premature closure of the mitral and tricuspid valves. *Circulation* 45:663, 1972.
47. Swanton, R. H., et al. Systolic and diastolic ventricular function in cardiac amyloidosis. *Am. J. Cardiol.* 39:658, 1977.
48. Taniguchi, T., et al. Jugular phlebogram in patients with idiopathic cardiomyopathy. *J. Cardiography* 9:11, 1979.
49. Tanioka, T., Sasada, T., and Ohta, N. Jugular phlebogram in patients with right ventricular overloading. *Cardiogr.* 4:409, 1974.
50. Vogel, J. H. K., Horgan, J. A., and Strahl, C. L. Left ventricular dysfunction in chronic constrictive pericarditis. *Chest* 59:484, 1971.
51. Wexler, L., et al. Pressure and velocity patterns in the venae cavae of normal human subjects. *Circulation* 36 (Suppl. 11):269, 1967.
52. Wiggers, C. J. *Modern Aspects of the Circulation in Health and Disease* (2nd ed.). Philadelphia: Lea & Febiger, 1923.
53. Wood, J. E. The mechanism of the increased venous pressure with exercise in congestive heart failure. *J. Clin. Invest.* 41:2020, 1962.
54. Wood, P. Chronic constrictive pericarditis. *Am. J. Cardiol.* 7:48, 1961.
55. Yanagisawa, N., et al. Non–invasive diagnosis of pleuropericardial defect. *J. Cardiogr.* 9:190, 1979.
56. Zelis, R. Contribution of local factors to elevated venous tone of congestive heart failure. *J. Clin. Invest.* 54:219, 1974.

5. *Inspection and Palpation of the Chest*

THE NORMAL APEX BEAT OR APEX IMPULSE

1. What is meant by the term *apex beat* or *apex impulse?*

   ANS.: The term was originally meant to refer to the palpable apex of the LV. During **isovolumic contraction** the heart rotates counterclockwise (as viewed from below), and part of the heart, usually the lower part of the anterior LV, strikes the anterior chest wall.

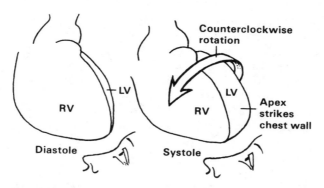

This counterclockwise rotation occurs during isovolumic contraction, i.e., before blood is ejected from the ventricles.

   Unfortunately, in the sitting or supine position, the part of the heart that strikes the chest wall is not necessarily the apex as seen on an x-ray or by direct examination of the heart. In patients with a large enough RV, the "apex beat" may be due to movement of the RV. Therefore, the apex beat really means the *most lateral palpable ventricular movement, or most lateral cardiac impulse.*

   In the **left lateral decubitus** position, however, the actual apex of the heart may be palpated, provided that the LV rather than the RV dominates that area.

2. What is the disadvantage of using the term *point of maximum impulse* (PMI) as a synonym for apex beat?

   ANS.: Maximum precordial pulsations may be due to such abnormalities as a dilated pulmonary artery, a ventricular **aneurysm,** or an aortic aneurysm. Therefore the term "apex beat" is preferable.

Boldface type indicates that the term is explained in the Glossary.

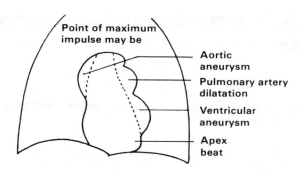

The point of maximum impulse (PMI) should not be equated with the apical impulse.

Palpability of the Apex Beat or Most Lateral Ventricular Impulse

1. How often is the normal apex beat palpable in the sitting position?

    ANS.: It is felt in about 1 out of 5 normal subjects over age 40. However, even in children and teen-agers, an apex beat is palpable in the sitting position in only about half the subjects [45A].

    Note: a) A cardiac impulse is more likely to be palpable in the sitting position than in the supine position because in the latter the heart falls away from the anterior chest wall.

    b) Vibrations of the first heart sound are often mistaken for a slight impulse. It may not be appreciated that heart sounds can be palpable.

2. How often is a normal LV impulse palpable in the left lateral decubitus position?

    ANS.: In about 4 out of 5 older adults and in almost all children or young adults.

3. Why does a thick chest in an obese normal young person not necessarily make the LV impulse impalpable?

    ANS.: Possibly because the heart is physiologically enlarged in obese people, which may make their LV impulse palpable.

4. What is the significance of finding a palpable apex beat in a thick chest or one with an increased anteroposterior diameter in a patient over age 50?

    ANS.: The mere palpability of the left ventricular impulse in such a chest suggests cardiomegaly.

5. What phase of respiration will bring the heart closest to the chest wall so that you can best feel the left ventricular impulse?

    ANS.: Whatever phase of respiration brings an impulse between the ribs. This may be fully held expiration, inspiration, or even halfway between inspiration and expiration.

6. Which part of the hand can best feel a slight or faint impulse?

    ANS.: The fingertips or the area just proximal to them are best for feeling faint localized movements (see figure on p. 162).

    Note: a) All chest palpation is best done from the right side of the bed, with the patient's bed as comfortably high as possible—ideally, at the level of the examiner's waist.

    b) Removing the stethoscope from the ears may help to sharpen the kinesthetic sense, enabling you to appreciate faint impulses more easily.

    c) Each hand should be tried separately. Some examiners find that the fingers of one hand are more sensitive than those of the other in detecting fine movements.

Site of the Most Lateral Cardiac Impulse and Its Normal Limits

1. Besides the greater likelihood of finding it palpable, what are the advantages of examining for the site of a lateral cardiac impulse with the patient sitting rather than in the supine position?

    ANS.: The site of a cardiac impulse is best measured in the sitting position with the feet up on the bed for the following reasons:

    a) The most lateral impulse often moves slightly more to the left and against the chest wall in this position, making it easier to ascertain its lateral extent.

    Note: This lateral shift in the sitting position with the legs up is probably due to the upward push by the compressed abdominal contents and diaphragm. In the standing position, for example, the most lateral cardiac movement does not shift to the left [38].

    b) It allows routine palpation from behind, which has several advantages. Occasionally a very subtle lateral impulse can be felt only when the hand palpates from a quiet, immobile area like the back. A hand on the anterior chest is often disturbed by left parasternal movements and heart sound vibrations that mask any slight motion at the tips of the fingers. Also, a frontal approach may mislead you into thinking that the movement on the front of the chest is the most lateral left ventricular impulse when in fact it may only be the right ventricular movement or an aneurysm, and the true most lateral left ventricular movement may be near the posterior axillary line.

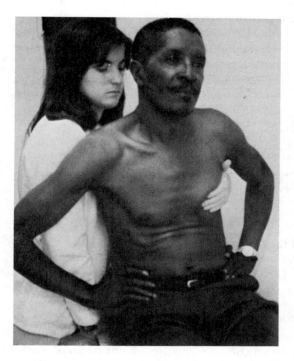

A posterior in addition to an anterior approach may allow you to feel more subtle movements, especially if your left hand is more sensitive than your right.

c) The sitting position is more like an x-ray position than the supine position, and we are more familiar with the site of the normal apex on x-ray in each individual type of chest in the upright position.

*d) It allows you to relate the most lateral impulse site to the circumference of the chest, thus offering the use of another method of establishing the normalcy of the impulse's position. This method requires you to imagine the chest as a circular structure with the base of the heart lying exactly in its center. If you draw an imaginary line from the center of the chest to the midsternum and another to the most lateral impulse, the angle thus produced is the heart or apex beat angle, whose upper normal limit is about 50 degrees [22].

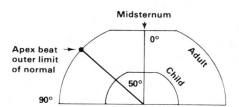

The outer normal limit for a heart angle in adults (with their legs up on a bed) is about 50 degrees.

This angle can be calculated from the formula:

$$\text{Heart angle} = \frac{\text{Distance from midsternum} \times 360}{\text{Chest circumference}}$$

The following nomogram, taken from the original study in 1941, will expedite the calculation [22].

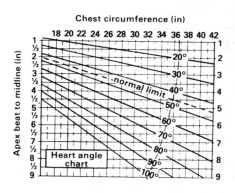

By encircling the chest with a tape measure with the zero mark at the midsternal line, you can measure in one step the circumference of the chest and the distance in inches of the apex impulse from the midsternal line.

2. With the patient in the sitting position, how can you judge most quickly whether or not the most lateral ventricular impulse is in the normal site?

ANS.: The most lateral ventricular impulse normally is at about the mid-left thorax, at the horizontal level of the fourth or fifth interspace. If it is more than 2 cm to the left of the mid-left thorax, cardiomegaly should be suspected.

Note: The midclavicular line is more popular as the site of the normal most lateral ventricular impulse. Unfortunately, medical dictionaries equate the midclavicular line with the nipple line, to which it may

*Material marked with an asterisk is for reference and for advanced students in cardiology.

bear no relation. The term also has a false aura of accuracy about it, as if the site of the most lateral impulse were not a rough measurement. Instead of trying to find the exact lateral end of the clavicle, which is often difficult to ascertain, it is quicker and easier simply to view the left thorax by standing at the foot of the bed with your head in line with the mid-left thorax. Find the mid-left thorax by the method used by artists to find the center of any object. Hold a ruler or pencil horizontally, with the left end flush with the mid-sternal line. Test for the mid-left thorax with a finger that you gradually shift across the ruler from a tentative midpoint of the left thorax. When the distance between the midsternal end of the ruler and your finger equals the distance between your finger and the left edge of the chest, your finger is at the midpoint of the left thorax. An apex impulse should not normally be over 2 cm to the left of the mid-left thorax.

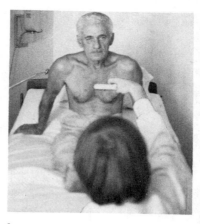 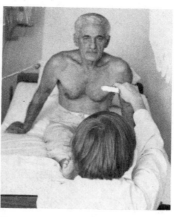

A   B

In A, the left edge of a tongue blade is on the midsternal line while the forefinger marks off an estimated site of the mid-left thorax. In B, the left edge of the tongue blade is now on the estimated site of the mid-left thorax. If the left edge is really in the center of the left chest, the forefinger will now be in a line with the edge of the left chest, as shown here.

3. How far from the midsternal line is the normal most lateral ventricular impulse?
   ANS.: The upper limit of normal is 10 cm from the midsternal line. This measurement is surprisingly useful, because a figure of more than 10 cm has a good correlation with cardiomegaly, even in a large chest. This may be due to the fact that when the chest is so large that, say, 11 cm would be normal for that chest, a ventricular impulse will not normally be palpable in such a chest—i.e., if it is palpable at all in a huge chest, cardiomegaly is probably present.
   Note: a) In the left lateral decubitus position, the normal ventricular impulse site is unknown because it then depends on mediastinal mobility.
   b) Determination of cardiac size by x-ray is usually calculated by cardiothoracic ratios. Fifty-five percent of the widest cardiac diameter is said to be the upper limit of normal. There are, however, many patients who have normal hearts but because of excess body

weight are falsely thought to have cardiomegaly due to an increased cardiothoracic ratio. Also, many short, underweight patients have a normal cardiothoracic ratio when the heart is actually enlarged. Use of Ungerleider and Clark's height and weight tables is the next best way of judging cardiac diameter.

Theoretical transverse diameters of heart for various heights and weights

Table for determining percent deviation from average

Height

(Light figures represent weights)

% Minus (−)   % Plus (+)

25	20	15	10	5		5	10	15	20	25
75	80	85	90	95	**100**	105	110	115	120	125
76	81	86	91	96	**101**	106	111	116	121	126
77	82	87	92	97	**102**	107	112	117	122	128
77	82	88	93	98	**103**	108	113	118	124	129
78	83	88	94	99	**104**	109	114	120	125	130
79	84	89	95	100	**105**	110	116	121	126	131
80	85	90	95	101	**106**	111	117	122	127	133
80	86	91	96	102	**107**	112	118	123	128	134
81	86	92	97	103	**108**	113	119	124	130	135
82	87	93	98	104	**109**	114	120	125	131	136
83	88	94	99	105	**110**	116	121	127	132	138
83	89	94	100	105	**111**	117	122	128	133	139
84	90	95	101	106	**112**	118	123	129	134	140
85	90	96	102	107	**113**	119	124	130	136	141
86	91	97	103	108	**114**	120	125	131	137	143
86	92	98	104	109	**115**	121	127	132	138	144
87	93	99	104	110	**116**	122	128	133	139	145
88	94	99	105	111	**117**	123	129	135	140	146
89	94	100	106	112	**118**	124	130	136	142	148
89	95	101	107	113	**119**	125	131	137	143	149
90	96	102	108	114	**120**	126	132	138	144	150
91	97	103	109	115	**121**	127	133	139	145	151
92	98	104	110	116	**122**	128	134	140	146	153
92	98	105	111	117	**123**	129	135	141	148	154
93	99	105	112	118	**124**	130	136	143	149	155
94	100	106	113	119	**125**	131	138	144	150	156
95	101	107	113	120	**126**	132	139	145	151	158
95	102	108	114	121	**127**	133	140	146	152	159
96	102	109	115	122	**128**	134	141	147	154	160
97	103	110	116	123	**129**	135	142	148	155	161
98	104	111	117	124	**130**	137	143	150	156	163
98	105	111	118	124	**131**	138	144	151	157	164
99	106	112	119	125	**132**	139	145	152	158	165
100	106	113	120	126	**133**	140	146	153	160	166
101	107	114	121	127	**134**	141	147	154	161	168
101	108	115	122	128	**135**	142	149	155	162	169
102	109	116	122	129	**136**	143	150	156	163	170
103	110	116	123	130	**137**	144	151	158	164	171
104	110	117	124	131	**138**	145	152	159	166	173
104	111	118	125	132	**139**	146	153	160	167	174
105	112	119	126	133	**140**	147	154	161	168	175
106	113	120	127	134	**141**	148	155	162	169	176
107	114	121	128	135	**142**	149	156	163	170	178
107	114	122	129	136	**143**	150	157	164	172	179
108	115	122	130	137	**144**	151	158	166	173	180
109	116	123	131	138	**145**	152	160	167	174	181
110	117	124	131	139	**146**	153	161	168	175	183
110	118	125	132	140	**147**	154	162	169	176	184
111	118	126	133	141	**148**	155	163	170	178	185
112	119	127	134	142	**149**	156	164	171	179	186
113	120	128	135	143	**150**	158	165	173	180	188
113	121	128	136	143	**151**	159	166	174	181	189
114	122	129	137	144	**152**	160	167	175	182	190
115	122	130	138	145	**153**	161	168	176	184	191
116	123	131	139	146	**154**	162	169	177	185	193
116	124	132	140	147	**155**	163	171	179	186	194
117	125	133	140	148	**156**	164	172	179	187	195
118	126	133	141	149	**157**	165	173	181	188	196
119	126	134	142	150	**158**	166	174	182	190	198
119	127	135	143	151	**159**	167	175	183	191	199
120	128	136	144	152	**160**	168	176	184	192	200
121	129	137	145	153	**161**	169	177	185	193	201
122	130	138	146	154	**162**	170	178	186	194	203
122	130	139	147	155	**163**	171	179	187	196	204
123	131	139	148	156	**164**	172	180	189	197	205

Actual   Predicted Diameter (mm)   Actual

The heart is usually enlarged if the width is 10 percent greater than the average prediction, which is shown in the boldface vertical column on the right. Subtract 8 mm for women, since this table was derived from thousands of male insurance applicants (personal communication from Dr. H. E. Ungerleider).

c) Because cardiac volume determination includes the lateral chest film and body surface area (BSA), it improves the accuracy of the diagnosis of cardiac size.

The length dimension (L) is measured in centimeters from the junction of the superior vena cava and right atrium to the cardiac apex. The broad diameter (B) is the measurement of the junction of the right atrium and diaphragm to the junction of the pulmonary artery and left atrial appendage. The lateral dimension (D) is the greatest horizontal cardiac diameter. Cardiac

$$\text{volume} = \frac{\text{L} \times \text{B} \times \text{D}}{\text{BSA}} \times 0.42.$$

The 0.42 is the correction factor for a 6-foot distance of the heart from the film. The upper normal values are 490 ccm^2 for females and 540 ccm^2 for males [34A].

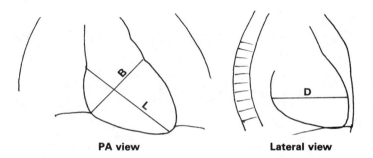

PA view   **Lateral view**

4. What is the present status of chest percussion in determining heart size?
   ANS.: It is not used by most cardiologists for the following reasons:
   a) A palpable ventricular impulse indicates the heart size quickly and easily and when a ventricular impulse is not palpable because of a thick chest or overaeration due to pulmonary disease, percussion is unreliable.
   b) Dressler, who devoted 20 pages of his book on clinical cardiology to percussion of the chest for cardiac abnormalities, begins by stating that he finds it impossible to percuss cardiac borders [13].
      Note: Dressler worked out a system for defining "areas of cardiac dullness," which gave him much information. However, it requires great skill, as well as a study of his findings, to make use of percussion to detect cardiac abnormalities.

CAUSES OF A DISPLACED LEFT VENTRICULAR IMPULSE

1. Does left ventricular hypertrophy (LVH) displace the LV impulse to the left?
   ANS.: No. There must be dilatation as well as LVH to displace an LV impulse. Pure LVH tends to encroach on the ventricular cavity by growing inward as

much as outward. Even if an LV free wall doubled its thickness from 1 to 2 cm (which would happen only with the most severe hypertrophy), and did not encroach on the volume, the border of the heart would not extend laterally more than 1 cm beyond normal.

Note: Dilatation without some hypertrophy of a ventricle is very rare. If a ventricle is dilated for a long enough period of time, it will nearly always show hypertrophy in obedience to Laplace's law, which states that pressure is proportional to tension and inversely proportional to radius or volume. This means that the larger the volume, the greater must be the wall tension to maintain pressure. The need for tension seems to stimulate hypertrophy, which in turn supplies the necessary tension. Exceptions are the acute dilatation that may occur with a ruptured aortic cusp and the chronic dilatation associated with the diffuse fibrosis seen in some severe **cardiomyopathies.**

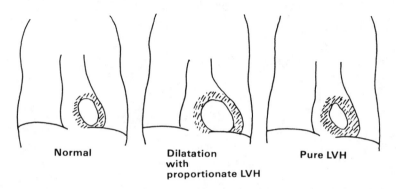

Normal   Dilatation with proportionate LVH   Pure LVH

Pure LVH causes an encroachment inward on the cavity and has been called "concentric" hypertrophy. Dilatation with proportionate hypertrophy has been called "eccentric" hypertrophy.

A heart that is primarily hypertrophied, as in aortic stenosis (AS) or hypertension, can become a dilated heart when cardiac decompensation occurs. Therefore, although AS or hypertension will not displace an LV impulse when only pure hypertrophy is present, the LV impulse may be displaced when the patient goes into failure.

2. What is meant by concentric and eccentric hypertrophy?

ANS.: Left ventricular hypertrophy without dilatation is called concentric hypertrophy. The term *concentric* implies the existence of an "eccentric" type of hypertrophy. Because, however, the latter term suggests that the ventricle is eccentrically hypertrophied but does not mean this at all, it is a poor term. Eccentric hypertrophy means that the chamber dilatation (usually with proportionate hypertrophy) has forced the geometric center of the heart to be shifted eccentrically to the left.

*3. What kind of cardiac **malposition** besides dextrocardia will cause a ventricular impulse to be palpable on the right chest?

ANS.: Dextroversion (see types of **malpositions of the heart**).

Note: To confirm the presence of mirror image dextrocardia by physical examination, percuss for the stomach bubble in order to reveal tympany on the right.

To confirm dextroversion by physical examination, palpate for aortic pulsations in the second right interspace; they may be present here because of the anterior position of the aorta caused by the rotation of the LV anteriorly.

*4. What can displace an LV impulse to the left in the absence of cardiomegaly in a patient with normal lungs?

ANS.: a) **Pectus excavatum.**

b) Congenital complete absence of the pericardium.

CHARACTER OF THE LEFT VENTRICULAR IMPULSE

The Normal Left Ventricular Impulse

1. What is the timing of movement of the normal LV impulse?

ANS.: The normal LV impulse is best observed with the patient in the left lateral decubitus position. The impulse rises and retracts quickly by the first half of systole. Listen with your stethoscope to the heart sounds while feeling with one finger. A normal impulse will fall on to the second sound or even before it. This is not a visual phenomenon, so do not compare what you see with what you hear. Compare what you feel with what you hear.

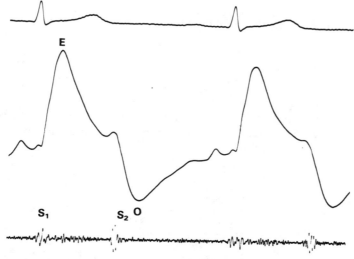

This depicts a normal apex impulse (apex cardiogram, or ACG) recorded over the apex beat with the subject in the left lateral decubitus position. The fingers feel the E-O slope as a purely systolic retraction. The S_2-O portion of the slope is so short and rapid that the O nadir is perceived as ending at the S_2. The end-systolic hump of the ACG is not perceived by palpation as interrupting the E-O slope.

2. What causes the initial outward movement that results in the heart striking the chest wall?

ANS.: During isovolumic contraction the heart rotates counterclockwise (as seen from below) and flings the apical area of the heart against the anterior chest wall. (See figure on p. 113.)

3. How can you explain the midsystolic retraction of the normal LV impulse?

ANS.: The retraction is probably due to the inferolateral LV wall's contracting and pulling away from the anterior chest wall. This retraction occurs after the initial counterclockwise rotation of the heart during isovolumic contraction has flung this part of the heart briefly against the chest wall.

Note: One theory holds that when ejection occurs, the circular muscle, which does not extend to the apex, pulls on the oblique muscle of the apex to cause precordial retraction [11]. This theory has two weaknesses: (a) The part of the heart that strikes the chest wall, especially in the supine position, is probably not the apex but a segment anterior and superior to the actual apex. (b) The outer surface of the apex probably does not really retract—i.e., the angiographic picture of retraction is really an illusion caused by the sides of the LV wall closing in during systole.

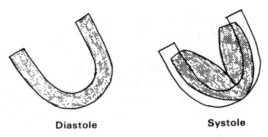

Diastole   Systole

The apparent upward movement of the apex on cineangiograms is an illusion caused by the drawing together of the side walls, closing off the apex from below upward.

4. How can you tell that the most lateral impulse is caused by the LV and not by a large RV usurping that area?

ANS.: a) Only the LV impulse feels like a localized thrust (i.e., as though a golf or ping-pong ball inside the chest were being pushed against your fingers). The RV usually has a more diffuse, poorly circumscribed movement.

b) The LV impulse usually manifests pure medial retraction. This means that as the heart rotates to thrust the LV outward, the medial aspect of the heart moves posteriorly and pulls the chest wall muscle and skin with it.

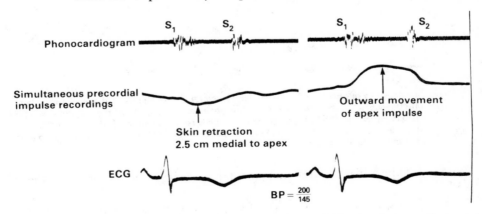

Note the retraction medial to the apex which shows a sustained impulse due to the effect of LVH. Although these tracings were taken in the supine position, medial retraction is best seen in the left lateral decubitus position.

Note: a) When both the outward and medial movements are large, the movements are sometimes called a ventricular rock.

b) Medial retraction is misunderstood by the novice to mean that the skin moves medially. Instead, it means that the skin medial to the apical impulse retracts or moves inward.

5. How can you best elicit medial retraction?

ANS.: The patient should be in the left lateral decubitus position. Place one finger on the most lateral impulse and note with your eyes whether the skin superomedial, medial, or inferomedial to the apical impulse retracts.

6. What cardiac diagnoses tend to be ruled out by the presence of a palpable LV impulse?

ANS.: a) Any abnormality that causes a dilated RV without concomitant dilatation of the LV. For example, secundum type **atrial septal defects** (ASDs) and **primary pulmonary hypertension** should not be readily diagnosed if a LV apex beat is found.

* *Note:* In **endocardial cushion defects** there may be severe mitral regurgitation (MR) that enlarges the LV. Therefore, this type of ASD may be suggested by identifying an LV impulse.

An LV impulse may occasionally be palpable in secundum ASDs even though the LV is often smaller than normal in patients with ASD [27]. The reason is unknown, but this may be due to the exaggerated counterclockwise rotation that occurs in ASDs [43].

b) The presence of a palpable LV apical impulse rules out any abnormality that causes pure right ventricular hypertrophy (RVH), such as pure pulmonary stenosis (PS). This is because a hypertrophied RV tends to rotate the heart clockwise (seen from below). This rotation places the LV more posteriorly, so that even if the RV is merely hypertrophied and not dilated, the LV is still usually not palpable.

* *Note:* In severe PS with a marked right-to-left shunt through an intra-atrial communication (ASD or patent foramen ovale), the LV may enlarge enough to become palpable in the left lateral decubitus position.

THE LEFT VENTRICULAR IMPULSE IN LEFT VENTRICULAR HYPERTROPHY

1. How does the character of the LV impulse in LVH differ from the normal LV impulse?

ANS.: a) It is sustained.

b) It may have an extra hump or dip on the upstroke.

2. What is meant by a sustained LV impulse?

ANS.: The sustained impulse continues its outward movement longer than normal throughout systole.

Note: To determine whether or not the impulse is sustained, you must time the bottom of the fall of the impulse and relate it to the second heart sound (S_2). If the movement falls onto or before the S_2, it is not sustained. If, however, the bottom of the fall occurs after the S_2, then it is sustained. To determine whether the outward movement is sustained, say a word such as *down* at the bottom of the fall. If the word follows the S_2, the impulse is sustained.

Note: Visible skin movements can be delayed over what is felt. It is preferable simply to feel the movement of a finger or stethoscope on the ventricular impulse in timing the fall or retraction.

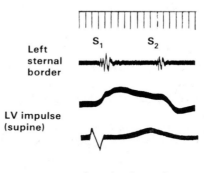

Sustained apex host

If you imagine a sound shortly after the S_2, the sustained apex beat will seem to fall onto it rather than onto the S_2.

* 3. In which kind of LVH is there no sustained LV impulse?

   ANS.: When the LVH is proportional to a mild or moderate amount of volume overload, as in moderate aortic regurgitation (AR), persistent ductus arteriosus, ventricular septal defect (VSD), or severe anemia, in which conditions the LV impulse may be overactive but not sustained.

   Note: The degree of AR can be roughly judged by the presence of a sustained impulse. In mild to moderate AR, there is an overactive (larger amplitude of movement) but nonsustained impulse. Only if AR is at least moderately severe is there a sustained impulse.

* 4. What can cause a sustained LV impulse in the absence of LVH?

   ANS.: Congenital complete absence of the pericardium. The LV impulse here is generally displaced into the midaxillary line.

The Atrial Hump in Left Ventricular Hypertrophy

1. How does a cineangiogram show the effect of a contracting atrium on the ventricle?

   ANS.: When contrast material is injected into the LV, a cineangiogram can show that the LV suddenly expands at the end of diastole in response to atrial contraction.

2. When is this end-diastolic or presystolic expansion of the LV palpable?

   ANS.: It is normally not palpable. Only a very strong left atrial contraction can expand the LV with enough force to cause a palpable presystolic hump on the LV impulse.

   Note: If the atrial hump effect is too close to the outward movement of the ventricular contraction, it may be impalpable even if it is very high. This can be caused by a short P-R interval.

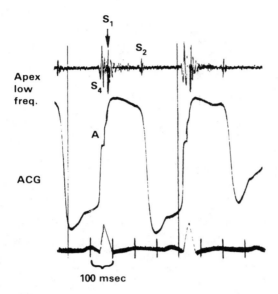

A short P-R of about 80 msec due to a preexcitation abnormality has caused the atrial hump (A) to be too close to the major ventricular movement to be palpable.

3. What is the cause of a left atrial contraction strong enough to make a palpable left ventricular hump at the LV impulse?

ANS.: Severe loss of LV **compliance** (i.e., loss of distensibility of the LV).

   Note: The strong atrial contraction effect on the LV is often called the atrial kick or booster–pump effect. The reason for this is that the expansion of the LV just before its contraction produces an increased energy of ventricular contraction, or **Starling effect.**

4. How does the left atrium "get the message" to contract harder when the LV is stiffer?

ANS.: In diastole, the mitral valve is open and the atrium and ventricle are in continuity (i.e., they are, in effect, an "atrioventricle"). When the ventricle is stiff, the atrioventricle is also stiff, and when blood pours into a stiff chamber, the pressure rises steeply. If the atrium is under high pressure at the end of diastole, then, due to the Starling effect, it will contract more strongly.

   Note: Eventually the atrium itself will hypertrophy in response to its continued strong contractions and will then contribute to the stiffness of the atrioventricle.

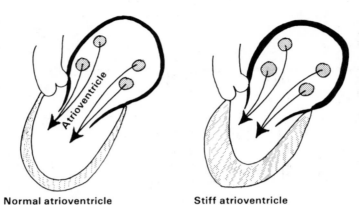

Normal atrioventricle   Stiff atrioventricle

A stiff ventricle must be transmitting its loss of compliance to the atrium during diastole when the AV valves open.

5. What is the most common cause of chronic increased stiffness (diastolic) of the LV?
   ANS.: Left ventricular hypertrophy secondary to hypertension. The next most common cause is LVH secondary to coronary disease (i.e., the confluent patchy areas of fibrosis or infarction plus the tendency to hypertrophy of the remaining healthy myocardium can cause a stiff LV).
*6. Which type of aortic stenosis (AS) is most likely to produce a palpable atrial presystolic hump (A wave) at the site of the LV impulse?
   ANS.: Hypertrophic subaortic stenosis (HSS), in which the septum is disproportionately hypertrophied in comparison with the free wall. Perhaps HSS tends to produce a palpable atrial hump because the extremely thick septum causes a marked loss of compliance, but the resulting strong atrial contraction can easily expand the rest of the LV, which, although thick, is not nearly as thick as the septum that caused the strong atrial contraction in the first place. In valvular AS the entire LV is equally hypertrophied and therefore resists the expansion of a left atrial contraction.
   Note: A palpable atrial hump or A wave in the presence of valvular AS is strongly correlated with a gradient of at least 75 mm Hg in patients without angina or past history of infarction [21]. In HSS no such correlation can be made. A palpable A wave in the presence of valvular AS is unusual enough to point to suspicion of the addition of a hypertrophic cardiomyopathy such as HSS [32].
7. Why is it especially important to palpate for an A wave in AS?
   ANS.: a) The S_4 may be inaudible, or the S_4 may be mistaken for an S_1, and the murmur that follows is thought to be midsystolic. You may be able to palpate an A wave but not hear an S_4 because the frequency of vibrations may be too low for audibility but not for palpation.
      b) An A wave tells you that there is no concomitant mitral stenosis (MS), because MS will not permit a large enough atrial hump to be palpable.
8. What does an atrial "kick" feel like to the palpating fingers?
   ANS.: When it is strong and far from the ventricular outward movement, it feels like a double outward movement. When it is slight or close to the ventricular outward movement, it feels like a notch or vibration on the apical upstroke.
      Note: These movements are best felt by the part of the hand near the fingertips with the patient in the left lateral decubitus position. Occa-

sionally a suspected faint atrial kick can be confirmed by observing a double outward movement of the patient's skin, your finger, or your stethoscope on the LV impulse.

Atrial Kick

Close to
LV movement

Far from
LV movement

What
you
feel

What
you
feel

What
you
feel

Notch or
hesitation
on upstroke

Double
outward
movement

If only a notch or slight hesitation is present on the upstroke, the tips of the fingers must be used to perceive it. If a large double movement is felt, it must be distinguished from a midsystolic dip.

THE LEFT VENTRICULAR IMPULSE IN LEFT VENTRICULAR DILATATION

1. When should you suspect that the LV is enlarged when displacement of the LV impulse is questionable?

   ANS.: In the left lateral decubitus position

   a) When the area of medial retraction is enlarged.
   b) When the LV impulse is felt in more than one interspace.

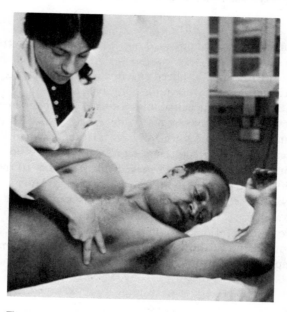

The normal apex beat is not felt through two interspaces during the same phase of respiration.

Note: This does not refer to the normal downward movement of the LV impulse with inspiration that may cause it to be palpable one interspace lower on inspiration than on expiration. An impulse is enlarged if it can be easily felt in two interspaces in the *same phase of respiration.*

c) When the apical impulse is more than one and a half fingertips (or 3 cm) wide in the X axis (i.e., if it is felt equally well with two fingers placed side by side perpendicular to the ribs).

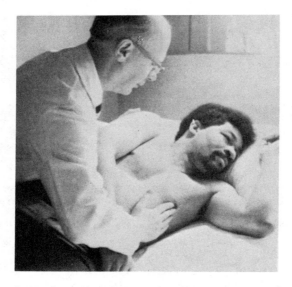

A normal apical impulse is no larger than about 1½ fingertip widths.

2. What is meant by a "heave" or "lift"?

ANS.: Any large area of sustained outward movement may be referred to as a heave or lift.

    Note: a) A "thrust" is a localized sustained movement (i.e., felt in a small area no larger than a ping-pong ball).

       *b) The LV is often palpable as a dilated chamber in the presence of severe MS for unknown reasons. About a third of subjects with the largest hearts and pure MS have a larger LV than RV without any heart failure to suggest a significant cardiomyopathy [52]. The large left atrium of MS may displace the LV to the left and anteriorly, giving a false impression of a large LV.

*3. When is congenital absence of the left pericardium suspected as the cause of an LV impulse in the left axilla?

ANS.: When there is an inferior or right axis deviation on an electrocardiogram together with an x-ray showing a prominent main pulmonary artery with marked displacement of the heart to the left of the vertebral column [44].

THE EARLY RAPID FILLING HUMP IN DILATED HEARTS

1. When does a ventricle expand rapidly, in early, middle, or end-diastole?

    ANS.: In early diastole there is a rapid expansion. This early diastolic rapid expansion suddenly halts and gives way to slow expansion. At the end of the slow expansion phase, the atrium contracts and produces a short period of rapid expansion again at the end of diastole.

    Note: The cause of the sudden change from early rapid to slow expansion of the LV is unknown. These phases of diastole are also known as rapid filling and slow filling phases.

2. What can exaggerate the change from early rapid to slow filling phases?

    ANS.: Anything that increases the rate of expansion of the LV. This is most marked when an increased volume of blood must be transported from the left atrium to the LV, as in MR.

    * *Note:* a) The point of change from the early rapid to the slow filling phase can become palpable in severe MR. This palpable hump or bump after the main rise and fall of the LV impulse is always associated with a third heart sound (S_3).

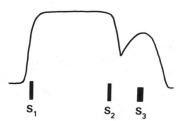

A slight outward movement following the major out-and-back movement suggests a palpable early rapid filling of the LV and is most commonly felt together with an S_3 in severe MR.

*3. What can cause a double outward movement besides an atrial hump (A wave) or rapid early filling hump?

    ANS.: A midsystolic dip. This is most often felt in patients with severe HSS. It is, however, occasionally palpable in patients with the prolapsed mitral valve syndrome or with acute myocardial infarction [54].

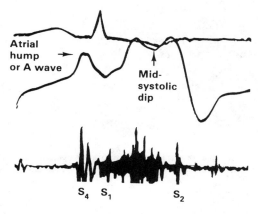

This apex impulse tracing (apex cardiogram) is from a 45-year-old man with HSS. The atrial hump and the midsystolic dip give an impression of a triple outward movement.

Note: A double *diastolic* outward movement is seen in some patients with sudden, severe AR [60]. The second movement occurs after the mitral valve has closed in mid-diastole, and further filling from the aortic valve occurs.

RIGHT VENTRICULAR OVERLOAD PARASTERNAL MOVEMENT

Normal Left Parasternal Movement

1. What is the normal movement at the lower left parasternal area?

   ANS.: The major movement is a very small retraction. The retraction may be preceded by a short, small-amplitude outward movement in young people or in those with thin chests [10, 15, 26].

   Note: Large areas of chest motion, as is usual with left parasternal movements, are often best palpated with the proximal part of the palm (thenar and hypothenar areas). This method transmits the movement to the entire arm, which may amplify the perception of palmar motion. All movement must be measured in relation to a fixed point in space; the above technique uses the shoulder as the fixed point, or fulcrum.

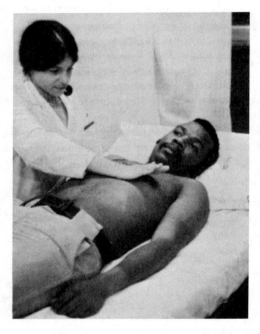

In this patient with MS, the physician is palpating the movement of a large RV, which was producing a right ventricular rock, i.e., a sustained left parasternal impulse and lateral retraction.

2. What can exaggerate the normal left parasternal retraction?

   ANS.: a) Any cause of a large LV, as in AR. This is really a large area of para-apical medial retraction that has extended as far medially as the sternum.

        b) A right ventricular volume overload without a pressure overload [3].

3. How can you tell that the left parasternal movement is due to an RV overload?

   ANS.: a) The presence of an RV rock (i.e., lateral retraction in the mid- or lateral thorax) occurring simultaneously with outward parasternal movement, suggests a large RV.

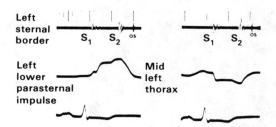

A sustained left parasternal impulse with lateral retraction is a sign of a volume overload of the RV (and probably also of a pressure overload).

        b) The presence of a second left interspace outward systolic movement due to a dilated pulmonary artery suggests a large RV because this degree of pulmonary artery dilatation is usually seen only with severe pulmonary hypertension or a large volume RV overload, as in ASD.

        c) The presence of an epigastric downward impulse suggests a large RV.

          Note: If you place the fingers or the pad of the left thumb pointing upward into the epigastrium during held inspiration you may feel an impulse coming down and striking the tips of the fingers or the thumb pad. This suggests the presence of a large RV [23]. If the fingers are used and the impulse strikes the pads of the fingers, it is due to an aortic or hepatic pulsation. This is an especially useful maneuver if an increased chest diameter hides left parasternal movements.

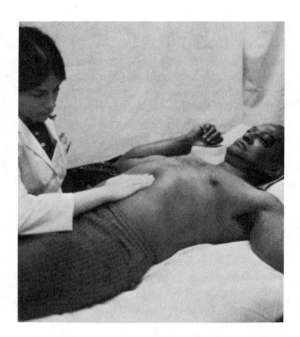

A large RV will come down and strike the tips (not the pads) of your fingers.

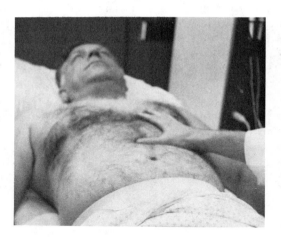

If your fingernails are long enough to cause discomfort if you push up into the epigastrium, you may use the pad of your thumb to test for RV pulsations during a held deep inspiration.

* d) The presence of an outward movement that is more marked to the right of the sternum than to the left is usually due to a huge right atrium and implies not only RV overload but severe tricuspid regurgitation (TR) [23].

  * *Note:* a) An exaggerated initial outward movement at the left lower sternal border with or without a mid- and late systolic retraction is common in high flow ASDs [24].

      b) A biventricular overload, as in VSD, may be manifest on the chest wall by a biventricular rock, that is, both the left parasternal and the apical areas may rise with systole, with an area of systolic retraction between them.

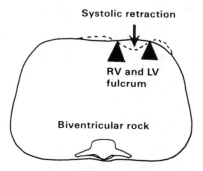

Systolic retraction

RV and LV
fulcrum

Biventricular rock

Retraction in the mid-left thorax, with sustained outward movements on either side, tells you that there is a biventricular volume overload.

*4. What conditions may produce large RV stroke volumes without either tricuspid or pulmonary regurgitation?

ANS.: Shunt flows such as occur in **ASD, VSD,** and **anomalous pulmonary venous connection** into the right atrium.

A shunt produced by partial anomalous pulmonary venous connection may not prevent palpation of the LV impulse because anomalous pulmonary veins usually must drain an entire lung before the RV enlarges enough to hide LV events.

5. List some causes of primary tricuspid regurgitation (TR) (i.e., not secondary to pulmonary hypertension) that are severe enough to create telltale precordial pulsations.

ANS.: a) Rheumatic heart disease (almost never without severe mitral disease as well).

*b) Congenital TR (i.e., either idiopathic or with endocardial cushion defects).

*c) **Carcinoid heart disease** (due to carcinoid plaques on the undersurface that fix the valves in the open position).

*d) Traumatic heart disease (i.e., due to ruptured chordae tendineae).
Note: All causes of primary TR are rare.

*e) Infective endocarditis in heroin addicts.

*6. How may severe TR affect the precordial movements in an unexpected fashion?

ANS.: a) The left parasternal area may retract instead of expand during systole, presumably because the RV, like an overdistended balloon in diastole, empties during systole and may cause the entire left parasternal area to retract.

b) The entire right precordium may expand during systole, while the entire left precordium retracts. This occurs because the right atrium may be so enlarged to the right, and the liver so expanded by the regurgitant volume, that systole may expand the entire right chest.

The Sustained Left Parasternal Impulse

1. How can you distinguish RVH from RV dilatation by palpation?

   ANS.: Pure RVH may produce a sustained impulse at the mid- to lower left parasternal area. It will not be very marked in amplitude or very extensive in area. On the other hand, RV dilatation, such as that seen in uncomplicated ASD, can produce an extensive area movement that may have a large amplitude and may not be sustained but instead may be overactive [26].

   * *Note:* a) In ASD the palpability of the RV at the left sternal border is partly due to the exaggerated counterclockwise rotation of the LV seen in these patients [43].

   b) A hyperkinetic impulse at the left lower sternal border (large initial outward movement followed by retraction) and a simultaneous late systolic outward movement at the right sternal border is a reliable sign of ASD [24].

   c) Eventration of the right diaphragm has been known to produce large and sustained left parasternal systolic movements by displacing the heart anteriorly and to the right.

2. List the most common causes of a sustained RV heave.

   ANS.: a) Pulmonary stenosis.

   * *Note:* The maximum impulse in PS is often found a few centimeters away from the parasternal area or even in the mid-left thorax, especially in older subjects [30].

   b) Pulmonary hypertension.

   * *Note:* a) Although a sustained parasternal movement in a patient with ASD suggests pulmonary hypertension, some patients with ASD have sustained RV heaves even without pulmonary hypertension [24]. Because there is no significant RVH in most patients with ASD unless there is pulmonary hypertension, the cause of the occasional sustaining is unexplained [17, 30]. However, trabecular hypertrophy occurs in ASD, which perhaps could change the pattern of RV contraction [36].

   b) In pulmonary stenosis and in primary pulmonary hypertension the left parasternal movement is a gentle systolic heave with a peak in early to mid- (not late) systole.

3. Why is there usually a sustained and often marked left parasternal movement in significant pure MS, despite the presence of only slightly elevated pulmonary arterial pressure?

   ANS.: This may be due to a combination of the RVH and dilatation plus the effect of a large left atrium that could hold the RV hard against the left parasternal area [14].

   Note: There may be a large volume in the RV in MS in the absence of pulmonary regurgitation or primary TR. Three theories may explain this.

   a) A sudden rise in pulmonary artery pressure occurs with exertion in patients with left atrial obstruction. One response of the RV to a sudden rise in resistance is dilatation. Perhaps, then, even at rest, it does not return to its normal size because in patients with left atrial obstruction there is always some slight increase in pulmonary artery pressure that may sustain the RV in its dilated state.

b) Pulmonary emboli may cause sudden episodes of dilatation on exertion, and the RV may never return to normal.

c) If the left atrial and pulmonary venous pressures rise high enough, some pulmonary venous blood may flow from the pulmonary veins into the bronchial veins and then by way of the azygos into the superior vena cava and RV, thus resulting in a significant left-to-right shunt, which may increase the RV volume. (This theory has not yet been proved.)

*4. How can palpation of RV pulsations tell you whether PS is valvular or infundibular?

ANS.: Because the transmitted systolic movement originates in the high pressure zone just *below* the stenosis, in valvular PS a parasternal impulse may be detected as high as the third left interspace; in infundibular stenosis the impulse may be confined to the fourth and fifth interspaces. The impulse in subinfundibular stenosis (rare) may be detected only in the fifth interspace.

Note: The dilated part of the poststenotically dilated pulmonary artery in pulmonary valve stenosis is not usually palpable, probably because the pulmonary artery above the valve tends to angulate sharply backward, away from the chest wall.

---

*Left Parasternal Impulse in Uncommon Congenital Heart Abnormalities

*1. What left parasternal movement should make you doubt the presence of an Ebstein's anomaly?

ANS.: A systolic movement in the fourth or fifth interspace (i.e., over the body of the RV).

Note: A movement in the third left interspace is not unusual. Apparently, a slight dilatation of the remaining RV due to the TR that is commonly present can cause left parasternal movement, but it will not be low, as with the usual dilated RV of TR or ASD. An impulse occurring below the third left interspace is strong evidence against an Ebstein's anomaly.

*2. What should you suspect if the murmur and LV impulse of a VSD are identified, but despite the absence of a low RV parasternal impulse there is a pulmonary artery pulsation in the second left interspace?

ANS.: A VSD with a large shunt that is ejecting its blood mostly into the pulmonary artery without creating much pulmonary hypertension.

Note: If, on the other hand, you think that the patient has a VSD and a *disproportionately hyperdynamic* parasternal impulse characteristic of a marked RV volume overload, these signs suggest that the VSD is shunting directly into the right atrium because a VSD usually causes only a mild RV volume overload for these reasons:

a) The LV usually ejects its blood high into the infundibular area and not into the body of the RV.

b) A VSD shunt occurs mainly during systole, when the RV is contracting.

*3. What precordial movements are expected in truncus arteriosus?

ANS.: Biventricular volume overload pulsations, unless the pulmonary arteries are small or absent, in which case only the RV impulse is palpable. If there is a short main pulmonary artery, that vessel may dilate and produce an impulse in the second left interspace.

*4. What should you suspect in a cyanotic child with a palpable LV and no RV impulse?

ANS.: Either pulmonary atresia (with an intact ventricular septum and small RV), tricuspid atresia, Ebstein's anomaly, or vena cava to left atrial communication.

Note: In one type of pulmonary atresia, however, there is a large right atrium and RV due to TR. This can cause a palpable RV impulse. There is also a rare type of tricuspid atresia with a palpable RV impulse due to the presence of a large VSD, which can cause an increase in RV blood flow.

*5. What precordial movements are felt in transposition of the great vessels?

ANS.: A biventricular overload impulse is expected because the pulmonary and systemic circuits operate in parallel and are relatively independent of each other. Further, each circuit has an excessive volume of blood. When, however, pulmonary flow is reduced by severe pulmonary hypertension or stenosis, only the RV impulses will be palpable. The RV is, of course, a systemic ventricle in patients with transposition.

LEFT-SIDED CAUSES OF LEFT PARASTERNAL MOVEMENT

1. When is mid- to lower left parasternal movement due to the LV in the absence of dextroversion?

ANS.: a) In young subjects with long, thin chests, the LV impulse may be very medial (i.e., at the left parasternal area).

b) In some subjects in whom the LV is markedly enlarged, the movement may extend medially to the left parasternal area (as well as laterally).

c) The movement may occur in the presence of a ventricular aneurysm, in which case it will be sustained with a late peak [3].

*d) Left parasternal movement may also occur in congenitally corrected transposition of the great vessels because the septum may be rotated to a position more perpendicular to the chest wall than normal, the dextroversion thus swinging the left-sided systemic ventricle (an anatomical RV) more medially than normal.

2. When is the left parasternal outward movement due to a left atrium? Why?

ANS.: In severe chronic MR. The left atrium is a midchest structure (i.e., it is not really a left atrium but a posterior atrium).

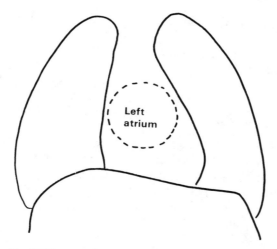

The "left" atrium is really a posterosuperior atrium, since it is behind and above the right atrium. Although it is slightly to the left of the right atrium, it is a midline structure.

If the posterior atrium expands markedly due to severe MR, it can push the RV (which is an anterior structure) against the chest wall [39].

*3. How can you tell whether or not an expanding left atrium is the cause of a marked left parasternal movement?

ANS.: a) You should suspect it only in the presence of severe *chronic* MR. Increased amplitude is not expected in acute MR because the healthy left atrium does not usually enlarge enough to push the RV forward significantly. However, an acute event such as ruptured chordae tendineae occurring as a complication of chronic MR is very likely to cause marked left parasternal movement.

Note: Any slight left parasternal movement that is felt in patients with ruptured chordae will be markedly sustained (i.e., it will rise to its peak at the S_2, and then fall to a nadir at the timing of an S_3).

b) Compare the LV apical movement with the left parasternal movement by placing a finger on each. A left atrial lift will begin and end slightly later than the LV thrust. Right ventricular movement will begin and end at the same time or even before the LV thrust.

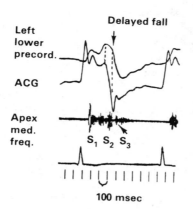

Left lower precord.

ACG

Apex med. freq.

S_1 S_2 S_3

Delayed fall

100 msec

The left lower parasternal area movement shows a delayed fall in comparison with the apical impulse in this patient with severe chronic rheumatic MR.

c) The left parasternal movement will fall so that it reaches its nadir with the S_3 that is commonly heard with severe MR [2].

   Note: A posterior ventricular aneurysm can also produce this late systolic parasternal bulge [3].

d) Place your hands on each posterior hemithorax and note whether or not the left side expands less than the right [48]. There may be less expansion on the left side because a large left atrium can cause partial obstruction of the left bronchus.

e) In the rare subjects who have extreme left atrial dilatation, sustained pulsations are seen and felt even in the right precordium [20].

*f) An enlarged aorta may be palpable in the second and third *left* interspace in corrected transposition of the great vessels, because the aorta is excessively anterior and to the left due to rotation of the septum. (See question 1d, p. 136, for explanation.)

MISCELLANEOUS CHEST PULSATIONS

Ventricular Aneurysms

1. What is felt on the chest wall with a ventricular **aneurysm**?

   ANS.: Surprisingly, the commonest sign of a ventricular aneurysm is a larger than normal area of LV apical movement. This is completely indistinguishable from the impulse of a dilated and hypertrophied LV. In other patients, an aneurysm is felt as a sustained systolic bulge, separate from an LV impulse but too low for a pulmonary artery and too lateral for the RV.

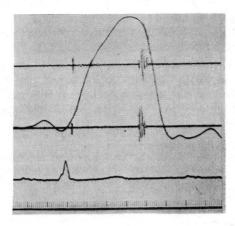

This precordial impulse was recorded at the level of the fourth intercostal space between the left sternal edge and mid-clavicular line. Note that it is a sustained impulse because it starts to fall with the S₂.

Note: a) The term *paradoxical pulsation* is often used to describe the precordial movement that is palpable with a ventricular aneurysm. This is a poor term for any precordial systolic bulge. The term refers to what is seen in an open-chested dog or by fluoroscopy during an acute infarction: the infarct area bulges outward with systole while the rest of the heart contracts [16].

   b) During acute infarction, the lower left sternal border area may bulge with systole, but when healing occurs, this bulging may cease. Such a bulge, when felt during life but not seen at autopsy, is sometimes called a physiological aneurysm.

2. When will the most lateral ventricular impulse retract deeply in systole without the initial outward movement that is seen in RV overload?

   ANS.: In constrictive pericarditis [6]. Here, the left parasternal area retracts slightly also, but the right parasternal area may rise in systole. It is usually followed by a diastolic outthrust [3, 18, 37].

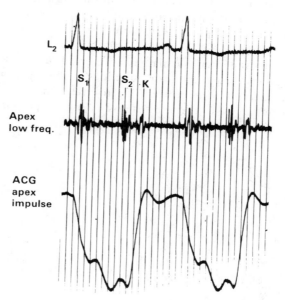

Apex cardiogram and phonocardiogram of a 25-year-old man with constrictive pericarditis due to uremic pericarditis and hemopericardium. Note the early S_3 or pericardial knock (K), the systolic apical retraction, and the diastolic outward movement.

Note: TR, if marked, will also produce the effect of apical area retraction [45]. This is really "lateral retraction" caused by a large RV movement.

Aortic and Arterial Pulsations on the Chest Wall

*1. How do you look for an aortic aneurysm by palpating the chest wall?

   ANS.: Look for pulsations in the right or left sternoclavicular joint area [18].

   Note: a) An aortic aneurysm may occasionally be suspected if it depresses the left bronchus with each pulsation. Depression of a left bronchus will in turn pull down the trachea. If you stand behind the seated patient and apply steady upward pressure on the cricoid cartilage with the tip of one forefinger, you will readily detect the downward pull on the trachea with each expansion. This phenomenon is known as the *tracheal tug*.

b) A dilated right aortic arch may also cause a right sternoclavicular pulsation. This, however, usually occurs only in the presence of cyanotic congenital heart disease because only then is the aortic arch likely to be both on the right and dilated. In the presence of cyanosis, a right aortic arch suggests tetralogy, especially with pulmonary atresia, because only severe tetralogy (i.e., with severe PS or atresia) can cause a right aortic arch to be dilated enough to produce a palpable impulse. The more severe the PS, the larger the shunt into the aorta and the greater the diameter of the aorta. This pulsation should be sought specifically just below the right sternoclavicular junction.

c) A large left coronary artery aneurysm can cause an abnormal systolic impulse at the left sternal border [61].

2. Where is coarctation most likely to produce pulsations on the chest wall? How are these brought out?

ANS.: The posterior intercostal arteries (enlarged collaterals) may be both visible and palpable. You can best make their pulsations visible by asking the patient to bend forward and let his arms dangle, to stretch the skin of the back. Project a light from above to create a shadow below the posterior ribs.

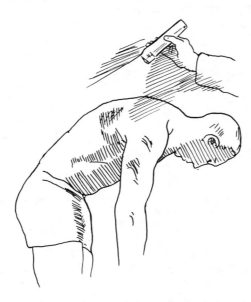

In the proper light, the dilated subcostal collateral arteries can be seen to pulsate.

3. What should you suspect if a patient with coarctation has no posterior chest-wall collateral vessel pulsations?

ANS.: Coarctation of the abdominal aorta [50].

Note: In the usual thoracic coarctation, there may also be no visible or palpable intercostal pulsations, no matter how severe the coarctation.

*4. What noncardiac condition can cause the entire left anterior chest wall to heave with systole?

ANS.: A large aneurysm of the descending aorta directly behind the heart.

GRAPHIC DISPLAYS OF CHEST MOVEMENTS

Methods

*1. What methods are most commonly used to show a visual record of chest movements on an oscilloscope or paper?

ANS.: The apex cardiogram, the kinetocardiogram, and the impulse cardiogram.

2. What is meant by an apex cardiogram (ACG)?

ANS.: It is a tracing of the movements of the chest wall, usually taken in the left lateral decubitus position by applying a chest piece (held on the chest by a hand or strap) that can transmit the movement to a transducer.

Note: A transducer is an instrument that can convert a mechanical signal into an electrical one or vice versa. The mechanical signal often comes from a funnel, cone, or small cup placed over the skin of the chest (chest piece) in which the air is displaced by movements of the chest wall. The change in air pressure is the mechanical signal that affects the transducer. Also in common use is a pressure-sensitive pin or disk whose movements affect a diaphragm that undergoes pressure changes that are transmitted to a transducer.

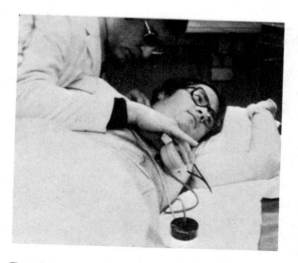

The pulse transducer is the black cylinder that is connected by a rubber tube to a side hole in a funnel held against the apical movement. The funnel is attached to a microphone, which the physician holds between his fingers. In this way, a simultaneous pulse tracing and phonocardiogram can be taken over the exact same area of the apex.

*3. What part of the ventricle is represented by a tracing of the movement of the cardiac "apex"?

ANS.: Apex cardiograms done on the exposed human heart during open heart surgery or on dogs on different layers from skin to pericardium show that the ACG represents the entire ventricular pulsation, not just movement of the apex itself. During ejection, the recoil of the ventricle against the chest wall is recorded as blood is ejected from the aorta. During ejection it is not surprising that the ACG follows Newton's second law and reflects the exact opposite of the forces of ejection. Only with the patient in the left lateral decubitus position are you close enough to the actual apex to record the opposing ballistic force of ejection. When the patient is in the supine position you are probably including the free-wall contraction in the tracing. Thus, in the supine position, the tracing is better called something other than an apex cardiogram. An *apex precordiogram* has been suggested as a suitable compromise. Perhaps we should use the term *impulse cardiogram* for supine recordings of ventricular motion, but even the latter term has already been given a specific meaning—it is a tracing of movements of the chest wall in the supine or 45-degree chest position taken by applying to the impulse a pin whose movement is transmitted in such a way that it can obstruct a photoelectric cell beam proportionate to the pin's displacement. The entire unit is fixed to a clamp on a bedside stand.

* 4. What is meant by a kinetocardiogram?

ANS.: It is a tracing of movements of the chest wall taken by applying to the chest wall a pin that is held in place by a rod fixed to the floor or bedstand; the chest movement is related to a fixed point in space. The chest movement is transmitted by way of the pin to a metal air-filled bellows and thence to a transducer.

* 5. Why is the ACG the most popular of the preceding methods?

ANS.: a) It is more easily and quickly applied to the cardiac impulse in all chest positions.

b) The same chest piece and transducer can be used for carotid or jugular tracings.

c) There is more literature on the information from an ACG.

The photoelectric technique provides the best representation of what the hand feels. However, there is very little information in the literature on its use, and what is felt by the hand is often of limited value for purposes in which apical movements have been helpful. For example, although the other methods exaggerate peaks and troughs, this exaggeration is often an advantage when the tracings are used as reference points for timing sounds and murmurs and when analyzing relative heights and rates and shapes of movements.

* 6. What element is necessary before an ACG or impulse cardiogram pulse unit can show a sustained cardiac impulse?

ANS.: The time constant should be at least three times the length of systole (i.e., at least 1.2 sec). Some investigators have recommended that it should be at least 2 or even 3 sec.

Note: a) The time constant is the rate at which a constant signal will drop down to the baseline or, to be more precise, the time needed for the signal to drop 36.6 percent of its original height. An ACG or an ECG taken with too short a time constant will overshoot all peaks and troughs and will be incapable of showing any sustained movements. It will act like a differential transducer, that is, it will begin to measure changes of rate or rates of velocity with time. Air leaks in crystal transducers may cause a short time constant [33]. It is also thought that too much air in a large funnel can shorten the time constant.

b) As long as the low-frequency cutoff point is at 0.15 Hz, different high-frequency cutoffs will have no effect on the timing of points or in wave configuration [47].

7. How can you distinguish outward from inward movement when looking at a graphic display of an ACG?

ANS.: Outward movements are the upward movements of a writing arm or oscilloscope beam. Inward movements are shown as downward movements below a baseline.

THE NORMAL APEX CARDIOGRAM

1. What are the disadvantages of the term *apex cardiogram?*

ANS.: a) The noncardiologist is led at first to believe that an ACG is some sort of an electrocardiogram taken at the site of the LV impulse.

b) It usually refers to a method of recording any precordial pulsations and not just to movement of the apex beat.

2. In the normal ACG what causes the first outward movement that begins after the onset of the QRS?

ANS.: The beginning of LV systolic movement, the onset of which is the C point.

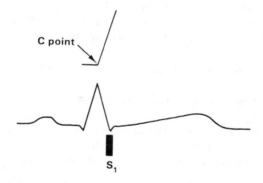

C point

S₁

The beginning of contraction of the LV on the ACG is called the C point.

*Note: a) The M_1 (or first heart sound component due to mitral closure events) occurs about 50 msec (0.05 sec) or less after the onset of the ACG movement. This interval is known as the C-1 interval.

b) The ACG outward movement rises either simultaneously with or slightly after the rise in intraventricular pressure [12]. The initial portion of mechanical systole may be associated with a change in ventricular configuration. If this change causes an outward thrust, the ACG may precede the rise in LV pressure, but if it results in retraction, the initial rise in pressure may not be perceived by the transducer and the ACG onset may follow the rise in LV pressure [48]. For all practical purposes, however, the ACG can be used to denote the onset of rise of ventricular pressure [40].

c) The C-1 interval is the "preisovolumic contraction period" because the mitral valve is still open and blood is flowing through it into the LV (i.e., the LV volume is still changing).

* 3. When in the outward phase of the ACG does the aortic valve open?

ANS.: Near the peak of the initial outward movement [7].

Note: a) The period between the closure of the mitral valve and the opening of the aortic valve (isovolumic contraction) is, on dual beam echocardiograms, about 48 ± 8 msec (from mitral valve apposition to the beginning of aortic valve opening). But the mitral component of the first heart sound occurs 20 to 40 msec after coaptation of the valve leaflets.

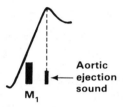

Aortic ejection sound

M₁

The interval between M₁ and any sound simultaneous with the opening of the aortic valve is isovolumic contraction time.

b) The end of the upstroke of the ACG or E point follows by a considerable interval the onset of ejection in the aorta. Therefore, it cannot be used as a marker for the exact time of opening of the aortic valve.

4. What does the normal ACG look like during ejection of blood through the aortic valve? Why?

ANS.: It looks like a sigmoid-shaped drop-off. The heart has struck the chest wall and is now retracting.

Note: The end–systolic shoulder represents the same point as the end-systolic part of the LV pressure curve and the beginning of ventricular relaxation; shortly after the end of the shoulder, the aortic valve closes.

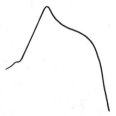

The only reason that this curve does not look like the sustained outward motion of the LV pressure curve is because the kind of transducer used to record it has a shorter time constant (see p. 142) than the ones used to record pressures at cardiac catheterization.

*5. What marks aortic valve closure and subsequent mitral valve opening on the ACG?

ANS.: Sometimes a slight notch on the downslope of the sigmoid curve marks aortic closure. The nadir of the ACG isovolumic relaxation phase is called the 0 point. This refers to the *opening* of the mitral valve.

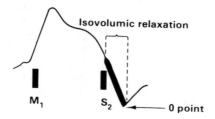

If the mitral valve makes a snapping sound when it opens, as in mitral stenosis, the opening snap will occur near the 0 point of the ACG.

Note: a) One study done with a pulse unit using a moderately short time constant showed that an S_2 to 0 point interval of less than 30 msec signified a high left atrial pressure [28]. In another study done with an infinite time constant ACG, a 2-0 interval of more than 110 msec was found in all subjects who had a reduced ejection fraction due to a cardiomyopathy regardless of left atrial pressure [40].

b) If you do not use a transducer with an infinite time constant, an accurate 0 point can be obtained if you record simultaneously a first derivative or dA/dt and use the point where it meets the baseline after ascending from its negative peak [41].

6. What happens to apical movement as the LV rapidly expands while it fills in early diastole?

ANS.: There is an outward movement, normally very rapid because it represents most of the phase of early rapid filling of the LV, when about 80 percent of the total diastolic blood volume enters the LV. This early diastolic wave has been called the rapid filling wave. The peak of the rapid filling wave is called the F point. (See figures on pp. 250, 256.)

7. What ACG movement follows the early filling wave (i.e., during the time of slow filling of the atrioventricle)?

ANS.: A slow rise called the slow filling wave or diastasis wave. (See figure on p. 367.)

8. How does atrial contraction at the end of slow filling in diastole affect the ACG, and what is this wave called?

ANS.: By suddenly expanding the LV, it produces an outward movement called an A wave or an atrial hump. (See figures on pp. 129 and 146.)

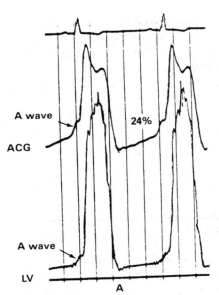 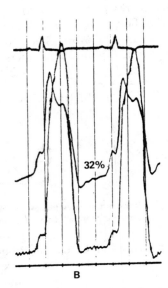

(A) Control LV pressure tracing and simultaneous apex cardiogram (ACG) in a patient with an abnormally high A wave. (B) After exercise there are parallel rises in LV end-diastolic and apex cardiographic A wave amplitude.

APEX CARDIOGRAM ABNORMALITIES

The following is a list of the ACG abnormalities that may aid in the diagnosis of heart disease.

*Atrial Hump or A Wave Abnormalities

1. In LVH or ischemic heart disease.
   a) The atrial hump may be greater than normal in amplitude. More than 12 percent of the total systolic deflection (A to EO or A/H) ratio is abnormal [4]. This abnormal ratio may appear only during angina or smoking and may become normal or disappear altogether with administration of sublingual nitrates.
   Note: 1) The A/H ratio may not correlate well with direct left atrial A wave pressures because the ACG A wave represents LV volume as well as pressure changes. If the A/H ratio is more than 14 percent, the atrial hump is almost always palpable if the P-R interval is not too short.
   2) The ratio of A wave to total amplitude of an ACG is not influenced by the time constant of the pulse unit unless it is extremely short (i.e., less than 0.05 sec) [32].
   b) When the A wave is longer in duration than normal (more than 50 msec), it is probably because atrial contraction is prolonged when the atrioventricle loses compliance [4]. In ischemic heart disease the time from onset to peak of the A wave is 60 ± 15 msec [35]. However, in hypertension it is 38 ± 7 msec because, for unknown reasons, in hypertension the A wave is more likely to be high and peaked than prolonged [35].

c) The A wave is likely to be notched in 40 percent of ACGs taken during early acute myocardial infarction [25].

*2. Over an aneurysm the A wave is very low [19].

*3. In MS the A wave is usually absent; if present, it is very low.

4. In one study in AS an A/H ratio of more than 16 percent always indicated an aortic valve area of less than 0.75 cm^2 and therefore severe AS [34].

*Rapid Filling Wave Abnormalities

*1. In MS the rapid filling wave is short or absent, so that during early filling there is often a shallow slope with no distinct change to show the onset of the slow filling phase; therefore, there is usually no distinct F point. When a rapid filling wave is present in significant MS, it is usually very short. The lowest normal duration is probably about 70 msec [9, 53].

*2. In severe MR there is often a marked overshoot in the rapid early filling wave. This overshoot may be palpable and is simultaneous with the S$_3$ (see figure on p. 256).

With combined MS and MR, a slow early filling wave strongly favors dominant stenosis [5].

Note: a) A short time constant of a transducer with an air leak may exaggerate the rapid filling wave.

b) A decrease in venous return, as occurs with a sublingual nitrate, may decrease the amplitude of the rapid filling wave.

*3. Over a ventricular aneurysm the rapid filling wave is either absent, very low in amplitude, or shorter in duration than normal. This appearance is probably due to the poor emptying of the sac in systole, with consequent poor filling in diastole.

*4. One study has shown that the duration of the slow filling wave divided by a rapid filling wave ratio of more than 2.8 indicates significant coronary disease in patients referred for angiography. This high ratio is presumably due to a shortened rapid filling wave secondary to loss of compliance of the LV. The ratio is surprisingly independent of the heart rate [51]. The short early filling duration is in accord with the finding that the filling volume during rapid filling of the LV is lower in patients with ventricular aneurysms [46]. This abnormal ratio of slow to rapid filling may also occur in AS and in hypertrophic cardiomyopathies [58].

*SYSTOLIC WAVE ABNORMALITIES

*Upstroke or C-E Interval Abnormalities

*1. In left atrial myxomas, large notching may occur on the upstroke [61].

Note: This same deep notch may occur on the upstroke in patients with MS and is probably associated with sudden deceleration of blood moving into the LV when the ring and pliable valves have reached their upper limit. It is possible that a deep notch may indicate good mobility of the mitral valves [61].

*2. In ischemic heart disease the C-E interval is prolonged. (The top normal limit is 90 msec.)

*3. If you are differentiating the ACG with the use of a differential transducer, the time from the beginning of the QRS to the peak of the first derivative during the preejection phase will correlate (R = 0.81) with the angiographic ejection fraction. The linear equation is: Ejection fraction = 142 − (0.952 × R to peak first derivative) [57].

* 4. In one study of AR, a C-E duration of more than 130 msec indicated a decreased ejection fraction [43].

    Note: In that study, the C-E duration did not correlate with the isovolumic contraction time because the E point occurred after the LV pressure curve crossed over the aortic pressure curve. The time after the crossover of the LV and aortic pressure curves appears to be the part of the C-E duration that is prolonged with decreased ejection fractions.

* 5. In AS a C-E duration of more than 10 msec denotes a decreased ejection fraction.

---

*Ejection Slope (E-S₂) Abnormalities

* 1. In ischemic heart disease

    * a) Instead of a good downstroke in late systole, a plateau or even an upward movement known as a late or midsystolic bulge may occur. This is also seen in LVH due to any cause.

    * b) There may be shortening of the early systolic downslope, so that the end-systolic shoulder begins earlier than normal (i.e., before midsystole). If we call the break in systolic slope between the early downslope and the shoulder "B," then the S_1-B is normally longer than B-S_2. An S_1-B that is shorter than B-S_2 may be due to asynergy between normal and abnormal muscle fibers, that is, the normal muscle shortening at higher velocity completes its contraction phase while the diseased muscle is still contracting [59].

        Note: This appearance may occur only during angina, after exercise, or after smoking a cigarette. It can improve or disappear with nitrates or coronary bypass surgery. In some patients with HSS, acute infarction or the prolapsed valve syndrome, the break in systolic slope becomes a midsystolic depression or dip and causes a double systolic impulse.

        The late systolic bulge occurs in up to 80 percent of patients with acute myocardial infarction and is thought to be due to asynergy [31]. Mid- or late systolic bulges are so common in the presence of right bundle branch block combined with anterior divisional block that conduction abnormalities must be considered one of the probable causes of the bulges and perhaps one of the causes of asynergy [8].

    * c) Over a ventricular aneurysm there is usually a monophasic wave with a poorly defined B point. It may rise to a peak in late systole (see Figure on p. 138).

        Note: If you are differentiating the ACG, you will see a sharp notch on the downslope that coincides with the aortic valve closure incisura. The distance from a sharp E point to this notch can be used to measure ejection times [25].

* 2. In constrictive pericarditis, you may see a small outward initial movement to a low E point, followed by a steep descent and wide trough during almost all of systole. A small positive wave follows the trough, ending with a peak just after the S_2 [18].

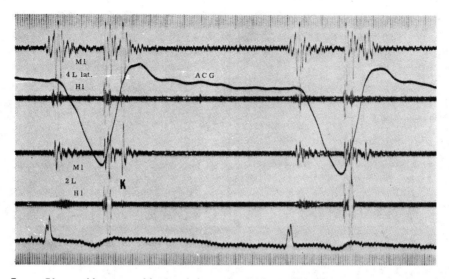

From a 51-year-old woman with constrictive pericarditis and atrial fibrillation. Note the systolic retraction on the apex cardiogram (ACG). Unlike an S_3, the pericardial knock (K) is loud even all along the left sternal border (2L and 4L). (From T. Hayashi, and T. Sakamoto. Phonocardiographic, mechanocardiographic and echocardiographic observations on pericarditis. *Cardiovasc. Bull.* 5:185, 1975.)

* 3. In patients with prolapsed mitral valves and both a click and a murmur there is often a systolic dip whose nadir varies from time to time in the same patient, coinciding exactly with the time of the systolic click [56].

* 4. An ACG may represent end-diastolic and end-systolic dimensions. These can be used to give you an ejection fraction.

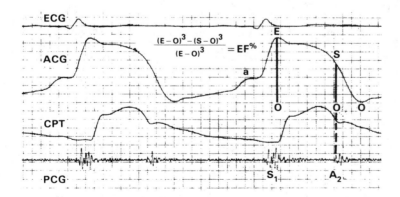

E-O coincides with the maximum outward deflection of the apex impulse. Because the ventricle is isovolumic up to this point, E-O can be used to represent the end-diastolic dimension. At the point of aortic valve closure, or A_2, the ventricle has completed ejection and is at its smallest dimension. If we call the A_2 downslope intercept S, then S-O may be used to represent the end-systolic dimension. Using the cube method for computing the ejection fraction, ejection fraction then equals $(E-O)^3 - (S-O)^3$ divided by $(E-O)^3$. The r value correlation with angiographic ejection fractions by this method is 0.89 in one study [1].

REFERENCES

1. Antani, J. A., Wayne, H. H., and Kuzman, W. J. Ejection phase indexes by invasive and noninvasive methods: an apexcardiographic, echocardiographic and ventriculographic correlative study. *Am. J. Cardiol.* 43:239, 1979.
2. Armstrong, T. G., Merran, J. K., and Gotsman, M. S. The left atrial lift. *Am. Heart J.* 82:764, 1971.
3. Basta, L. L., and Bettinger, J. J. The cardiac impulse: A new look at an old art. *Am. Heart J.* 97:96, 1979.
4. Benchimol, A., and Dimond, E. G. The apex cardiogram in ischaemic heart disease. *Br. Heart J.* 24:581, 1962.
5. Benchimol, A., et al. Diastolic movements of the precordium in mitral stenosis and regurgitation. *Am. Heart J.* 3:417, 1960.
6. Boicourt, O. W., Nagle, R. E., and Mounsey, J. P. D. The clinical significance of systolic retraction of the apical impulse. *Br. Heart J.* 27:379, 1965.
7. Braunwald, E., and Frahm, C. J. Studies on Starling's law of the heart. *Circulation* 24:633, 1961.
8. Byahatti, V., DePasquale, N. P., and Crampton, R. S. Indirect graphic studies in bilateral bundle branch block. *Chest* 58:223, 1970.
9. Coulshed, N., and Epstein, E. J. The apex cardiogram. *Br. Heart J.* 25:697, 1963.
10. Craige, E., and Schmidt, R. Precordial movements over the right ventricle in normal children. *Circulation* 32:232, 1965.
11. Deliyannis, A. A., et al. The cardiac impulse and the motion of the heart. *Br. Heart J.* 26:396, 1964.
12. Diendone, J. M. Tissue-cavitary difference pressure of dog left ventricle. *Am. J. Physiol.* 213:101, 1967.
13. Dressler, W. *Clinical Aids in Cardiac Diagnosis.* New York: Grune & Stratton, 1970.
14. Dressler, W., Kleinfeld, M., and Ripstein, C. B. Physical sign of tight mitral stenosis. Aid in selection of patients for valvulotomy. *J.A.M.A.* 154:49, 1954.
15. Eddleman, E. E., Jr. Kinetocardiographic changes as a result of mitral commissurotomy. *Am. J. Med.* 25:733, 1958.
16. Eddleman, E. E., Jr., and Langley, J. O. Paradoxical pulsation of the precordium in myocardial infarction and angina pectoris. *Am. Heart J.* 63:579, 1962.
17. Edwards, J. E., et al. *Congenital Heart Disease.* Philadelphia: W. B. Saunders, 1965. P. 197.
18. El-Sherif, A., and El-Said, G. Jugular, hepatic, and praecordial pulsations in constrictive pericarditis. *Br. Heart J.* 33:305, 1971.
19. El-Sherif, A., Saad, Y, and El-Said, G. Praecordial tracings of myocardial aneurysms. *Br. Heart J.* 31:357, 1969.
20. El-Sherif, N., and El-Ramly, Z. External left atrial pulse tracings in extreme left atrial dilatation. *Am. Heart J.* 84:387, 1972.
21. Epstein, E. J., et al. The "A" wave of the apex cardiogram in aortic valve disease and cardiomyopathy. *Br. Heart J.* 30:591, 1968.
22. Eve, F. C. Measurement of the heart in angular degrees. *Lancet* 1:659, 1941.
23. Feinstein, A. R., et al. Glossary of cardiologic terms related to physical diagnosis and history. *J.A.M.A.* 209:1693, 1969.
24. Fukumoto, T., et al. Right parasternal lift in atrial septal defect. *Am. Heart J.* 94:699, 1977.
25. Gabor, G., Porubszky, I., and Kalman, P. Determination of systolic time intervals using the apex cardiogram and its first derivative. *Am. J. Cardiol.* 30:217, 1972.
26. Gillam, P. M. S., Deliyannis, A. A., and Mounsey, J. P. D. The left parasternal impulse. *Br. Heart J.* 26:726, 1964.
27. Graham, T. P., Jr., Jarmakani, J. M., and Canent, R. V., Jr. Left heart volume characteristics with right ventricular volume overload. *Circulation* 45:389, 1972.
28. Gray, W., and Bell, H. 2-0 interval as an indicator of left atrial pressure. *Chest* 62:553, 1972.
29. Hayashi, T., and Sakamoto, T. Phonocardiographic, mechanocardiographic and echocardiographic observations on pericarditis. *CV Sound Bull.* 5:185, 1975.
30. Holt, J. H., Jr., and Eddleman, E. E., Jr. The precordial movements in adults with pulmonic stenosis. *Circulation* 35:492, 1967.

31. Jain, S. R., and Lindahl, J. Apex cardiogram and systolic time intervals in acute myocardial infarction. *Br. Heart J.* 33:578, 1971.
32. Johnson, A. D., Lonky, S. A., and Carleton, R. A. Combined hypertrophic subaortic stenosis and calcific aortic valvular stenosis. *Am. J. Cardiol.* 35:706, 1975.
33. Kastor, J. A., et al. Air leaks as a source of distortion in apexcardiography. *Chest* 57:163, 1970.
34. Kavalier, M. A., Steward, J., and Tavel, M. E. The apical A wave versus the fourth heart sound in assessing the severity of aortic stenosis. *Circulation* 51:324, 1975.
34A. Keats, T. E., and Enge, I. P. Cardiac mensuration by cardiac volume method. *Radiology* 85:850, 1965.
35. Kikawa, K., et al. The difference in apexcardiographic A-wave pattern between hypertension in ischemic heart disease. *J. Cardiogr.* 8:141, 1978.
36. Kjellberg, S. R., et al. *Diagnosis of Congenital Heart Disease.* Chicago: Year Book Medical Publishers, 1959. P. 411.
37. Lindsay, J., Jr., Crawley, I. S., and Callaway, G. M., Jr. Chronic constrictive pericarditis following uremic hemopericardium. *Am. Heart J.* 79:390, 1970.
38. Mainland, D., and Gordon, E. J. The position of organs determined from thoracic radiographs of young adult males with a study of the cardiac apex beat. *Am. J. Anat.* 68:457, 1941.
39. Manchester, G. H., Block, P., and Corlin, R. Misleading signs in mitral insufficiency. *J.A.M.A.* 191:99, 1965.
40. Manolas, J., et al. Time relation between apex cardiogram and left ventricular events using simultaneous high-fidelity tracings in man. *Br. Heart J.* 37:1263, 1975.
41. Manolas, J., and Rutishauser, W. Relation between apex cardiographic and internal indices of left ventricular relaxation in man. *Br. Heart J.* 39:1324, 1977.
42. Manolas, J., and Krayenbuehl, H. P. Comparison between apexcardiographic and angiographic indexes of left ventricular performance in patients with aortic incompetence. *Circulation* 57:692, 1978.
43. Mirro, M. J., et al. Angular displacement of the papillary muscles during the cardiac cycle. *Circulation* 60:327, 1979.
44. Morgan, J. R., Rogers, A. K., and Forker, A. D. Congenital absence of the left pericardium. *Ann. Intern. Med.* 74:370, 1971.
45. Mounsey, P. Praecordial pulsations in health and disease. *Postgrad. Med. J.* 44:134, 1968.
45A. Niehaus, F. W., and Wright, W. D. Facts and fallacies about the normal apex beat. *Am. Heart J.* 30:604, 1945.
46. Nosaka, H., et al. Diastolic left ventricular volume curve of ventricular aneurysm by left cineventriculogram with simultaneous recording of phonocardiogram: With a study of atrial fibrillation. *J. Cardiogr.* 7:187, 1977.
47. Pigott, V., and Spodick, D. H. The effects of high frequency filter cut-offs on the apexcardiogram. *Chest* 59:240, 1971.
48. Reddy, P. S., et al. High-fidelity, infinite time constant calibrated pressure apexcardiogram and its correlation with high-fidelity left ventricular pressure. *Br. Heart J.* 44:194, 1980.
49. Rivero-Carvallo, J. M. The left bronchial compression syndrome. *Am. J. Cardiol.* 9:521, 1962.
50. Shapiro, M. J. Coarctation of the abdominal aorta. *Am. J. Cardiol.* 4:547, 1959.
51. Silvestre, A., et al. Slow filling period/rapid filling period ratio in the apexcardiogram: Relation to the diagnosis of coronary artery disease. *Am. J. Cardiol.* 42:377, 1978.
52. Soloff, L. A., and Zatuchni, J. Cardiac chamber volumes and their significance in rheumatic heart disease with isolated mitral stenosis. *Circulation* 19:269, 1959.
53. Spodick, D. H., and Kumar, S. Rapid filling period of the left ventricle: Measurement by apexcardiography. *Aerosp. Med.* 39:1351, 1968.
54. Stapleton, J. F., and Groves, B. M. Precordial palpation. *Am. Heart J.* 81:409, 1971.
55. Tafur, E., Cohen, L. S., and Levine, H. D. The normal apex cardiogram, its temporal relationship to electrical, acoustic, and mechanical cardiac events. *Circulation* 30:381, 1964.
56. Towne, W. D., et al. The apex cardiogram in patients with systolic prolapse of the mitral valve. *Chest* 63:569, 1973.
57. Vetter, W. R., Sullivan, R. W., and Hyatt, K. H. Assessment of quantitative apex cardiography. *Am. J. Cardiol.* 29:667, 1972.

58. Vidal, J. M., and de la Calzada. Apexcardiographic index in ischemic heart disease. *Am. J. Cardiol.* 46:348, 1980.
59. Wayne, H. H. *Noninvasive Technics in Cardiology.* Chicago: Year Book Medical Publishers, 1973.
60. Wigle, E. D., and Labrosse, C. J. Sudden severe aortic regurgitation. *Circulation* 32:708, 1965.
61. Zitnik, R. S., and Giuliani, E. R. Clinical recognition of atrial myxoma. *Am. Heart J.* 80:689, 1970.

6. *The Stethoscope*

THE BELL CHEST PIECE

1. What is the relation between the tautness (stiffness) of a membrane that collects sound from the chest wall and the ability of the membrane to transmit high or low frequencies?

   ANS.: The more taut the membrane, the higher its natural frequency of oscillation and the more efficient it is at higher frequencies.

2. What is the ideal membrane to apply to a chest wall in order to bring out low frequencies?

   ANS.: A membrane that is as loose and flabby as possible.

3. How does the use of a bell chest piece fit into these acoustical laws?

   ANS.: The bell allows you to use the skin as a flabby diaphragm. The skin can be turned into a taut diaphragm if enough pressure is applied to the skin to produce pain.

4. Which chest piece diameter picks up the most sound, a very small one or a very large one?

   ANS.: A very large one. The ability of a chest piece to collect sound is proportional to its diameter.

5. Which chest piece diameter picks up low frequencies better, a small one or a large one?

   ANS.: A large one.

6. How much pressure should be applied with a bell chest piece?

   ANS.: Just enough to prevent room-noise leak. Any more pressure will tighten the skin and tend to damp out the low frequencies.

   Note: An exception to this occurs when you are listening for an S_4. (See page 270.)

7. What is the relationship between the internal volume of a stethoscope (air space enclosed by the chest piece and tubing) and the loudness of the transmitted sounds?

   ANS.: There is an inverse relationship—i.e., the smaller the internal volume, the greater the loudness of the sound.

8. What bell design will give the smallest internal volume and the largest diameter?

   ANS.: A shallow shell rather than a deep cone.

9. What then is the ideal chest piece for low frequencies?

   ANS.: A shallow bell with as large a diameter as is consistent with a reasonable seat on the chest wall when only a minimal amount of pressure is applied.

   * *Note:* It is believed by some cardiologists, with no explanation or testing other than their own ears, that a third chest piece consisting of a large-diameter corrugated diaphragm applied with light pressure (actually only the weight of the three-headed stethoscope) is sometimes best for hearing low frequencies. They still advise having a bell handy, however, both because it is needed for auscultation in small places

---

*Material marked with an asterisk is for reference and for advanced students in cardiology.

such as the supraclavicular fossa or between the ribs on a bony chest and because the bell is occasionally superior for certain low frequencies.

10. What kind of murmurs and sounds are best heard with the bell?

ANS.: Murmurs: diastolic murmurs through atrioventricular valves (mitral and tricuspid).

Sounds: the diastolic sounds known as the S_3 and S_4.

Note: The kettledrum (tympany) is bell-shaped and is also used to bring out the low-frequency, booming tones.

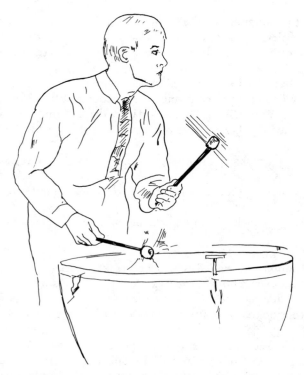

The diastolic rumble and deep, low groan
Needs the bell to magnify it.
For the third heart sound, like the kettledrum's tone,
There's nothing like a bell, so try it!

Note: Adults can hear frequencies up to 14,000 cycles per second (cps). However, since cardiac sound does not extend much above 1,000 cps, loss of ability to hear frequencies above 3,000 cps, which is the usual type of hearing loss in older physicians, should not interfere with hearing any cardiac sounds or murmurs [1, 2].

THE SMOOTH DIAPHRAGM

1. What is meant by "masking" of sounds?

   ANS.: Masking of sounds refers to the inability to hear a sound well because of interference by another loud sound occurring just before it or just after it.

2. Do low frequencies mask high ones easily?

   ANS.: Yes, unless the lower frequencies are very widely separated in pitch from the higher frequencies or are relatively soft [3, 6].

3. Do high frequencies mask low ones easily?

   ANS.: No, unless the high frequencies are relatively loud.

4. What is the purpose of the smooth, stiff diaphragm?

   ANS.: To damp out low frequencies and unmask high frequencies. If the resonance frequency of the diaphragm happens to be the same as that of the murmur, it may actually amplify the murmur.

   Note: a) Amplification of sound may also be due to the summation of reflected or standing waves in the tubing. Different tubing lengths therefore may amplify different frequencies [2].

   b) Although a bell will bring out low frequencies considerably better than a diaphragm, high frequency sounds and murmurs are actually heard just as well with the bell as with the diaphragm [10]. The major purpose of a diaphragm is to distinguish splitting of sounds and to make it easier for high frequency murmurs to be perceived without interference by lower frequencies.

5. Why not use the bell chest piece as a diaphragm by merely applying pressure, thus eliminating the need for two chest pieces?

   ANS.: The stretched skin is an inefficient diaphragm for filtering out low frequencies. The skin does not become stiff enough to be a good filter.

   Note: a) Many bells transmit high frequencies better than does the diaphragm of the same stethoscope [7]. This is especially true if it is a small-diameter, deep trumpet-shaped bell [3, 4]. Therefore, if there are not too many low frequencies present to mask the highs, it may be profitable to use the bell to hear high-pitched murmurs.

   b) Do not use x-ray film as a substitute for a damaged diaphragm. X-ray film has been shown to be about as good as no diaphragm at all for filtering out low frequencies. It is not stiff enough.

   c) A greater degree of pressure variation with the diaphragm has been attained through prestressing a nylon diaphragm by bowing it slightly forward. A small raised area in the center of the diaphragm can further increase the tension by exerting pressure against the skin [8].

   d) If the diaphragm is too thick, there is too much loss of amplitude (volume).

6. Which murmurs and sounds are usually heard well only with the stiff, smooth diaphragm?

   ANS.: Murmurs: the soft aortic and pulmonary diastolic murmur and the soft mitral regurgitation murmur. Sounds: splitting of first or second heart sounds and nonejection clicks.

   *Note: The rigid, wooden, monaural stethoscope invented by Laennec will decrease about tenfold the loudness of sound in the 60 to 700 cps range. This encompasses the medium- and high-frequency range of cardiac sounds and murmurs.

7. Why is it very difficult to hear the splitting of heart sounds with a bell?

ANS.: Because there are so many low-frequency "reverberations" surrounding each component that the ear cannot separate them if the splitting is close. The ear can separate two short, high-frequency sounds placed close to each other more easily that it can separate two prolonged low- or medium-frequency sounds.

*8. How can a diaphragm help in localizing a murmur?

ANS.: Because high-frequency sounds do not spread as widely across the chest wall as do low frequencies, the diaphragm may help you to localize sounds to their point of origin [2].

THE TUBING

1. Which frequencies are attenuated (damped) by too long a tubing?

ANS.: High frequencies. The low frequencies are relatively unaffected by tube length [9].

2. What is the shortest compromise length that will bring out high frequencies and still not be too short for comfort?

ANS.: A length of 12 inches (30 cm).

Note: It has not yet been proved that an additional 3 or 4 inches of length for tall physicians' comfort makes much difference.

*3. What frequencies are best carried by very narrow or very wide tubing?

ANS.: Very narrow tubes carry low frequencies best, and high frequencies are best carried by wide tubing.

Note: An internal diameter of 1/8 inch (3 mm) was once recommended as the ideal compromise for carrying both low and high frequencies. The average commercial stethoscope has an internal diameter of 3/16 inch (4.6 mm), which has been found recently to be even better than 1/8 inch. The Littman, Harvey, Leatham, and the Rappaport and Sprague stethoscopes are 1/8 inch in diameter. The Harvey three-headed stethoscope (one head with a corrugated diaphragm) has a metal head-piece 3/16 inch in diameter.

4. How can the thickness of the tubing affect auscultation?

ANS.: The thicker the tube, the better is the elimination of room noise. A vinyl tube has been found to be better than rubber for this purpose.

5. Why is a dull-surfaced rubber tubing inefficient for stethoscopes?

ANS.: This type of tubing increases internal frictional resistance.

6. Which is more efficient, a single tube or a double tube?

ANS.: The single-tube stethoscopes appear at first glance to be more efficient because they eliminate the necessity for binding parallel tubes together to prevent collision sounds, and they are more flexible and portable. However, tests have shown that *the double tube is more efficient for high frequencies* because it allows less interference from reflected waves [2, 4]. However, a single tube attenuates only frequencies of over 400 cps, which suggests that only the very softest and highest-pitched murmurs will be missed by using a single tube [10]. A single tube plus a shallow bell can attenuate the high frequencies by as much as 50 decibels [4]. This is the difference between a shout and a whisper.

AIR LEAKS AND EAR TIPS

1. How important are air leaks at either the earpieces, changeover valve, or chest piece?
   ANS.: The greatest impairment of the efficiency of a stethoscope is an air leak [5]. Room noise due to air leaks tends to mask high frequencies more than low ones.

2. How can you test for air leaks at the chest piece or changeover valve?
   ANS.: a) Blow into one tube while occluding the opposite earpiece and tubing. Your fingers will feel the air escaping. Blowing cigarette smoke into the tube will enable you to detect even smaller leaks but will be very disillusioning because few stethoscopes are made to pass this test.

   b) If withdrawing the chest piece quickly from the precordium produces a change in pressure that is painful to the ear, an air leak, if present, is probably unimportant.

3. Which kind of earpieces are most likely to cause air leaks, small ones that enter the canal or large ones that merely occlude the external canal?
   ANS.: Small ones are most likely to cause a leak (and so mask high frequencies). Small ones are also the least comfortable.

4. Why may small ear tips become partially obstructed when being inserted into the ear?
   ANS.: The external auditory meatus points slightly forward and then backward, forming an angle. The usual stethoscope headpieces are designed to point the ear tips slightly anteriorly. If the ear tips are too small, their aperture may impinge partially or completely against the cartilaginous meatus, which points backward [6].

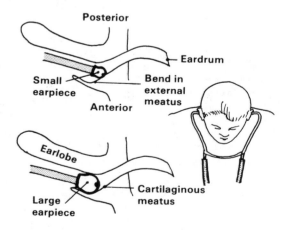

Headpieces are designed to point the ear tips slightly anteriorly. Small ear tips can therefore be partly occluded against the backward-directed meatus.

SUMMARY OF GOOD STETHOSCOPE CHARACTERISTICS

1. A shallow bell with a large diameter for low frequencies.
2. A smooth, stiff, thin diaphragm for high frequencies.
3. A pediatric-sized bell and diaphragm accessories.
4. An internally smooth vinyl tubing, not over 12 inches (30 cm) long and 3/16 of an inch (4.6 mm) in internal diameter.
5. Double tubing with some method of binding the tubes together.
6. The largest ear tips possible.
7. Metal headpieces that can be rotated so that the ear tips can be pointed in the most comfortable direction.

REFERENCES

1. Dawson, J. B. Auscultation and the stethoscope. *Practitioner* 193:315, 1954.
2. Ertel, P. Y., et al. Stethoscope acoustics I. The doctor and his stethoscope. *Circulation* 34:889, 1966.
3. Ertel, P. Y., et al. Stethoscope acoustics II. Transmission and filtration patterns. *Circulation* 34:899, 1966.
4. Ertel, P. Y., Lawrence, M., and Song, W. How to test stethoscopes. *Med. Res. Eng.* 8:7, 1969.
5. Groom, D. Comparative efficiency of stethoscopes. *Am. Heart J.* 68:220, 1967.
6. Groom, D., and Chapman, W. Anatomic variations of the auditory canal pertaining to the fit of the stethoscope earpieces. *Circulation* 19:606, 1959.
7. Hampton, C. S., and Chaloner, A. Which stethoscope? *Br. Med. J.* 4:388, 1967.
8. Howell, W. L., and Aldridge, C. F. The effect of stethoscope-applied pressure in auscultation. *Circulation* 32:430, 1965.
9. Johnston, F. D., and Kline, E. M. An acoustical study of the stethoscope. *Arch. Intern. Med.* 65:328, 1940.
10. Kindig, J. R., et al. Acoustical performance of the stethoscope: a comparative analysis. *Am. Heart J.* 104:269, 1982.
11. Ongley, P. A., et al. *Heart Sounds and Murmurs.* New York: Grune & Stratton, 1960. P. 32.

7. Diagramming and Grading Heart Sounds and Murmurs (The Auscultogram)

A **graphic method** for illustrating auscultatory findings is offered here not only as a means of keeping records as conveniently and efficiently as possible but also as an aid in learning auscultation. It has been shown that one such "auscultogram" (see figures) can equal a 629-word description of the auscultatory findings [5]. The graph can tell the story at a glance once the symbols are understood [2].

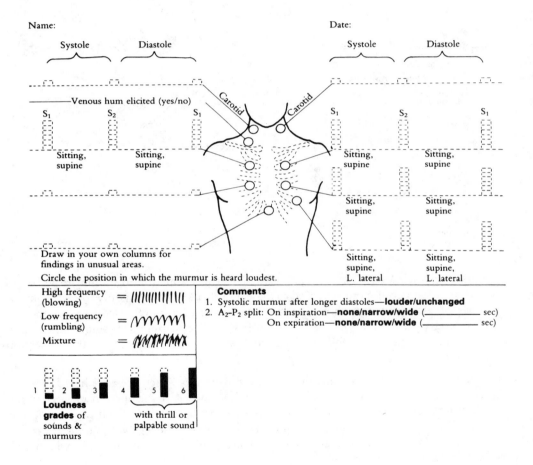

Name: Date:

| Systole | Diastole | | Systole | Diastole |

——————Venous hum elicited (yes/no)

S_1 S_2 S_1 Carotid   Carotid S_1 S_2 S_1

Sitting, supine   Sitting, supine   Sitting, supine   Sitting, supine

Sitting, supine   Sitting, supine

Draw in your own columns for findings in unusual areas.

Circle the position in which the murmur is heard loudest.

Sitting, supine, L. lateral   Sitting, supine, L. lateral

High frequency (blowing)	=	‖‖‖‖‖‖‖‖‖‖‖
Low frequency (rumbling)	=	⋁⋁⋁⋁⋁⋁
Mixture	=	⋀‖⋀‖⋀‖⋀

Comments

1. Systolic murmur after longer diastoles—**louder/unchanged**
2. A_2-P_2 split: On inspiration—**none/narrow/wide** (_____ sec)
   On expiration—**none/narrow/wide** (_____ sec)

1   2   3   4   5   6

Loudness grades of sounds & murmurs

with thrill or palpable sound

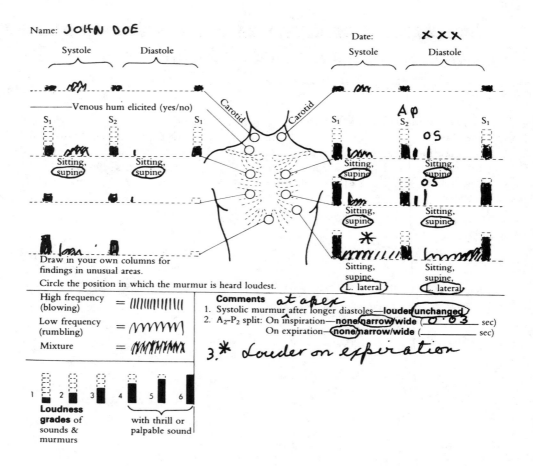

Name: **JOHN DOE**   Date: **× × ×**

Filling in such auscultograms serves a self-teaching function in training a person in auscultation because one is forced to dissect out and listen separately to each component of the cycle, a method that is the hallmark of a good auscultator. Although listening to the total effect of all the sounds and murmurs as a single unit is also important, beginners tend to listen this way to the exclusion of the dissection method.

We customarily describe murmurs in the position in which they are heard loudest, so that if we say that a diastolic murmur is "grade 4 at the apex in the left lateral decubitus position," we do not find it necessary to state in which position it was heard as grade 3 at the apex. The multiple choices of *sitting, supine,* and *left lateral* in the auscultogram are given to enable one to indicate the position in which that particular murmur was loudest.

The auscultogram uses widely spaced wavy lines for low frequencies and closely spaced straight lines for high frequencies because this resembles the way they look on a phonocardiogram. We show medium or mixed frequencies by means of low-frequency wavy lines with diagonal lines drawn through them. An explanatory example of the frequency symbols is necessary on each auscultogram.

The loudness of sounds and murmurs is indicated by their height on a vertical column that is divided into six parts to represent six grades of loudness. Drawing sounds and murmurs of different heights to indicate loudness instead of describing or numbering them is analogous to the difference between looking at a complicated column of numbers and looking at a simple bar graph.

Grading amplitude on a scale of 6 is acceptable if we can separate grades 3 and 4. When Freeman and Levine [3] in 1933 introduced the grading of murmurs up to 6, only grades 1, 2, and 6 were described in detail. Grade 6 was a murmur heard with the stethoscope off the chest, and grade 1 could be missed on first applying the stethoscope. Grade 2 was an easily heard, faint murmur. By 1959 Levine [4] had proposed that grade 5 was a murmur that could be heard when the edge of the chest piece (preferably the diaphragm) was applied to the precordium. However, he left the distinction between grades 3 and 4 to be made by the listener. This problem may be solved by using the thrill as a means of separating them; that is, if the murmur is accompanied by a thrill, it is grade 4 or more. With this system it appears possible that high–frequency murmurs may be very loud but not become palpable. However, in actual experience, the two typical high-frequency murmurs, those of aortic and mitral regurgitation, are associated with thrills often enough to convince one that when these murmurs become loud, they acquire low frequencies. In 1959 Bruns [1] helped to explain this phenomenon when he showed that according to the vortex theory of the production of murmurs, a high-pitched murmur from a small orifice acquires low frequencies as the orifice enlarges. The low frequencies tend to travel in the direction of flow (i.e., downstream from the source of the murmur).

Note: a) A grade 1 murmur is best defined as one that requires "tuning in." *Tuning in* is a term used to describe a psychological state in which you must first have an expectation (i.e., you must know what you are listening for), and then you eliminate room noise by an act of concentration.

b) It is not necessary to add *palpable* to the word *thrill* because all thrills are palpable.

Using palpability to separate grade 3 from grade 4 murmurs has many advantages:

1. It facilitates the teaching of grading by 6, because grades 3 and 4 are the only stumbling blocks.
2. It teaches the student the relation between a thrill and a murmur, making him realize that a long thrill is never felt in the absence of a loud murmur. (Widely split components of loud heart sounds or a slight bisferiens pulse may feel like *short* thrills.)
3. It lends itself to the grading of heart sounds.

A grading chart incorporated in one corner of every auscultogram teaches the system at a glance.

Note: Thrills and sounds are best perceived with the distal palm. One hand may be more sensitive than the other, so test each hand on a patient with a faint thrill or palpable sound to find your better hand.

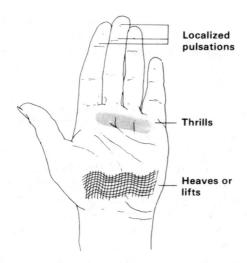

Localized
pulsations

Thrills

Heaves or
lifts

Although small localized movements are best perceived by the distal finger pads, thrills are best felt with the distal palm.

The auscultogram can serve as a means of training the cardiology student to acquire any habits of auscultation that a cardiology teaching service desires. For example, providing a place on the graph for noting the width and movements of the second sound split with respiration serves as a constant reminder to listen for such splits. Since we wish to teach our students the value of listening in the neck for heart sounds and murmurs, we include the neck on our diagram. We also provide a place for noting the effects of intermittent long diastoles.

The writing and listening should be done simultaneously (i.e., with the stethoscope in one hand and a pen in the other, the auscultator fills in the auscultogram). The auscultogram is used for the purpose of improving the ability to auscultate and providing an accurate record; the art of fine auscultation is not a memory test. Performing auscultation is one of the few times when it is best for a right-handed physician to carry out his examination from the patient's left side because this position allows him to hold the stethoscope with the left hand while writing with the right.

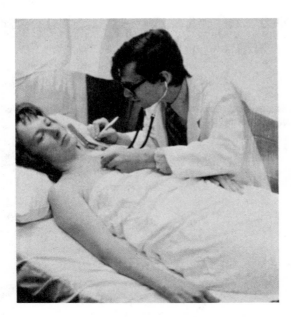

Simultaneous writing and listening is the key to this method of ear training and accuracy of recording.

It is convenient to print auscultogram pads that are small enough to fit on about half a hospital chart page. A sticky backing makes for easy attachment. The auscultogram illustrated on page 159 is the actual size.

REFERENCES

1. Bruns, D. L. A general theory of the causes of murmurs in the cardiovascular system. *Am. J. Med.* 27:360, 1959. Classic article.
2. Constant, J., and Lippschutz, E. J. Diagramming and grading heart sounds and murmurs. *Am. Heart J.* 70:326, 1965.
3. Freeman, A. R., and Levine, S. A. The clinical significance of the systolic murmur. *Ann. Intern. Med.* 6:1371, 1933.
4. Levine, S. A., and Harvey, W. P. *Clinical Auscultation of the Heart.* Philadelphia: Saunders, 1959.
5. Segall, H. N. A simple method for graphic description of cardiac auscultatory signs. *Am. Heart J.* 8:553, 1932-1933.

8. The First Heart Sound (The S_1)

PHYSIOLOGY OF FIRST SOUND COMPONENTS

1. Draw a left ventricular (LV) pressure curve.

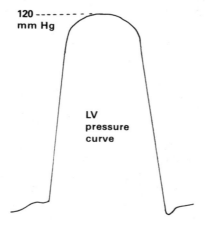

120 mm Hg

LV pressure curve

An LV pressure curve begins at a pressure of about 0 mm Hg and rises to the same systolic pressure as in the aorta, i.e., normally about 120 mm Hg.

2. Draw a left atrial pressure curve on the ventricular pressure curve and show where the mitral valve closes. Why does it close here?

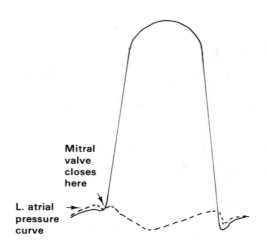

Mitral valve closes here

L. atrial pressure curve

The most important component of the S_1, which is the mitral component or M_1, occurs as the result of this valve closure, but the sound should not be thought of as due to the slapping together of leaflets. It is more probably due to sudden cessation of mitral valve flow at the time of maximum leaflet tension that occurs immediately after leaflet apposition setting the entire cardiohemic system into vibration.

ANS.: The mitral valve closes when LV pressure rises above left atrial pressure, which is about 10 mm Hg. If the left atrial pressure at the beginning of ventricular contraction is 10 mm Hg, then as soon as the LV reaches a pressure of slightly more than 10 mm Hg, the mitral valve will close.

3. Draw an aortic pressure curve on the ventricular pressure curve and show where the aortic valve opens.

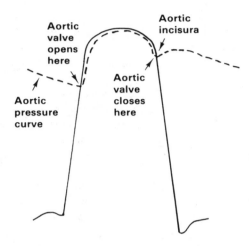

When the LV pressure reaches aortic diastolic pressure (about 80 mm Hg), the aortic valve opens, and an aortic valve-opening sound may be produced and become the second component of a split S_1. When aortic recoil power becomes stronger than LV ejection, the aortic valve closes to prevent regurgitation. The S_2 occurs at this time.

4. When does the aortic valve open if the aortic diastolic pressure is 80 mm Hg?
ANS.: The aortic valve opens when the LV pressure exceeds aortic diastolic pressure (80 mm Hg).
Note: The time between the closure of the mitral valve and the opening of the aortic valve is the **isovolumic contraction** period.

5. How do these pressure curves relate to the first heart sound, or S_1?
ANS.: The events associated with closure of the mitral valve and ejection of blood into the aorta are considered by some cardiologists to be responsible for the two major components of the S_1. Many other cardiologists believe that the second major component of the split S_1 is due to closure of the tricuspid valve, especially if the split is narrow [29].
*Note: The vibrations that are heard as heart sounds have been attributed to the effect of blood flow acceleration or deceleration caused by valves opening or closing [29]. We should not consider the mere coaptation of valve cusps as the cause of the sounds. The sounds are produced by the vibrations of the apposed cusps as the upward movement of the cusp bellies is suddenly checked when they reach their full extent of movement [68]. The first high-frequency component of the S_1 occurs about 20 msec after echocardiographic valve closure (apposition) and after the crossover of pressure pulses in the LV and left atrium [29,

Boldface type indicates that the term is explained in the Glossary.
*Material marked with an asterisk is for reference and for advanced students in cardiology.

51]. The echocardiogram on page 249 shows that the major component of the S_1 occurs well after (usually 20–30 msec after) coaptation of the mitral valve cusps [37]. Mitral valve closure is a continuous movement; the leaflets make contact near their leading free edge, after which the area of contact spreads toward the basal attachments as both leaflets are propelled toward the left atrium until restrained by the chordae to produce the M_1 [44]. This sudden tension of the elastic coapted cusps causes them to stretch and recoil in a rapid vibratory movement that produces the M_1. When the mitral valve is removed experimentally, the M_1 is absent [36].

* 6. How many components or discrete vibrations can be found in the S_1 of a phonocardiogram?

   ANS.: If low frequencies are being displayed and the paper speed is such that the heart sound components are spread out, four discrete vibrations can be described. If, however, only high frequencies are used, or the paper speed is not very fast, there may be only two or three distinct vibrations.

7. In what percentage of normal subjects is splitting of the S_1 audible?

   ANS.: In about 85 percent.

8. Which of the four phonocardiographic distinct vibrations are audible?

   ANS.: The S_1 commonly has two distinct components, that is, the first heart sound is said to be split. The following description is a synthesis of many theories:

   The first audible component of S_1 (simultaneous with the second phonocardiographic component), is called the M_1 because it is caused by events associated with mitral closure. The origin of the second audible (third phonocardiographic) component depends on the width of the split. When the split is narrow, the origin is probably tricuspid closure, and the sound is called the T_1. When the split is wide, the second audible (fourth phonocardiographic) component may be caused by the opening of a stiff aortic or pulmonary valve, as occurs with systemic or pulmonary hypertension or aortic or pulmonary valve stenosis. This second component of a wide split is called an ejection sound, but if the semilunar valves are stiff enough, the sound may be so short and sharp that it has the quality of a click. It may then be called an "ejection click." (See figure on page 173.)

M_1 T_1 A_1

Inaudible low-frequency component

Narrow splitting of S_1

M_1 T_1

Wide splitting of S_1

M_1 A_1

Narrow splitting of S_1 (less than the usual isovolumic contraction time of about 50 msec [0.05 sec]) may be due to M_1, T_1 components. Wide splitting (50 msec or longer) is probably due to the M_1, A_1 components, unless there is a right ventricular volume or pressure overload.

Note: a) Although the initial low-amplitude vibration of S_1 is occasionally due to atrial contraction, it sometimes occurs in atrial fibrillation. It may be audible in the presence of a mitral prosthetic valve [2]. Because it occurs before any anterior movement of the posterior left ventricular wall on echophonocardiography, it must occur during pre-isovolumic contraction and may emanate from the ventricular wall as it becomes taut.

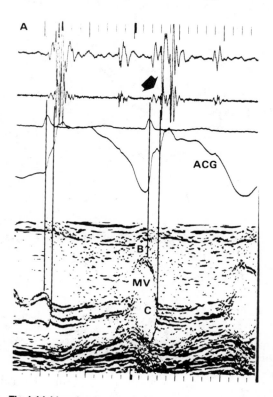

The initial low frequency component of the S_1 recorded in this patient with atrial fibrillation occurs during the pre-isovolumic contraction period of the left ventricle as seen on the apex cardiogram (ACG) and before mitral valve closure (C) on the mitral valve echocardiogram.

b) A root sound theory has been proposed to explain the second component (A_1) of a widely split S_1 in subjects with no valvular abnormalities—that is, it is caused by a change in the rate of pressure rise in the LV that suddenly tenses the aortic root structures just as the aortic valve begins to open [53]. However, all aortic ejection sounds that have been correlated with echocardiograms have been timed to be simultaneous with the peak of opening of the aortic or tricuspid valves [32, 42].

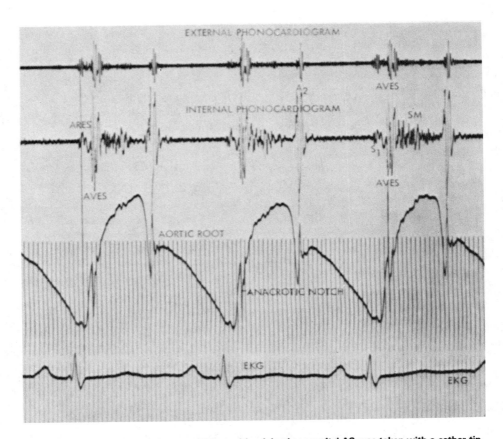

This aortic root tracing from a 16-year-old boy with minimal congenital AS was taken with a cather tip electromanometer to avoid any delays due to tubing. An aortic root ejection sound (ARES) is present, coincident with the onset of pressure rise in the aortic root. There is no M_1 in this area. An aortic valve ejection sound (AVES) is also present, occurring 40 msec (0.04 sec) later and simultaneously with the anacrotic notch. (From Whittaker, Shaver, Gray, and Leonard [63].)

c) The arguments against attributing the usual easily heard second component of a split first sound to tricuspid valve closure are as follows:

1) When the right ventricule (RV) is completely bypassed and destroyed, so that it cannot contract, the S_1 may still be split.

2) If the heart is explored with a microphone placed directly on the myocardium, all components of the S_1 become softer over the RV, and there is no amplification of any component of the first heart sound over the RV [35].

3) In subjects with left bundle branch block (LBBB), the S_1 often shows the same degree of splitting and the same number of components despite the marked delay in the onset of M_1 in LBBB [47]. Whenever wide splitting is heard in right bundle branch block (RBBB), the second component can often be shown to be due to an ejection sound and not a T_1 [74]. However, in one series 40 percent of patients with RBBB showed no clearly detectable split of S_1 (by auscultation), and in another 44

percent, the usual narrow physiological splitting was observed [65].

d) In a study of 16 normal subjects by echophonocardiography, the first major component of the S_1 coincided with mitral closure in all, and it coincided also with tricuspid valve closure in the majority. The second major component of the S_1 coincided with aortic valve opening in all, and with tricuspid valve closure in one-third [56].

*9. When is it likely that tricuspid closure *does* contribute to the S_1 in the presence of a normal tricuspid valve?

ANS.: Whenever the RV has a volume or pressure overload (e.g., in atrial septal defect (ASD) or in pulmonary hypertension). This is supported by the following findings:

a) In subjects with an ASD, the second major component of the S_1 coincides with the peak of the right atrial C wave.

b) In 75 percent of children with an ASD, the second component of a split S_1 at the apex occupied by the RV is louder than the M_1 [34, 64]. This relationship of component loudness is unusual in normal children.

c) In one study, among subjects with an ASD, only those with a complete RBBB were found to have a widely split S_1 [30]. (Although this suggests that the second component was a T_1, it may have been a pulmonary ejection sound.)

Note: a) In at least one report, it has even been shown that the second loud component of the split S_1 in ASD is not always due to T_1 because by intracardiac phonocardiography it was found that the second component was absent in the RV in half the patients tested, often occurred after the rise in pulmonary artery pressure, and showed a constant time relationship with the onset of rise of aortic pressure [55].

b) In mitral stenosis (MS) a tricuspid component may precede the delayed M_1 [28, 50]. Intracardiac phonocardiography has shown that a right-sided S_1 component precedes a left-sided S_1 component in about a fourth of patients with MS.

c) If the second component of a split S_1 increases on inspiration, you may then be justified in calling it a T_1. If it is more than 40 msec from the M_1 (in the absence of RBBB), it is probably an aortic ejection sound.

THE M_1 PLUS AORTIC EJECTION SOUND AS THE CAUSE OF A SPLIT S_1

1. How long after the M_1 does the aortic ejection sound (A_1) occur in normal subjects?

ANS.: The usual A_1 occurs at the end of isovolumic contraction (i.e., about 40–60 msec [0.04–0.06 sec] after the M_1 [14, 33]). To help you judge this normal split of the first sound interval, a 40-msec split takes as long as it does to say "pa-da" as quickly as possible. The 60-msec split can be imitated by saying "pa-ta" as quickly as possible. (A 40–60 msec split is a moderately wide split.)

Note: It may be easier to hear a split in the S_1 in older subjects because isovolumic contraction times tend to lengthen with age [3].

    a) The differentiation of an M_1 ejection sound interval from an S_4–S_1 is described on page 273, and from a pacemaker click-M_1 on pages 278, 279.

   * b) About two-thirds of acute myocardial infarction patients have very widely split first sounds (more than 60 msec) in the first 3 days, especially if heart failure is present. The isovolumic contraction time may not be prolonged in the first few days of acute infarction because of an excess of catecholamines and sympathetic outflow.

2. Which valvular abnormalities are the usual causes of an aortic ejection sound (or click)?

    ANS.: a) A bicuspid aortic valve without stenosis. (Bicuspid valves may or may not become stenotic.)

    b) A stiff aortic valve, such as that occurring in AS or hypertension.

    Note: Hypertension may stretch the aortic root, causing the cusps to become taut and therefore to open with a sound.

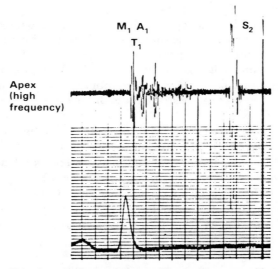

This phonocardiogram is from a 40-year-old woman with mild hypertension. The third component is probably an aortic ejection sound. This sounded simply like a widely split S_1, probably because the T_1 was too close to the M_1 to be audible.

3. What features suggest that the aortic ejection sound or click, as in AS, is due to an opening snap of the aortic valve and not merely to forceful ejection into the aorta?

    ANS.: a) It disappears with severe calcification of the aortic valve; conversely, the louder the sound, the more mobile the valve can be shown to be.

    b) It is not a feature of supravalvular AS or of obstruction below the valve (**hypertrophic subaortic stenosis** [HSS]) or discrete subvalvular stenosis [45].

*c) The ejection sound of AS occurs at the time of the anacrotic notch or onset of the anacrotic shoulder on the upstroke of the aortic pulse [29]. The onset of the anacrotic shoulder and the ejection sound have both been shown to be synchronous with the maximum open position of the stiff aortic leaflets.

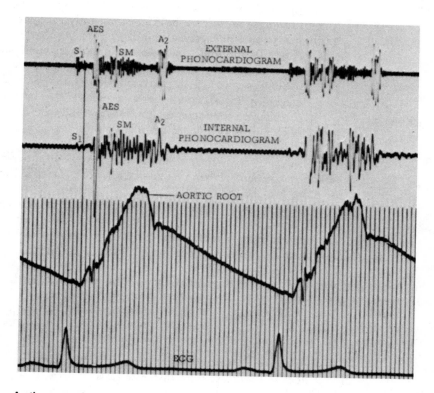

Aortic root tracing from a 23-year-old man with congenital AS taken with a catheter tip electromanometer (so that there are no tubing delays). The onset of the aortic ejection sound (AES) is coincident with the anacrotic notch, which occurs at the moment of peak doming of the stiff valve, in this case 38 msec from the onset of the aortic pressure rise. (From Whittaker, Shaver, Gray, and Leonard [79].)

*Note: In AS the flow, and therefore the murmur, begins after the stiff valve has reached the peak of its upward doming action, which occurs at the same time as both the ejection sound and the anacrotic notch. Therefore, the time between the onset of the aortic pressure rise and the anacrotic shoulder represents the time taken to raise the valve into its maximum domed position. This time has been found to be about 10 msec shorter when the valves are stiff than when the valves are mobile and explains why anacrotic shoulders are low in severe AS. The loudness of the ejection click is not correlated with the rate of rise of LV pressure but is correlated with both leaflet mobility and their distance of excursion.

4. Where is the aortic ejection sound best heard?

ANS.: The ejection sound is well heard wherever aortic events are best heard, i.e., anywhere in a straight line or "sash area" from the second right interspace to the apex. (See figure on page 296.) The ejection click of AS, however, is most often heard best at the apex because the AS murmur may be loud enough at the second left interspace and left sternal border to obscure the click.

5. Why is the aortic ejection sound of diagnostic help in the presence of AS?

ANS.: a) It helps to locate the site of the AS because only valvular AS characteristically has an audible ejection sound.

* *Note:* A small-amplitude phonocardiographic ejection sound may be present at any level of AS and is of no diagnostic help. In some patients with HSS an aortic ejection sound (as well as a dilated ascending aorta) is occasionally present [77]. This is not surprising considering the increased rate of flow into the aorta in early systole. This is also the cause of the ejection sounds heard in AR and thyrotoxicosis.

b) The absence of an ejection sound in valvular AS implies a calcified aortic valve. A calcified valve of that degree is highly correlated with a **gradient** of more than 50 mm Hg [23].

Note: The absence of an ejection sound warns you of two possibilities: either there is no valvular stenosis, or there is valvular stenosis with heavy calcification. The latter possibility can be ruled out by fluoroscopy or echocardiography. (Calcification is also likely if the A_2 is soft or absent.)

6. What features may suggest that an aortic ejection sound is due to a nonstenotic bicuspid aortic valve?

ANS.: a) If it is loud, especially if it is louder than the M_1, and is associated with a louder A_2 than normal.

b) If it is associated with AR, usually of only mild to moderate degree. (AR is commonly associated with a bicuspid aortic valve.)

c) If it does not increase with inspiration. (If it does, it is probably due to tricuspid closure.)

Note: A bicuspid aortic valve may calcify in patients over 50 years old and lead to aortic stenosis of any degree, or it may remain nonstenotic permanently [41A].

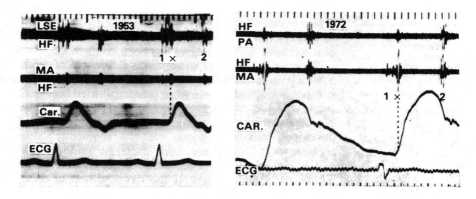

This patient was first seen in 1953 at age 28. The triple first sound is the M_1, T_1, and A_1. Note that twenty-five years later the late aortic ejection sound (labelled X) is still present and that it is louder than the M_1. No stenosis had developed by 1978. Note that aortic ejection sounds are simultaneous with the onset of the upstroke of an external carotid tracing.

THE PULMONARY EJECTION SOUND

The Ejection Sound in Pulmonary Stenosis

1. What is responsible for the ejection sound heard in valvular pulmonary stenosis (PS)? What proof can be offered?

   ANS.: It is an opening sound of the pulmonary valve. The evidence is as follows:

   a) The ejection sound is not present in pure infundibular stenosis.

   b) It is not present if the valve is severely dysplastic.

   c) It occurs at the peak of opening of the pulmonary valve on echophonocardiography.

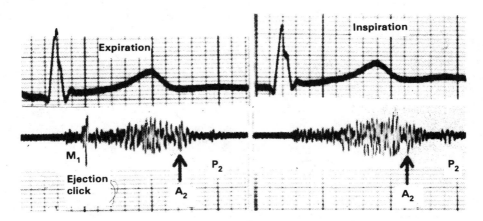

High-frequency tracing from the third left interspace of a patient with PS and a RV pressure of 100 mm Hg. The ejection click that disappears on inspiration shows that the site of obstruction is at the valve. The A_2–P_2 interval increases slightly from 100–120 msec (0.10–0.12 sec) on inspiration.

2. Why does the pulmonary ejection sound tend to disappear with inspiration in valvular PS?

ANS.: The sudden upward movement of a dome-shaped pulmonary valve produces the sound. If the valve is already in the domed or near-domed position when the RV contracts, there will be no sound or only a soft sound. On inspiration, the increased blood drawn into the right atrium causes it to contract more strongly. The stronger atrial contraction on inspiration at the end of diastole (the tricuspid valve is still open) raises the pressure in the RV just before the ventricle contracts. This rise in end-diastolic pressure in the RV may be higher than the pulmonary artery pressure. This is easy to understand if you realize that pulmonary artery diastolic pressure in PS may not be much more than 7 mm Hg, and RV end-diastolic pressure in PS can easily exceed 7 mm Hg. Thus, the pulmonary valve will be raised into the domed position at the end of diastole if the end-diastolic pressure in the RV rises to 8 mm Hg with a strong right atrial contraction.

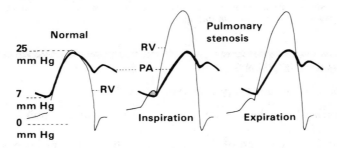

These RV and pulmonary artery pressure tracings show how inspiration can raise the end-diastolic RV pressure above pulmonary artery pressure because of a strong right atrial contraction plus a thick RV.

On expiration, the end-diastolic pressure in the RV falls, and the pulmonary valve is now in the *down* position at the beginning of RV systole. Ventricular contraction can now balloon the pulmonary valve upward into a dome, causing a click.

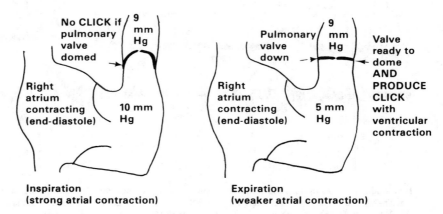

On the left is shown how right atrial contraction is assisted by inspiration in raising RV pressure higher than pulmonary artery pressure. This causes the pulmonary valve to dome up before the RV contracts. On the right is depicted the effect of a reduction in RV diastolic pressure caused by expiration, resulting in a downward position of the pulmonary valve when the RV begins to contract.

Note: Further proof that the pulmonary ejection sound in PS is a valvular sound and is due to the dome snapping upward is offered by the following facts:

    a) A click or sound can occur *before the QRS* at the end of diastole if the RV end-diastolic pressure is higher than the pulmonary artery diastolic pressure due to atrial systole. (It can even occur in early diastole at the peak of early rapid ventricular filling if the RV pressure exceeds pulmonary artery pressure at that time.)

    b) It occurs simultaneously with the anacrotic notch on the pulmonary artery pressure curve (as seen by intracardiac phonocardiography and simultaneous micromanometer pressure tracings), at which time the maximum upward position of the pulmonary cusp opening movement occurs, and the ejection murmur begins.

3. Why does the aortic ejection click not change significantly with respiration?

    ANS.: The end-diastolic pressure in the LV in AS, even when very high (the normal end-diastolic pressure is not much higher than 10 mm Hg), can never exceed the usual diastolic pressure in the aorta (which is rarely ever lower than 50 mm Hg). Therefore, expiration alone can never force the aortic valve into an upward domed position at the end of diastole.

*4. Why may the pulmonary ejection sound or click of PS show respiratory variation only in the sitting position?

    ANS.: If the PS is moderately severe, the supine pressure in the RV may be high enough at the end of diastole to keep the valve in the domed position even in expiration, and respiration will have no effect on the click. However, in the sitting position the decrease in venous return may cause a lower RV pressure at the end of diastole and may allow the pulmonary valve to fall to the downward position with expiration.

    Note: a) In very mild PS, there may be a pulmonary ejection click in both inspiration and expiration, with only a little attenuation on inspiration.

        b) If the pulmonary ejection sound is still present on inspiration, it may be seen to move closer to the M_1 with inspiration as long as the pulmonary valve is moved into even a slightly higher position with inspiration. It may even summate with the M_1 at the apex on inspiration, making the S_1 louder at this site (if the apex is occupied by the RV).

5. Where is the pulmonary ejection sound best heard?

    ANS.: Wherever pulmonary sounds and murmurs are best heard (i.e., anywhere along the left sternal border). The pulmonary ejection click may be heard well toward the mid-left thorax if the RV is enlarged.

*6. What does the presence of an ejection click tell you about the severity of PS?

    ANS.: An ejection click tends to occur more often in mild to moderate stenosis (i.e., with RV pressures of not over 70 mm Hg). Occasionally, however, it can be present with stenosis that is severe enough to produce an RV systolic pressure of 120 mm Hg [80]. (Normal RV systolic pressure is about 25 mm Hg.)

*7. Why is there a good correlation between ejection clicks and poststenotic dilatation beyond a valvular stenosis (i.e., dilatation of the pulmonary artery just beyond the valve)?

ANS.: Most patients with ejection clicks have systolic murmurs due to turbulent blood flow through the stenosed valve. The turbulence causing the murmur may disrupt the elastin structure of the artery just beyond the valve [5, 7]. One theory of poststenotic dilatation is based on the principle that turbulent blood flow increases the forces that tend to drag the lining of a vessel downstream. The distorted endothelial cells then initiate changes in the subjacent layers that can modify the lumen [60].

Low-frequency vibrations, even if inaudible, can cause dilatation of an artery, especially if the artery is young [5].

Note: a) The absence of poststenotic dilatation beyond a purely infundibular PS has not been explained. Perhaps the turbulence that produces the murmur here is dissipated before it can reach the pulmonary artery walls with enough force to destroy the molecular structure.

b) Poststenotic dilatation is so common in the presence of an ejection click that it was originally believed that all ejection clicks were caused by distention of the dilated segment.

*8. What is the likely cause of an ejection sound heard in patients with tetralogy of Fallot?

ANS.: If there is severe enough tetralogy (tetralogy that is almost pulmonary atresia, also known as pseudotruncus arteriosus), there is usually an aortic ejection sound that is due to the dilated and volume-overloaded aorta receiving the blood volume shunted from right to left by way of the ventricular septal defect (VSD). In mild (acyanotic) tetralogy it is probably a pulmonary ejection sound due to pulmonary valve stenosis [38].

Note: a) About one-third of patients with tetralogy have pure valvular stenosis. (Embryologically, this is not true tetralogy.) The others have either pure infundibular or mixed infundibular and valvular stenosis. If it is purely valvular and not severe (acyanotic type), there may be not only an ejection sound but also an audible pulmonary second sound (P_2). (The latter is unusual in cyanotic tetralogy because of low distending pressures and flow beyond the stenotic valve.)

b) The rare pulmonary ejection sound with mild tetralogy does not usually decrease with inspiration because the VSD does not allow the stronger right atrial contraction to increase the RV diastolic pressure—that is, the right atrium may contract very strongly with inspiration but instead of doming the pulmonary valve, its energy is dissipated through the VSD [38].

*9. Which early sounds or clicks are neither aortic nor pulmonary?

ANS.: a) A persistent truncus arteriosus quadracuspid valve almost always produces an ejection sound, often louder than any of the heart sounds, and is not influenced by respiration [75].

b) The nonejection click of the prolapsed valve syndrome (see p. 329) may come so early that it imitates an aortic or pulmonary ejection click. With these early prolapsed valve clicks, however, a systolic regurgitant murmur can nearly always be elicited [24].

c) Ventricular septal defects often close spontaneously by developing a membranous septal aneurysm (a windsock-like pouch with a small opening at the end). This aneurysm may produce an early systolic click as it is abruptly distended under high pressure from the LV [54].

Note: These VSD clicks are loudest on expiration, are usually localized to the left lower sternal border, and are not loud. They are usually present with the pansystolic crescendo murmur of the pinhole VSD. Since their Q to click intervals are in the range of 100–130 msec, these M_1-click intervals are much the same as those with pulmonary or aortic ejection clicks.

Ejection Sounds in Pulmonary Hypertension

1. Why is an ejection sound heard in pulmonary hypertension?

   ANS.: The pulmonary valve cusps are made stiff and taut by the stretching of the pulmonary valve ring—that is, the high pressure in the pulmonary artery may cause a dilated pulmonary artery root, which stretches the valve ring. The tautened cusps, opening at a very rapid rate, probably produce the sound or click. Simultaneous echophonocardiography has shown that the click occurs at the peak of opening of the pulmonary valve [42].

   Note: The pulmonary ejection click noted in bilateral pulmonary artery stenosis probably has an etiology similar to that heard in pulmonary hypertension [10].

2. How does an ejection sound heard in pulmonary hypertension differ from one heard in PS?

   ANS.: In pulmonary hypertension the ejection sound is
   a) Often heard better lower down on the chest.
   b) Rarely changed by respiration.

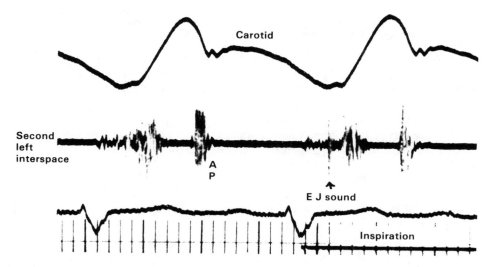

This high-frequency phonocardiogram and simultaneous carotid tracing is from a patient with severe pulmonary hypertension secondary to a VSD *(Eisenmenger syndrome)*. Note that the pulmonary ejection sound does not diminish with inspiration.

*Note: a) Primary pulmonary hypertension often produces a vibratory S_1, which is thought to be due to a loud T_1 [72].

b) The ejection sound of pulmonary hypertension is often followed by a short murmur that ends in midsystole. The end of the murmur coincides with the end of the semiclosure movement of the pulmonary valve seen on an echocardiogram [63].

c) Both the $Q–P_1$ interval and the $M_1–P_1$ interval become longer in pulmonary hypertension because isovolumic contraction is prolonged as the RV takes longer to reach a high pulmonary diastolic pressure. The intervals are usually more than 140 msec.

---

*The Q to Pulmonary Ejection Click ($Q–P_1$) Interval

*1. What happens to RV isovolumic contraction time and the $Q–P_1$ interval with increasing PS? Why?

ANS.: They become shorter because as PS becomes more and more severe,

a) The rate of RV pressure rise becomes faster [21].

b) The pulmonary diastolic pressure becomes lower.

Note: a) The $Q–P_1$ interval in mild PS (RV pressure not higher than 60 mm Hg) is about 110 msec or more. The $Q–P_1$ interval in severe PS (RV pressure 120 mm Hg or more) is about 60 to 100 msec. This refers to the rate-corrected $Q–P_1$ (i.e., the interval must be corrected to a heart rate of 60 by dividing by the square root of the R–R interval [17].

b) If the stenosis is severe, the ejection sound may merge with the M_1. A clue to its presence, however, may be detected by a respiratory variation in S_1 loudness [21].

c) The earliness of an aortic ejection click does not correlate with the degree of AS.

Ejection Sounds in Idiopathic Dilatation of the Pulmonary Artery

1. How can you explain the ejection sound in idiopathic dilatation of the pulmonary artery if high pressure in the artery is not present to tighten the valve ring, and the pulmonary valve is not stenosed and therefore unable to produce an opening snap?

ANS.: Idiopathic dilatation of the pulmonary artery implies an abnormal artery with marked loss of elasticity. A jerky expansion of this lax pulmonary artery may cause a sound or a click.

*Note: a) Sudden expansion of a dilated pulmonary artery was the only reasonable explanation for the ejection click heard in a patient with an absent pulmonary valve and dilated pulmonary artery in whom intracardiac phonocardiograms showed that the ejection murmur preceded the click by 50 msec [1].

b) The ejection sounds of idiopathic dilatation of the pulmonary artery tend to be far from the M_1, suggesting that a distal event, such as dilatation of a lax pulmonary artery, may be the cause of the click.

c) Simultaneous pulse tracings and intracardiac phonocardiograms show that the ejection sound heard in idiopathic dilatation occurs slightly later than the onset of rise of pulmonary artery pressure [2].

2. What lesion produces rapid ejection into a dilated pulmonary artery without an ejection sound or click?

ANS.: An **atrial septal defect** (ASD) produces rapid flow through the pulmonary artery, but there is often no audible ejection sound unless pulmonary hypertension is present or the pulmonary artery is markedly dilated. If the dilatation is due only to extra volume and there is no destruction of the pulmonary artery tissue to reduce its elasticity, there is apparently no mechanism to produce the ejection sound.

*Note: a) With most ASDs, a split first sound is recorded on the phonocardiogram with the second component at the time compatible with a pulmonary ejection sound. The second component is louder than the first component of the split S_1 at the apex, which is usually usurped by the RV in patients with ASDs, and this reversal of normal loudness of the S_1 components has been proposed as a helpful clue to the presence of an ASD [34]. Although it has been timed on echocardiograms with closure of the tricuspid valve (T_1), it is still possible that it is sometimes a pulmonary ejection sound (P_1). (The T_1/M_1 loudness ratio has not correlated well with either the degree of pulmonary hypertension or the pulmonary-systemic flow ratio.)

b) In the rare patients who have an ASD plus pulmonary hypertension, there is a good correlation between the $Q–P_1$ or $M_1–P_1$ interval and the degree of pulmonary hypertension. If the $Q–P_1$ is more than 140 msec or the $M_1–P_1$ more than 60 msec, the pulmonary artery systolic pressure is probably more than 80 mm Hg.

THE LOUDNESS OF THE M_1

1. What factors besides chest wall shape or thickness control the loudness of the M_1?

ANS.: a) The rate of rise of ventricular pressure. The faster the rise at the time that the LV pressure exceeds left atrial pressure, the louder the M_1 [19].

b) The duration of LV contraction before it exceeds left atrial pressure. Because the LV accelerates in the early phase of its contraction, the longer the LV must contract before it can close the mitral valve, the louder the M_1 [66].

c) The pressure in the left atrium at the moment that LV pressure exceeds it to close the valve. This is synonymous with the degree of opening of the mitral valve when the LV begins to contract because the higher the left atrial pressure in relation to LV pressure at the onset of LV contraction, the wider will the mitral valve be open.

d) The stiffness of the mitral valve bellies. An immobile valve can produce little sound.

e) The distance of the heart from the chest wall. With large pericardial effusions the heart is suspended by the great vessels and swings in a pendular arc whose period is twice the heart rate. Therefore, the heart is closer to the stethoscope during every other cycle and produces an auscultatory (as well as electrical) alternans of the loudness of S_1 [11A].

Ventricular Pressure Rise and M_1 Loudness

1. What is the physiologist's way of expressing the rate of rise of pressure?
   ANS.: Delta P/delta t = change of pressure/change of time. This is usually shortened to dP/dt.
2. What is the relationship between the dP/dt of the LV and M_1 loudness?
   ANS.: The greater the dP/dt (i.e., the faster the rate of LV pressure rise), the louder the M_1 [62].
3. What can cause an increased dP/dt of the LV and therefore make the M_1 louder?
   ANS.: Increased contractility due either to the Starling effect of a large volume or to positive inotropic agents such as catecholamines, sympathetic stimulation, digitalis, or thyroxine. Sympathetic stimulation is probably the cause of the loud M_1 in sinus tachycardia and in exercise [22].
4. What can decrease the dP/dt of the LV and therefore make the M_1 softer?
   ANS.: a) Drugs such as beta blockers that decrease contractility [22].
   b) Any myocardial damage such as that due to myocardial infarction or chronic cardiomyopathy.
   Note: a) These soft first sounds are often described as muffled because they have lost most of their high frequencies [59].
   * b) For some unknown reason, the M_1 was in one study more likely to be softer in posterior than in anterior myocardial infarction [57].
   c) The M_1 is said to be soft in acute myocardial infarction because the acutely infarcted area tends to balloon outward paradoxically with systole so that part of the energy developed by the LV is absorbed. This argument is weakened by the finding that in most patients with ventricular **aneurysms** the S_1 is no softer than it is in patients with a previous infarction and no aneurysm [40]. Also, in some patients with anteroseptal aneurysms the S_1 may actually be loud. This has been explained by the fact that a sudden tensing of the tissue of a ventricular aneurysm (suspended between two rubber stoppers in a tank of water) can produce as loud a sound as tensing of mitral valve leaflets, especially in the low-frequency range [14].
   * d) In acute myocardial infarction the softness of the S_1 correlates with a prolonged preejection period by systolic time intervals. As patients recover from the infarction, the S_1 becomes louder and the preejection period becomes shorter [70].
   e) An increased cardiac muscle mass such as that seen in athletes also tends to make low frequencies dominant in the S_1 [59].

The P–R Interval and M_1 Loudness

1. Why does a short P–R interval cause a loud M_1?
   ANS.: The P controls the timing of atrial contraction, which raises left atrial (LA) pressure. The force of the contraction opens the mitral valve further at the end of diastole. The R controls the timing of ventricular contraction. If the P–R interval is short, ventricular contraction occurs so quickly after the atri-

um has contracted that the LA has not had time to relax (short X descent). Therefore, atrial pressure is still at a high level when the pressure in the LV exceeds it, closing the mitral valve [66]. This means that the ventricle has a long time to contract before it can overcome LA pressure. Therefore, the LV has had time to accelerate to a rapid dP/dt part of its pressure curve by the time it closes the mitral valve. (See the following figure for Question 2.)

2. Why does a long P–R interval cause a soft M_1?

ANS.: The delayed LV contraction gives the LA pressure a chance to drop to low levels (deep X descent) by the time the LV begins to contract. Thus, LV pressure will exceed LA pressure at the very early and slow part of its acceleration curve [66].

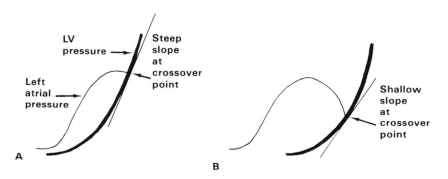

(A) If the P-R interval is short, the LV contracts before the left atrium has had a chance to relax and drop its pressure. Therefore, the LV pressure will not exceed left atrial pressure until it has contracted for a long enough time to accelerate to a stage of rapid pressure rise by the time the mitral leaflets are closed. This produces an abrupt deceleration of forward flow and a loud sound. (B) If the P-R interval is long, the LV contracts later than at A, so that the left atrium has had time to drop to a low pressure when the LV pressure exceeds it. The pressure cross-over point is on the slow part of the LV acceleration curve, and the valves are closed at a relatively slow rate, producing a soft sound.

Note: a) If the above thesis is true, then the shorter the P–R interval, the longer it should take for the LV contraction to close the mitral valve and therefore, the longer will be the Q-mitral closure interval. The truth of this thesis is illustrated in the following figure.

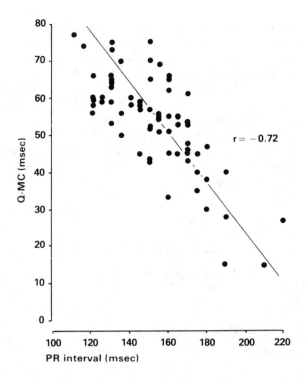

This shows the relation between Q-mitral valve closure on echocardiography (Q-MC) and the P-R interval. The longer the P-R, the shorter the Q-MC.

b) It has usually been taught that the reason for the loud M_1 with a short P–R is that the mitral leaflets are wide open at the time of the LV contraction onset—that is, atrial relaxation, which is known to be able to close mitral valves by a kind of suction effect, has not had much time to act [32]. The analogy of a wide-open door making more noise when it closes than does a slightly open door is not valid unless the door is made to accelerate as it closes. It should be noted that the degree of valve opening and LA pressure at the onset of LV contraction are direct variables; therefore, to say that the LV has more time to accelerate when the valve is wider open at the onset of ventricular contraction is the same as saying that LA pressure is highest at the onset of LV contraction and there will be more time for the ventricle to accelerate by the time it reaches LA pressure.

In one study the S_1 showed little correlation with the degree to which the valve is open when the LV begins to contract [66]. This is true because the time needed for a valve to move from fully open to closed is so rapid that there is not enough time for a significant amount of LV acceleration to occur. If, however, the mitral valves are closed or nearly closed when the LV begins to contract, then no matter what the LV dP/dt is at the time of closure, the M_1 sound will be soft or absent.

c) Echocardiograms show that at the end of diastole the mitral valve undergoes an immediate semiclosure movement after atrial contraction causes it to reach peak opening. Thus, the beginning of mitral valve closure may be said to be atriogenic. When P–R intervals are very long (0.2 to 0.5 sec), as in complete AV block, it has been noted that the AV valves are actually brought into apposition entirely by atrial systole, and ventricular contraction may not be followed by the high-frequency components of the S_1 [32]. The soft S_1 occurs because the ventricular pressure rise simply stretches the closed valve to its elastic limits. With a P–R of more than 0.5 sec, the AV valves reopen again during diastole after closure by atrial systole, probably due to the rising LA pressure caused by continued inflow of blood from the pulmonary circuit into the LA. This explains the secondary accentuation of the S_1 that occurs with very long P–R intervals [8].

d) The paradox of a short P–R interval and a normal or soft M_1 is seen in the Wolff-Parkinson-White (W-P-W) syndrome, type B, in which pre-excitation activates the RV first, but conduction over the His bundle reaches the LV at a normal interval as if the P–R interval were normal.

e) The paradox of a long P–R interval and a loud S_1 is seen in mitral stenosis (MS) and also in Ebstein's anomaly. In the latter, the M_1 may actually be very soft, but the second component of the S_1 may be loud, short, and clicking because it is caused by closure of a large deformed anterior leaflet of the tricuspid valve. Because this leaflet has been likened to a large sail flapping in the breeze, this loud T_1 has been called a sail sound [15]. It may come either soon after the M_1 or so late that it occurs near midsystole. It is presumably late because of the very slow initial rise in RV pressure that occurs in Ebstein's anomaly. The sail sound has been shown to occur at the transition between the slow and the rapid rise in RV pressure. It often increases with inspiration and is usually associated with a very late tricuspid opening snap.

f) In sudden, severe aortic regurgitation the mitral valve may be closed in mid-diastole and is associated with a soft or inaudible S_1 [41, 46].

3. Which situations can be diagnosed by hearing the effect of a changing P–R interval on the M_1?

ANS.: Any **atrioventricular (AV) dissociation,** as in complete AV block or some ventricular tachycardias. (If the ventricular tachycardia has retrograde VA conduction into the atria, there will be no AV dissociation.)

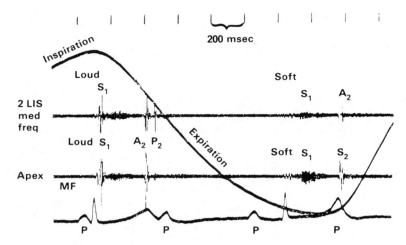

This medium-frequency (MF) phonocardiogram is from a patient with complete AV block, i.e., the P waves and QRS complexes are independent, thus causing the P-R intervals to vary. Note the loud S_1 after the short P-R (first one) and the soft one after the long P-R both at the apex and second left interspace (2 LIS).

*Note: a) Type 1 second degree AV block (Wenckeback periods) also has gradually longer P–R intervals until complete AV block occurs and a beat is dropped. The gradually longer P–R interval has been said to cause a softer and softer first sound until a pause occurs. However, if the longest P–R is very long (e.g., about 360 msec), the valves may reopen owing to continued pulmonary venous return, and so produce a slight increase in loudness. Usually, though, the P–R changes are so small (from 120–140 msec) that no perceptible M_1 changes may occur.

b) The first heart sound will not change despite complete AV block if there are no P waves (e.g., if the atria are fibrillating or fluttering).

c) There is no correlation between the ejection fraction or the duration of isovolumic contraction and M_1 loudness in AV dissociation. The maximum ejection fraction occurs at a P–R interval of 180–200 msec, but at 200 msec the M_1 may disappear altogether [8]. As the P–R becomes either longer or shorter than this range, the ejection fraction decreases [4]. This suggests that the intensity of the S_1 cannot be taken as an indicator of ventricular function.

The S_1 Loudness in Arrhythmias and in Bundle Branch Blocks

*1. In atrial fibrillation, how will the different lengths of diastole and the absence of atrial contraction control the loudness of the M_1 if the mitral valve is normal?

ANS.: Because there is no atrial contraction there is also no atrial expansion to draw the mitral leaflets up into a closed position before ventricular contraction occurs. Only changes in LV contractility can affect the loudness of the M_1. A series of short cycles can cause an increase in contractility due to a **postextrasystolic potentiation** effect and will produce a loud M_1. A short diastole, on the other hand, will modify the loudness by causing a decrease in LV stretch and a decrease in the Starling effect. A series of short diastoles followed by a long diastole should, therefore, produce a loud M_1 (postextrasystolic potentiation plus Starling effect [16]).

Note: a) Although the preceding R–R interval controls contractility and therefore the loudness of the S_1, it has been shown that the pre-preceding (penultimate) R–R interval controls it also, by a postextrasystolic potentiation effect, i.e., the shorter the cycle length before the preceding R–R interval, the greater the contractility and S_1 loudness. This is the major reason why at the bedside it is difficult to relate the observed intensity of the S_1 to cycle length.

b) In atrial fibrillation the loudest M_1 occurs when the M_1 coincides with or occurs just after an S_3 [61]. This suggests that when a ventricle contracts just after it has been expanding rapidly, it either accelerates more rapidly or takes longer than usual to reverse the forward flow, so there is more time for acceleration by the time the mitral valve is closed.

*2. How can S_1 loudness during normal heart rates suggest the cause of paroxysmal tachycardias?

ANS.: If the S_1 is very loud, it suggests a short P–R interval, a normal QRS type of preexcitation, and therefore a Lown-Ganong-Levine syndrome with episodes of atrial tachycardia.

*3. How does LBBB affect the loudness of the M_1?

ANS.: It tends to cause a soft M_1 because

a) The dP/dt of early contraction is often decreased in LBBB [12], probably because initial conduction is almost entirely septal, and therefore the main LV mass may not participate in preisovolumic contraction (i.e., in pre-M_1 contraction [8]).

b) The onset of left ventricular contraction may be delayed so that the effect is the same as that of a long P–R interval.

The M_1 Loudness in Valvular Heart Disease

1. Why does the M_1 in severe AS tend to be soft?

ANS.: When the systolic gradient exceeds 50 mm Hg, LV contractility has been shown to decrease, especially in patients over age 40 [67].

2. How does a forward gradient across the mitral valve at the end of diastole affect the loudness of the M_1? Why?

ANS.: It makes the M_1 loud because the gradient at the end of diastole requires the ventricle to reach a higher pressure before it can close the valve. The LV therefore has more time to accelerate before it closes the valve.

3. How does a stiff mitral valve, as in mitral stenosis, affect the duration and pitch of the M_1? Why?

ANS.: It makes the M_1 short and snapping. The resistance of the fibrotic and tethered edges to movement may cause the still flexible bodies or bellies of the leaflets to billow upward with a sudden motion like that of a snapping sail.

Note: a) The posterior leaflet usually has relatively little "belly" to billow unless it has redundant tissue, as in the prolapsed mitral valve syndrome (see p. 329). Therefore, the anterior leaflet is mainly responsible for this snapping effect of the M_1.

*b) As porcine mitral valves become fibrosed, the high frequencies become dominant [69].

4. What is the short, snapping M_1 of MS often called?

ANS.: The closing snap.

> *Note:* a) The apical impulse in MS has often been characterized as "tapping." Since this term also describes a palpable first sound, it should not be used to describe a movement or impulse.
>
> *b) The normal M_1 is simultaneous with a notch on the upstroke of the apex cardiogram, but in MS the major loud, snapping sound occurs later than the notch, which is deeper than normal and simultaneous with a soft component of the S_1 [52]. This suggests that the major loud component of the M_1 in MS is indeed a "closing snap." The softer, earlier component may be a T_1.
>
> A left atrial myxoma may also have a deeper notch than normal on the upstroke of the apex cardiogram coincident with the M_1, and this lesion often mimics MS on auscultation.

5. When will a stiff mitral valve produce no unusually loud, snapping M_1?

ANS.: When the belly of the anterior leaflet is very stiff and immobile due to either calcium or fibrosis.

*6. In MS, how does the M_1 loudness vary if atrial fibrillation is present?

ANS.: At least three types of M_1 loudness are seen:

> *Type 1:* If the MS is mild, there is softening with short diastoles that is the same as that heard with a normal valve. However, there is less tendency for the M_1 to become louder after long diastoles.
>
> *Type 2:* If the valves are severely stenosed and calcified (i.e., no opening snap is present), the M_1 depends entirely on end-diastolic volume and on the preceding and pre-preceding R–R intervals (Starling and postextrasystolic potentiation effect). Thus, the S_1 becomes louder in proportion to the length of the previous diastole and inversely to the length of the R–R preceding the previous diastole.
>
> *Type 3:* If the valves are moderately stenosed, the S_1 loudness varies inversely with the duration of the previous diastole—i.e., the shorter the previous R–R interval, the louder the M_1 because of dependence on the end-diastolic left atrial to LV gradient [58].

*THE M_1 IN MITRAL REGURGITATION

1. How does the duration of the forward diastolic gradient across a mitral valve due to torrential flow across the mitral valve (as in mitral regurgitation [MR]) differ from that of MS?

ANS.: The torrential flow may cause a gradient only in early and mid-diastole, whereas a stenotic valve, even with less-than-normal flow, causes a gradient across the mitral valve throughout all of diastole. (See page 366 for illustration of mitral valve gradient.)

*2. What should happen to the rate of rise of ventricular pressure before the mitral valve closes (the preisovolumic contraction period) if a ventricular leak such as a VSD or MR is present? How should this affect the loudness of the M_1?

ANS.: The rate of pressure rise and therefore the loudness of the M_1 should be decreased [71]. In actual fact, however, only about half the patients with pure MR have a soft M_1 because the extradiastolic stretch of the volume overload compensates for the leak and allows a rate of rise of pressure that is even faster than normal [20]. Therefore, if the LV is not damaged, the M_1 may even be loud.

Note: The finding that about 70 percent of patients with papillary muscle dysfunction murmurs have a loud S_1 may mean that because these murmurs often crescendo to the S_1, there may be only trivial regurgitation at the onset of the LV contraction.

*3. In what type of MR will there be almost no forward flow across the mitral valve during the last part of diastole?

ANS.: In sudden, severe MR, such as occurs with ruptured chordae, the LV resists the sudden increase in volume load [41], probably because of the inability of the pericardium to stretch adequately in response to a sudden volume overload. The LV diastolic pressure may rise rapidly enough to exceed momentarily the left atrial pressure by mid- or late diastole, and the mitral valves may close. This will make the M_1 soft or inaudible.

Note: It seems improbable that a measurable reversed gradient could occur across the mitral valve in diastole for more than a moment if the ventricular pressure rise is due entirely to flow from the left atrium, because as soon as the pressure rises high enough in the LV to close the mitral valve, the forward flow and LV pressure rise ceases. However, a slight momentary reversed gradient probably can occur.

Sudden, severe AR, however, such as occurs when a sinus of Valsalva ruptures, can easily cause a reversed gradient between the LV and the left atrium, eliminating the M_1.

*THE Q–1 INTERVAL

*1. What is meant by the Q–1 interval?

ANS.: The Q–1 interval is the time from the onset of the QRS complex to the M_1, i.e., the Q–M_1 interval. (The upper limit of normal is 70 msec.)

*2. What important factors prolong the Q–1 interval?

ANS.: Left bundle branch block, hypertension, a poorly functioning myocardium, a high atrial pressure (as in MS and MR), or a shunt flow through a VSD or a persistent ductus arteriosus [26].

Note: a) There is a close correlation between the prolongation of the Q–1 interval and the size of the left-to-right shunt through a VSD [26].

b) There is a poor correlation between the Q–1 interval and the severity of MS, although almost all subjects with significant MS have a Q–1 beyond the upper limit of normal, and successful mitral surgery will shorten the Q–1 interval [27, 31].

       c) Valvular AS prolongs the Q–1 slightly, but HSS prolongs it markedly to about 70 msec or more, possibly because the unusual LVH delays spread of septal activation [25].

*3. How does the Q–1 vary with various diastolic lengths in atrial fibrillation in (a) MS and (b) normal subjects?

    ANS.: a) In MS, the shorter the previous diastole, the higher the left atrial pressure and the longer the Q–1.

        b) In normal subjects the Q–1 intervals change very little with varying diastoles.

    Note: a) In patients with MS and atrial fibrillation we can judge the severity of the LA–LV gradient at the end of diastole by the length of diastole needed to equalize the end-diastolic gradient. The end-diastolic pressure will equalize in about 700 msec with mild MS, and in about 1 sec with severe MS. Therefore, if the Q–1 requires at least 1-sec cycles to stabilize, the disease is probably severe [73].

        b) How the Q–1 is used in combination with the opening snap to judge the severity of MS is discussed on page 241 [71].

        c) The C–1 interval probably correlates better than the Q–1 with the severity of MS. (See the following section.)

*THE C–M₁ (C–1) INTERVAL

*1. What is meant by the C–1 interval?

    ANS.: It is the interval between the onset of ventricular contraction on the apex cardiogram and the mitral closure sound. This is the preisovolumic contraction period.

    Note: a) Some factors that control the C–1 interval besides inotropism are:

        1) The heart rate. The faster the rate, the shorter the C–1.

        2) The stiffness or resistance of the mitral valve. A stiff valve produces a longer C–1

        3) The height of the left atrial pressure.

        b) You can use the C–1 interval to help in diagnosing the presence or absence of MS because if the C–1 interval is less than 30 msec, MS is very unlikely. If, on the other hand, the C–1 interval is more than 50 msec, MS is very likely [40].

*2. How can the C–1 interval be used to estimate the mean LA pressure in MS?

    ANS.: The greater the MS, the longer the LV must contract before it can close the mitral valve. Isovolumic contraction time (i.e., the time between the M_1 and the opening of the aortic valve [roughly the E point on the apex cardiogram]) is unchanged by MS or by MR plus MS as long as the MS is predominant [49]. When C–E is relatively constant, the ratio of

$$\frac{C{-}1}{C{-}E}$$

correlates with the degree of MS with an r of approximately 0.85 [9].

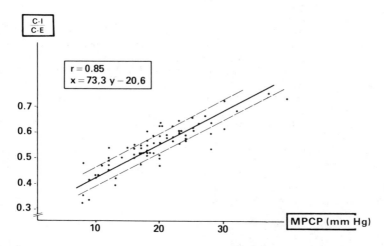

The longer the C-1 is relative to the C-E, the higher the mean pulmonary capillary pressure (MPCP) and the more severe the mitral stenosis. (From Comhaire and Uyttenhove [9].)

REFERENCES

1. Ahuja, S. P., and Coles, J. C. Further observations on the genesis of early systolic clicks. *Am. J. Cardiol.* 17:291, 1966.
2. Armstrong, T. G., and Gotsman, M. S. Initial low frequency vibrations of the first heart sound. *Br. Heart J.* 35:691, 1973.
3. Aronow, W. S. Isovolumic contraction and left ventricular ejection times. *Am. J. Cardiol.* 26:238, 1970.
4. Bashour, T. T., Naughton, J. P., and Cheng, T. O. Systolic time intervals in patients with artificial pacemakers. *Am. J. Cardiol.* 32:287, 1973.
5. Boughner, D. R., and Roach, M. R. Effect of low frequency vibration on the arterial wall. *Circ. Res.* 29:136, 1971.
6. Brockman, S. K. Dynamic function of atrial contraction in regulation of cardiac performance. *Am. J. Physiol.* 204:597, 1963.
7. Bruns, D. L., et al. Experimental observations on poststenotic dilatation. *J. Thorac. Cardiovasc. Surg.* 38:662, 1959.
8. Burggraf, G. W., and Craige, E. The first heart sound in complete heart block: Phonoechocardiographic correlations. *Circulation* 50:17, 1974.
9. Cheng, T. O. Early systolic ejection click associated with supravalvular pulmonary stenosis. *Am. J. Cardiol.* 18:2, 1966.
10. Cheng, T. S. Some new observations on the syndrome of papillary muscle dysfunction. *Am. J. Med.* 47:924, 1969.
11. Comhaire, E., and Uyttenhove, P. Evaluation of mitral stenosis. *Am. Heart J.* 81:443, 1971.
11A. Costeas, F. X., et al. Acoustic, mechanical and electrical alternans in hemopericardium of occult leukemic origin. *Chest* 60:460, 1971.
12. D'Cunha, G. F., Friedberg, H. D., and Jaume, F. The first heart sound in intermittent left bundle branch block. *Am. J. Cardiol.* 27:447, 1971.
13. DiBartolo, G., Nunez-Dey, D., and Bendezu-Prieto, J. Left heart studies in mitral stenosis with special reference to intracardiac phonocardiography. *Am. J. Cardiol.* 10:93, 1962.
14. Dock, W. The genesis of diastolic heart sounds. *Am. J. Med.* 50:178, 1971.
15. Fontana, M. E., and Wooley, C. F. Sail sound in Ebstein's anomaly of the tricuspid valve. *Circulation* 46:155, 1972.
16. Frank, M. N., and Kinlaw, W. B. Indirect measurement of isovolumic contraction time and tension period in normal subjects. *Am. J. Cardiol.* 10:800, 1962.

17. Gamboa, R., Hugenholtz, P. G., and Nadas, A. S. Accuracy of the phonocardiogram in assessing severity of aortic and pulmonic stenosis. *Circulation* 30:35, 1964.

18. Gibson, D. G., Broder, G., and Sowton, E. Effect of varying pulse interval in atrial fibrillation on left ventricular function in man. *Br. Heart J.* 33:388, 1971.

19. Gould, L., Belletti, D., and Lyon, A. F. The genesis of the first heart sound with varying P–R intervals. *Dis. Chest* 52:817, 1967.

20. Gould, L., and Shariff, M. Comparisons of the left ventricular, aortic, and brachial arterial first derivative. *Vasc. Surg.* 3:34, 1969.

21. Hultgren, H. N., et al. The ejection click of valvular pulmonic stenosis. *Circulation* 40:631, 1969.

22. Hume, L., and Reuben, S. R. The effects of exercise on the amplitude of the first heart sound in normal subjects. *Am. Heart J.* 95:4, 1978.

23. Hunt, D., et al. Quantitative evaluation of cineaortography in the assessment of aortic regurgitation. *Am. J. Cardiol.* 31:696, 1973.

24. Hutter, A. M., Jr., et al. Early systolic clicks due to mitral valve prolapse. *Circulation* 44:516, 1971.

25. Ibrahim, M., et al. Systolic time intervals in valvular aortic stenosis and idiopathic hypertrophic subaortic stenosis. *Br. Heart J.* 35:276, 1973.

26. Karnegis, J. N., and Wang, Y. The Q–1 interval of the phonocardiogram. *Am. J. Cardiol.* 11:452, 1963.

27. Kelly, J. J., Jr. Diagnostic value of phonocardiography in mitral stenosis: Mode of production of first heart sound. *Am. J. Med.* 19:862, 1955.

28. Lakier, J. B., et al. Tricuspid component of first heart sound. *Br. Heart J.* 35:1275, 1963.

29. Laniado, S., et al. Temporal relation of the first heart sound to closure of the mitral valve. *Circulation* 47:1006, 1973.

30. Leatham, A. Heart murmurs, mechanism, intensity, and pitch. *Lancet* 2:757, 1958. (Classic article.)

31. Lee, Y., Scherlis, L., and Singleton, R. T. Mitral stenosis, hemodynamic, electrocardiographic and vectorcardiographic studies. *Am. Heart J.* 69:559, 1965.

32. Leech, G., et al. Mechanism of influence of PR interval on loudness of first heart sound. *Br. Heart J.* 43:138, 1980.

33. Leech, G., Mills, P., and Leatham, A. The diagnosis of a non-stenotic bicuspid aortic valve. *Br. Heart J.* 40:941, 1978.

34. Lopez, J. F., Linn, H., and Shaffer, A. B. The apical first heart sound as an aid in the diagnosis of atrial septal defect. *Circulation* 26:1296, 1962.

35. Luisada, A. A., et al. Normal first heart sounds with nonfunctional tricuspid valve of right ventricle. *Circulation* 35:119, 1967.

36. Luisada, A. A., and MacCanon, D. M. Functional basis of heart sounds. *Am. J. Cardiol.* 16:631, 1965.

37. Luisada, A. A., and MacCanon, D. M. The physiologic basis of the heart sounds. *Dis. Chest* 49:258, 1966.

38. Martin, C. E., et al. Genesis, frequency, and diagnostic significance of ejection sound in adults with tetralogy of Fallot. *Br. Heart J.* 35:402, 1973.

39. Martin, C. E., et al. Ejection sounds of right-sided origin. *Am. Heart Assoc. Monograph* 46, 1975.

40. McGinn, F. X., Gould, L., and Lyon, A. F. The phonocardiogram and apexcardiogram in patients with ventricular aneurysm. *Am. J. Cardiol.* 21:467, 1968.

41. Meadows, W. R., et al. Premature mitral valve closure. *Circulation* 28:251, 1963.

41A. Mills, P., et al. The natural history of a non-stenotic bicuspid aortic valve. *Br. Heart J.* 40:951, 1978.

42. Mills, P. G., et al. Echocardiographic and hemodynamic relationships of ejection sounds. *Circulation* 56:430, 1977.

43. Mills, P. G., et al. Echophonocardiographic studies of the contribution of the atrioventricular valves to the first heart sound. *Circulation* 54:944, 1976.

44. Morgan, M. T., and Criley, J. M. Mitral valve closure and first heart sound. *Am. J. Cardiol.* 34:878, 1974.

45. Oakley, C. M., and Hallidie-Smith, K. A. Assessment of site and severity in congenital aortic stenosis. *Br. Heart J.* 29:367, 1967.

46. Oliver, G. C., Jr., Gazetopoulos, N., and Deuchar, D. C. Reversed mitral diastolic gradient in aortic incompetence, *Br. Heart J.* 29:239, 1967.

47. Oravetz, J., et al. Dynamic analysis of heart sounds in right and left bundle branch blocks. *Circulation* 36:275, 1967.

48. Oreshkov, V. I. Q–1 or C–1 interval in the diagnosis of mitral stenosis. *Br. Heart J.* 29:778, 1967.

49. Oreshkov, V. I. Isovolumic contraction time and isovolumic contraction time index in mitral stenosis. *Br. Heart J.* 34:553, 1972.

50. O'Toole, J. D., et al. The contribution of tricuspid valve closure to the first heart sound: An intracardiac micromanometer study. *Circulation* 53:752, 1976.

51. Parisi, A. F., and Milton, B. G. Relation of mitral valve closure to the first heart sound in man. *Am. J. Cardiol.* 32:779, 1973.

52. Perosio, A. M. A., Silva, M. A. C., and Ricci, G. J. The first heart sound: Its relation with the apex cardiogram. *Am. J. Cardiol.* 32:283, 1973.

53. Piemme, T. E., Barnett, G. O., and Dexter, L. Relationship of heart sounds to acceleration of blood flow. *Circ. Res.* 18:303, 1966.

54. Pieroni, D. R., et al. Auscultatory recognition of aneurysm of the membranous ventricular septum associated with small ventricular septal defect. *Circulation* 44:733, 1971.

55. Plass, R., Schmidt, K. H., and Guenther, K. H. Intracardiac sounds and murmurs in atrial septal defect. *Am. J. Cardiol.* 28:173, 1971.

56. Prakash, R. Genesis of heart sounds. *J.A.M.A.* 240:2732, 1978.

57. Price, W. H., and Brown, A. E. Alterations in intensity of heart sounds after myocardial infarction. *Br. Heart J.* 30:835, 1968.

58. Ravin, A., and Bershoff, E. The intensity of the first heart sound in auricular fibrillation with mitral stenosis. *Am. Heart J.* 41:539, 1951.

59. Renner, W. F., and Renner, G. W. The quality of resonance of the first heart sound after myocardial infarction: Clinical significance. *Circulation* 59:1144, 1979.

60. Rodbard, S., Ikeda, K., and Montes, M. An analysis of mechanisms of post-stenotic dilatation. *Angiology* 18:349, 1967.

61. Rytand, D. A. The variable loudness of the first heart sound in auricular fibrillation. *Am. Heart J.* 37:187, 1949.

62. Sakamoto, T., et al. Hemodynamic determinants of the amplitude of the first heart sound. *Circ. Res.* 16:45–57, 1965.

63. Sakamoto, T., et al. Echocardiogram and phonocardiogram related to the movement of the pulmonary valve. *Jap. Heart J.* 16:107, 1975.

64. Sanchez, J., et al. Diagnostic value of the first heart sound in children with atrial septal defect. *Am. Heart J.* 78:467, 1969.

65. Segall, H. N., and Sharp, A. Heart sounds in bundle branch block. *Jap. Heart J.* 8:468, 1967.

66. Shah, P. M., Kramer, D. H., and Gramiak, R. Influence of the timing of atrial systole on mitral valve closure and on the first heart sound in man. *Am. J. Cardiol.* 26:231, 1970.

67. Simon, H., et al. The contractile state of the hypertrophied left ventricular myocardium in aortic stenosis. *Am. Heart J.* 79:587, 1970.

68. Stein, P. D., and Sabbah, H. N. Origin of the second heart sound: Clinical relevance of new observations. *Am. J. Cardiol.* 41:108, 1978.

69. Stein, P. D., et al. Frequency of the first heart sound in the assessment of stiffening of mitral bioprosthetic valves. *Circulation* 63:200, 1981.

70. Stein, P. D., Sabbah, H. N., and Barr, I. Intensity of heart sounds in the evaluation of patients following myocardial infarction. *Chest* 75:679, 1979.

71. Surawicz, B., et al. Role of the phonocardiogram in evaluation of the severity of mitral stenosis and detection of associated valvular lesions. *Circulation* 34:759, 1966.

72. Tanaka, K., et al. Diagnostic significance of phonocardiography and apex cardiography in patients with primary pulmonary hypertension. *CV Sound Bull.* 5:385, 1975.

73. Tavel, M. E., Feigenbaum, H., and Campbell, R. W. A study of the Q–1 interval in atrial fibrillation with and without mitral stenosis. *Circulation* 31:429, 1965.

74. VanBogaert, A. A new concept on the mechanism of the first heart sound. *Am. J. Cardiol.* 18:253, 1966.

75. Victorica, B. E., et al. Persistent truncus arteriosus in infancy. *Am. Heart J.* 77:13, 1969.

76. Vogel, J. H. K., and Blount, S. G., Clinical evaluation in localizing level of obstruction to outflow from left ventricle. *Am. J. Cardiol.* 15:782, 1965.
77. Weintraub, A. M., et al. Poststenotic dilatation of the aorta with muscular subaortic stenosis. *Am. Heart J.* 68:741, 1964.
78. Wexler, L. F., et al. The relationship of the first heart sound to mitral valve closure in dogs. *Circulation* 66:235, 1982.
79. Whittaker, A. V., et al. Sound-pressure correlates of the aortic ejection sound. *Circulation* 39:475, 1969.
80. Yahini, J. H., Dulfano, M. J., and Toor, M. Pulmonic stenosis. *Am. J. Cardiol.* 5:744, 1960.

9. The Second Heart Sound

1. What produces the normal second heart sound (S_2)?

   ANS.: Events associated with closure of the aortic and pulmonary valves.

   *Note: a) Valve "closure" itself probably produces no noise. Echocardiography shows that the sounds occur slightly after the apposition of the leaflets. Shortly after apposition the sealed cusps are made tense and then to vibrate (stretch and recoil) due to the rapid force of aortic or pulmonary artery recoil [40].

   b) Closure of the aortic valve causes a sudden deceleration of forward flow. In dogs the peak of this sudden deceleration is associated with the simultaneous occurrence of the A_2 and the aortic incisura [77].

2. Which valve normally closes first, the aortic valve or the pulmonary valve?

   ANS.: The aortic valve. (It is crucial to remember this.) The sequence is A, P (i.e., aortic and pulmonary), as in Atlantic & Pacific. The A comes first, as in the alphabet. We shall call the aortic component of the second sound A_2 and the pulmonary component P_2.

*3. What is the old meaning of A_2 and P_2 (to which we shall *not* refer in this book)?

   ANS.: A_2 used to mean the total S_2 in the "aortic area" (second right interspace). P_2 used to mean the total S_2 in the "pulmonary area" (second left interspace). We now use A_2 to mean only the *aortic component* of the S_2, and P_2 to mean the *pulmonary component* of the S_2.

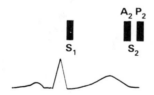

A_2 is the aortic valve closure component of the S_2. P_2 is the pulmonary valve closure component of the S_2. Note that the S_2 occurs near the end of the T wave of the ECG; i.e., the T wave is a systolic event.

---

*Material marked with an asterisk is for reference and for advanced students in cardiology.

EXPLANATION OF NORMAL SPLITTING SEQUENCE OF S₂

1. Draw a separate ventricular pressure curve and aortic pressure curve.

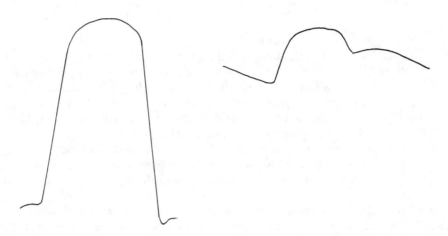

2. Superimpose the aortic pressure curve on the ventricular pressure curve.

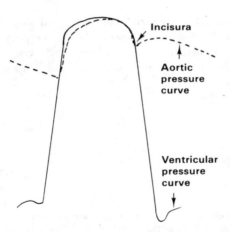

Incisura

Aortic
pressure
curve

Ventricular
pressure
curve

Note that when the LV pressure rise exceeds aortic pressure, the aortic valve will open and produce a single chamber effect or an "aortoventricle." The point at which ejection is finished and the aortic and LV pressure curves separate is called the incisura and is simultaneous with the aortic second sound, or A₂.

3. At what pressure in the left ventricle (LV) would you expect the aortic valve to open, assuming a normal blood pressure of 120/80 mm Hg?
   ANS.: When pressure in the LV rises to just above aortic diastolic pressure (about 80 mm Hg), the aortic valve will open.
4. After the aortic valve opens, what is the difference in pressure between the LV and the aorta?
   ANS.: Almost none. The LV and the aorta are almost a single pressure chamber as soon as the aortic valve opens. (It may be called an "aortoventricle" at this

time.) Only in the presence of aortic stenosis (AS) is there a significant pressure difference **(gradient)** between the aorta and the ventricle.

*Note: In actual fact, there is a slight positive gradient between the LV and the aorta during the first two-thirds to three-quarters of systole. It has been called an impulse gradient. This can be accurately measured only by a special electromanometer type of catheter.

5. What do we call the notch on the carotid or aortic pressure tracing that occurs roughly at the time of aortic valve closure? How is it related to the heart sounds?

ANS.: In the external carotid tracing taken by putting a pressure-sensitive pickup on the neck, it is called the *dicrotic notch*. In aortic pressure tracings, it is called the *incisura*. The incisura is simultaneous with the A_2 if aortic root pressure tracings are used for timing. (See figure on page 196.)

6. At what pressure does the A_2 occur—i.e., does it occur at aortic systolic, diastolic, or some intermediate pressure?

ANS.: The aortic valve closes when the force of ventricular ejection decreases, and the peripheral resistance plus the elastic recoil of the expanded aorta overcomes the decreasing pressure in the LV. This occurs at just below aortic systolic pressure (e.g., if the systolic pressure in the aorta is 120 mm Hg, the A_2 probably occurs at a pressure of about 110 mm Hg). (See figure on page 194.)

Note: The pulmonary artery pressure tracing also has a dicrotic notch or incisura where the P_2 occurs. The normal pulmonary artery pressure is about 25/10 mm Hg.

*7. How is the actual aortic valve closure related in time to the incisura and the A_2?

ANS.: The actual closure or coaptation (apposition) of the aortic and pulmonary valves has been shown by echophonocardiography to occur usually slightly before (0 to 20 msec) their respective incisuras and sounds [4]. This is because forward blood flow (which is due to inertia of the ejected blood) continues even after LV pressure has dropped below aortic pressure and the valve has closed. Forward flow continues for a short time after the onset of the sound [52].

Note: The duration of forward flow after aortic pressure exceeds LV pressure is controlled by the impedance of the system of blood flow and the vessels into which flow is occurring. That is, it comprises the forces that tend to resist forward flow, namely, the size of the vascular bed (capacitance), the resistance of the vascular bed, the compliance or distensibility of the vascular bed into which the blood is ejected, and the inertia of the mass of blood flowing into the vascular bed. Thus, if impedance is low, forward flow will continue for a long time after the pressure crossover point, and the A_2 and P_2 will occur very late. The leaflet coaptation-to-A_2 interval has been called the "hangout" interval [65].

Boldface type indicates that the term is explained in the Glossary.

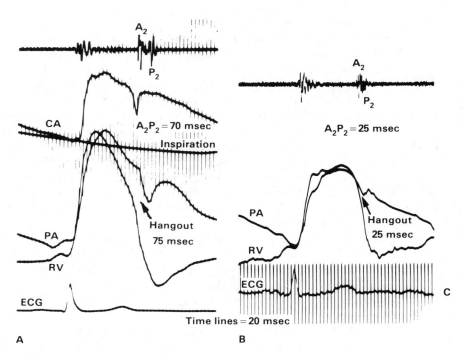

(A) The RV and PA pressure curves during inspiration from a normal 20-year-old man. (B) The same pressure curves also during inspiration, from a normal 61-year-old male. The distance separating the pulmonary incisura from the RV pressure curve is called the "hangout interval," and is seen to be nearly equal to the A_2P_2 interval in each patient. This interval is the time necessary to overcome the inertia of forward flow.

8. If the aortic valve closes at a pressure of about 100 mm Hg, and the pulmonary valve closes at about 20 mm Hg, why will aortic closure occur first?

   ANS.: The second heart sounds occur simultaneously with the incisuras of the pulmonary artery and aorta. The timing of the incisuras, in turn, has been shown to be related to the impedance to flow. For example, the less the arteriolar resistance and elastic recoil and the greater the capacity of the pulmonary arteries, the longer will forward flow continue and the later will the incisura occur on the pressure curve of the pulmonary artery [67]. The pulmonary vascular resistance is about a tenth that of the systemic resistance. The elastic recoil of the normal pulmonary artery is probably less than that of the aorta, and capacitance of the pulmonary vascular bed is greater than that of the aorta. Therefore, forward flow continues longer in the pulmonary circuit than in the aortic circuit after their respective pressure crossovers. This causes the pulmonary pressure and closure sound (P_2) to occur later than the aortic incisura and A_2 [66].

   Note: a) The conduction system of the heart feeds the LV before the right ventricle (RV). Therefore, contraction begins slightly earlier in the LV than in the RV. However, this contributes very little to the relative timing of the respective closure sounds.

   *b) In truncus arteriosus the single truncal valve theoretically should be incapable of causing a split S_2. However, when the cusps are abnormal or when there are more than three, the S_2 is likely to be split and may even increase in width on inspiration. The cause of this split is unknown. It seems to be the "true reduplicated second sound" that all split sounds were called before it was recognized that they came from the aortic and pulmonary valves separately. The split may be a double movement of the valves due to a different impedance of the pulmonary and aortic circuits.

  * c) Split P_2s have been recorded in some normal subjects; the cause of this is also unknown.

PHYSIOLOGY OF THE NORMALLY MOVING SPLIT

1. Does the normal split of the S_2 widen on inspiration or expiration?
   ANS.: It widens on inspiration, so that the A_2P_2 becomes an A_2–P_2.
2. Does the split movement of the S_2 occur because of the movement of the A_2 or the movement of the P_2?
   ANS.: Both. The P_2 moves out, away fom the A_2, and the A_2 moves inward, away from the P_2.
3. Which component moves more, the A_2 or the P_2?
   ANS.: The P_2. In all age groups, but especially over age 40, there are normal subjects in whom the A_2 does not move at all [30]. When it does move, it can contribute up to 30 percent of the total movement [30].

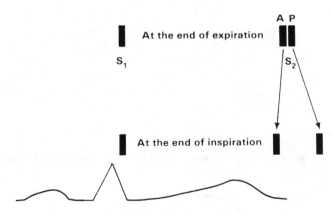

The P_2 outward movement contributes more to the inspiratory widening of the S_2 than does the inward movement of the A_2.

4. Why does the P_2 occur later with inspiration?
   ANS.: There are at least two explanations:
     a) The RV becomes larger with inspiration [66] because inspiration lowers the intrathoracic pressure (makes it more negative), and this acts to draw more blood from the superior and inferior venae cavae into the right side of the heart. The lungs act as bellows—i.e., when they expand, they function like a suction apparatus, which sucks blood from the inferior and superior venae cavae into the right atrium and ventricle. This in-

creased RV volume on inspiration delays pulmonary closure because when a ventricle increases its volume and has only one outlet for systole, it takes longer to eject that extra volume.

b) On inspiration the pulmonary impedance falls because the capacitance of the pulmonary vasculature is increased [66]. (See page 195 for explanation.) This also contributes to the delay in pulmonary valve closure.

*Note: The Q–P$_2$ interval is prolonged with inspiration even though the isovolumic contraction time as measured by the preejection period is shortened [42A].

5. Why does the A$_2$ occur earlier with inspiration?

ANS.: Because the LV becomes smaller with inspiration [65]. This occurs because inspiration, by enlarging the chest volume, also enlarges the vascular capacity of the lungs so much that they cannot compensate by drawing enough blood from the RV. In other words, the lungs do not fill from the RV in proportion to their increase in blood space potential during inspiration. This excessive increase in lung capacity withholds some blood from the LV.

*Note: Maximum widening of the split A$_2$–P$_2$ occurs at the peak of inspiration. Maximum narrowing occurs almost equally between mid- and end-expiration [47].

6. Does the normally moving split phenomenon (i.e., widening on inspiration and narrowing on expiration) refer (a) to held expiration and inspiration or to moving respiration, and (b) to deep respiration or to normal respiration?

ANS.: a) It refers to moving respiration.

b) It refers to normal depth of respiration.

Note: a) Held expiration results in a steady state in which the split remains fixed somewhere between the width on inspiration and expiration, with the A$_2$ coming first as usual.

b) A split S$_2$ at end-expiration is so rare after age 50 that it should be considered abnormal. The causes of expiratory splitting of the S$_2$ will be discussed under the headings of wide splitting, fixed splitting, and reversed splitting.

LOUDNESS OF COMPONENTS OF THE S$_2$

The Psychology and Physics of Loudness

1. What is the difference between the intensity, loudness, and amplitude of a sound or murmur?

ANS.: Intensity refers to the energy of the sound, whereas loudness refers to the subjective sensation produced by that energy on the ear. Amplitude refers to the size of the waves or movement produced by the sound energy. On a phonocardiogram, amplitude refers to the height of the sound or murmur.

2. Is the greatest amplitude or loudness of the components of the S$_2$ in the low-, medium-, or high-**frequency** range?

ANS.: In the low- and medium-frequency range.

3. Since the bell is best for bringing out low and medium frequencies, why is it usually better to listen to the splitting of the S$_2$ with the diaphragm?

ANS.: The diaphragm separates the two components of the split better. Soft, high-frequency components are masked by louder and longer low and medium frequencies unless they are markedly separated in pitch and width. Because the diaphragm damps out the louder low and medium frequencies, which reverberate around the high ones, volume is sacrificed for clarity in separating the components. Therefore, if one of the components of S_2 is very soft, the bell may actually bring it out better.

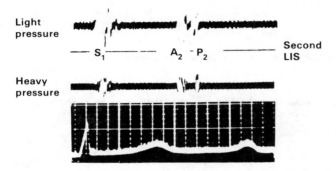

Light pressure
— S_1 — A_2 - P_2 ——   Second LIS

Heavy pressure

With light pressure, the low and medium frequencies dominate and cause the split sounds (about 50 msec [0.05 sec] apart) to run together. Heavy pressure, by turning the skin into a diaphragm, attenuates the reverberations of the low and medium frequencies and helps to separate the components of the split.

4. What makes an A_2 or a P_2 loud when there is more volume going through the valve?
   ANS.: If the aortic or pulmonary artery root is distended by an increased volume, the distended aorta or pulmonary artery beyond the valve has a greater recoil velocity, which closes the valve with more energy.
   *Note: The distention-recoil vibrations of the elastic valve leaflets have a greater amplitude if the rate of change of aortic-LV or pulmonary artery pressure gradients at the time of valve closure is rapid.

Sites of A_2 and P_2 Loudness

1. What was originally meant by the expression "A_2 is louder than P_2"?
   ANS.: The A referred to the "aortic area" (second right interspace), and the P meant "pulmonary area" (second left interspace). The expression meant that the entire S_2 in the second right interspace is louder than the entire S_2 in the second left interspace.
2. What is wrong with using the expression "A_2 is louder than P_2" or vice versa?
   ANS.: Now that A_2 and P_2 refer to the aortic and pulmonary components of the S_2, an altogether different meaning is implied.

   If you consider the S_2 as a single entity (whether split or not), it may normally be louder, in both children and adults, in *either* the second left or second right interspace [81].
3. Which *component* of the S_2 is best heard in normal subjects at the second left interspace (formerly called the "pulmonary area")? What is the clinical significance of this?

ANS.: Not only is the A_2 louder than the P_2 in the second left interspace in 70 percent of normal subjects in all age groups, but also in subjects over age 20, *the A_2 is always normally louder than the P_2 in the second left interspace* [57]. Even with severe pulmonary hypertension, as in **Eisenmenger reactions,** the A_2 is often louder than the P_2 in the second left interspace. This, together with the fact that the P_2 is often best heard in the third or fourth left interspace, rules out the second left interspace as truly a pulmonary area. Because this term is misleading, we encourage use of the term *second left interspace* instead.

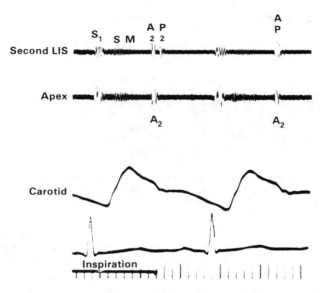

This simultaneous carotid pulse tracing and phonocardiogram is from a normal 16-year-old with a normal split of S_2 on inspiration. Note that (1) only the A_2 would be audible at the apex, and (2) the A_2 has a greater amplitude than the P_2 at the second left interspace (2nd LIS).

Note: a) The second left interspace may be called the "classic" or "traditional" pulmonary area.

*b) Normally, the rate of change of the aortic-LV gradient at the time of aortic valve closure is greater than the pulmonary artery-RV gradient at the time of pulmonary valve closure. This helps to explain why the P_2 is softer than the A_2 in the second left interspace.

4. Where is the A_2 normally heard on the chest wall?
   ANS.: Anywhere that one would normally listen to hear heart sounds.
5. Where is the P_2 normally heard on the chest wall?
   ANS.: In adults the P_2 is normally heard all along the left sternal border, often only a few centimeters to the left of the sternum. In infants and young children, and in young adults with a thin chest wall and a narrow anteroposterior chest diameter, it may also be heard at the apex.
   Note: This implies that if the P_2 (split S_2) is also heard to the right of the sternum or at the apex in a thick-chested adult, the P_2 is probably louder than normal. When the P_2 is heard unexpectedly at the apex, you will usually find that the RV is enlarged and the apex beat is not

due to the LV but entirely to the RV. Thus, in **atrial septal defects** (ASDs), it is expected that the large RV will make the P_2 audible at the apex, even though there may be no pulmonary hypertension.

6. Where is the splitting of the S_2 most often appreciated on the chest wall?

ANS.: At the second or third left interspace parasternally.

Note: a) In obese patients the split S_2 is often best appreciated at the *first* left interspace [48].

  *b) The split second sound may be best heard to the right of the sternum in dextrocardia, persistent truncus arteriosus, or in transposition of the great vessels whether they are congenitally corrected or not [78].

  c) In cyanotic tetralogy of Fallot, the S_2 is usually single and consists entirely of the A_2 because the P_2 is attenuated by

    1) A deformed pulmonary valve when there is valvular stenosis (this occurs in only about one-third of tetralogies).

    2) The anterior placement of the aorta relative to a posteriorly placed pulmonary artery.

    3) The low pulmonary artery pressure resulting from the diversion of RV blood through the high subaortic **ventricular septal defect** (VSD) directly into the aorta.

7. Where is the aortic component of the S_2 usually heard best in normal subjects of all ages?

ANS.: At the second and third left interspaces, probably because the aortic valve is situated behind the sternum, close to this area. This fact further denies that the second right interspace should be called *the* "aortic area," as it is in most of the auscultation literature.

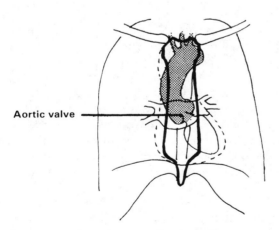

Aortic valve

The root of the aorta with its aortic valve is behind the middle of the sternum.

Causes of a Loud A_2 or P_2

1. What conditions tend to make the aortic component of the second sound louder than normal?

ANS.: a) Conditions that raise aortic systolic pressure (e.g., systemic hypertension). Systemic hypertension occasionally produces a drumlike or "tambour" S_2.

b) Conditions that produce a hyperkinetic systemic circulation (e.g., youth, thyrotoxicosis, and aortic regurgitation).

Note: The loudness of the aortic closure depends on the recoil of the aorta and the rate of diastolic expansion of the LV. Therefore, it is related to ventricular performance [69]. It follows, then, that a hypertensive patient in heart failure may not have a loud A_2.

2. What conditions, besides a thin chest wall, tend to make the P_2 louder than normal?

ANS.: a) Conditions that cause pulmonary hypertension.

b) Conditions that produce increased blood flow into the pulmonary artery, as in ASD or VSD.

Note: a) In VSD with normal or slightly elevated pulmonary artery pressures, the P_2 may be accentuated slightly, but it is difficult to detect this because it may still be softer than the A_2 in the second left interspace. Even if it is louder, it is not heard at the apex because the volume overload on the left heart accentuates the A_2 and also enlarges the LV, so that pulmonary events cannot be transmitted well to the apex.

b) The increased pulmonary flow due to an ASD does not necessarily make the P_2 louder than the A_2 unless the pulmonary artery pressure is at least 50 mm Hg [43]. If pulmonary stenosis (PS) is present with the ASD, the P_2 will probably be even less than 50 percent of the A_2 and will usually split to 60 msec or more [42].

c) In mitral stenosis (MS) the absolute loudness of the P_2 is a good sign of pulmonary hypertension only if it is loud. A soft P_2 may be present despite severe pulmonary hypertension. A P_2 that is louder than the A_2 in the second left interspace is also a good sign of pulmonary hypertension, but it does not tell you the degree of pulmonary hypertension.

d) The P_2 is as loud as or louder than the A_2 in pulmonary hypertension even though pulmonary artery pressure may not be quite as high as aortic pressure because

1) The pulmonary valve is more distensible and has a larger surface area than the aortic valve.

2) The pulmonary valve is anterior to the aortic valve [70].

3. Why does the A_2 tend to be loud in hyperkinetic states such as thyrotoxicosis and aortic regurgitation (AR)?

ANS.: The intensity of the A_2 is increased if the aortic valve closes when the aorta is energetically recoiling from the violent stretch due to the increased volume flung into it during systole. This occurs because the loudness of the A_2 is proportional to the energy present when the closure of the aortic valves decelerates the forward flow through the valve.

Note: a) With severe AR the A_2 may be soft, presumably because of the absence of adequate valve substance to cause a sudden deceleration of forward flow. Also, when AR is severe, the peripheral resistance may be so low that the aortic recoil energy may be dissipated peripherally.

*b) One study using an intracardiac phonocatheter placed across the aortic valve found a softer than normal A_2 with all degrees of AR. This finding contradicts clinical experience with a stethoscope and must be considered to be due to a technical artifact that occurs when a phonocatheter is placed above a regurgitant valve [56].

4. How does inspiration affect the loudness of each component of the S_2?

ANS.: The P_2 commonly becomes louder because extra blood in the pulmonary artery on inspiration causes more energetic elastic recoil. The A_2, on the other hand, becomes softer because inspiration decreases the volume ejected into the aorta and also places the aorta farther from the stethoscope.

Note: All sounds become softer on inspiration if you listen over the upper chest, where excess lung space is interposed between the stethoscope and the heart on inspiration.

Causes of a Softer A_2 or P_2

1. What can make either the A_2 or the P_2 softer than normal, besides the effect of respiration and abnormal chest shapes and thickness?

ANS.: a) Conditions that lower systolic pressure. The P_2 will soften if there is severe pulmonary stenosis, which is associated with low pulmonary artery pressure, especially if there is a right-to-left shunt through an ASD or a VSD.

b) Conditions that decrease the elastic recoil power of the aortic or pulmonary roots such as
   1) Poor myocardial contractility.
      *Note: With an ejection fraction of less than 50 percent the S_2 is softened and correlates with a prolonged pre-ejection period and short ejection time by systolic time intervals. During recovery from acute infarction, the S_2 increases in loudness as the pre-ejection period shortens and the ejection time lengthens [72].
   2) Poststenotic or idiopathic dilatation of the pulmonary artery that is caused by damage to the elastic tissue of the main pulmonary artery.

c) Conditions that stiffen the **semilunar valves** (e.g., calcification, sclerosis, or fusion of the cusps, as in AS or PS).
   *Note: a) In PS the pulmonary valve is thick and leathery. It is often adherent at its base to the surrounding pulmonary artery. This not only makes the P_2 soft but also adds to its lateness, because the RV pressure must drop considerably below the pulmonary artery pressure before it can move the relatively immobile valve.
      *b) A massive pulmonary embolus that touches the pulmonary valve will make the P_2 soft even in the presence of pulmonary hypertension.
      * c) Conditions that place the pulmonary artery farther from the stethoscope (e.g., transposition of the great vessels, congenitally corrected or not) will soften the P_2 even in the presence of pulmonary hypertension.
      *d) If the PS is purely subinfundibular due to a hypertrophic cardiomyopathy (very rare), the P_2 may be of normal loudness

  although delayed [45]. In congenital infundibular PS the P_2 may be inaudible [45].

  * e) Supravalvular AS can soften the A_2. Fibrous attachments to the aortic valves may partly account for this. In supravalvular PS the P_2 is either normal or increased in loudness [51].

  * f) When the aortic or pulmonary valves are calcified or fibrosed, the low frequencies tend to be attenuated, that is, the dominant frequencies are higher than they are when the valves are normal [71]. Similarly, with porcine xenograft aortic prostheses the low frequencies are lost over the years, probably due to degenerative changes [71].

Relative Loudness, Pitch, and Duration of the S_1 and S_2

1. When is it difficult to distinguish an S_1 from an S_2 by stethoscope alone?
   ANS.: When systole equals diastole in duration. This is called a "ticktack" rhythm (like the ticking of a clock) or embryocardia (like the fetal heart sounds).

2. What causes ticktack rhythm?
   ANS.: Anything that shortens diastole more than it does systole, as in tachycardias. As the heart rate increases, both systole and diastole are shortened, but diastole is shortened relatively more than systole.
   * *Note:* Severe AR may also produce a ticktack rhythm because it can prolong systole in relation to diastole.

3. How may the relative loudness of the S_1 and S_2 help to distinguish one from the other?
   ANS.: The S_2 is normally louder than the S_1 at the second right or left interspace (i.e., at the **base of the heart**), possibly because this is where the aortic and pulmonary valve structures are closest to the chest wall. At the apex the S_1 is usually louder than the S_2.
   Note: The apex area is not as reliable as the base for distinguishing an S_1 from an S_2 by loudness, because with a long P–R interval or with myocardial damage, the S_1 may be very soft.

4. If the S_1 is louder than the S_2 at the base, what does this suggest?
   ANS.: It suggests that an extra-loud S_1 is present, as in MS, or that there is an extra-soft S_2.

5. How can you tell at the bedside which heart sound is the S_2 when relative loudness is of no help?
   ANS.: a) The S_2 is higher in pitch, sharper, and shorter than the S_1 because it is usually single on expiration. The S_1 is relatively muffled and rough because of its three components. This is implied by the term *lub-dup* that is often used to mimic the sound of the S_1–S_2.

   b) Palpate the carotid while listening with the stethoscope. The S_1 will be heard just before the carotid impulse is felt. The carotid has the same relationship to the S_1 as an early systolic murmur (i.e., if we use the letter C to represent the carotid impulse, then the rhythm goes "1–C–2, 1–C–2"). This is due to the slight delay between the beginning of ventricular contraction, which produces the S_1, and the arrival of the carotid impulse in the neck.

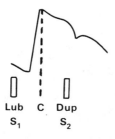

Lub C Dup
S₁   S₂

The tap of the carotid pulse on your fingers is felt _after_ and _not with_ the first heart sound.

c) Place the stethoscope or a finger over the apex beat, and note the outward impulse that occurs during systole. It should bulge outward with or just after the S_1. The stethoscope itself will rise during systole, and this will tell you which sound is the S_1. The S_1 will appear to "produce" the rise in apical impulse.

d) If you hear inspiratory splitting of one sound at the left sternal border and therefore know which sound is the S_2 there, then "inch" toward the apex. Inching means keeping the rhythm intact by moving the stethoscope rhythmically a few inches at a time exactly in time with the heart sounds.

NARROW AND WIDE SPLITTING DEFINED

*1. What do physiologists often call heart sounds in contrast to heart murmurs?
ANS.: Transients. This merely implies noises of short duration.

*2. What is the smallest time interval between transients that the ear is capable of distinguishing as two separate sounds?
ANS.: 20 msec. This narrow interval will allow a distinction as two separate sounds only if they are very short and high in frequency, as, for example, the sound of a camera shutter or a snare drum. For practical purposes, a split of 20 msec sounds merely like an impure or dirty sound rather than a sharp and clean one. This means that the narrowest split of heart sounds that the ear can clearly separate is about 30 msec.

3. What is meant by a wide split of the S_2?
ANS.: There are two ways of defining a wide split.

a) A sound that splits widely on inspiration—i.e., to at least 60 msec (0.06 sec), even if it is single on expiration.

b) A persistent split of S_2 on expiration that widens still more on inspiration.

Note: The concept of wide and narrow splitting is best understood if you practice the vocal imitation of splitting widths as follows. A normal narrow split on inspiration is 30–40 msec (0.03–0.04 sec). Imitate this by rolling the tongue as in a Spanish _dr_ or _tr_. For a slightly wider split of 50–60 msec (0.05–0.06 sec) say "pa–da" quickly. For a wide split of 70–80 msec (0.07–0.08 sec) say "pa–ta" quickly. Articulate both the _p_ and the _t_ sharply. A very wide split is 90–100 msec (0.09–0.10 sec). For this say "pa-pa" as quickly as possible.

THE WIDELY SPLIT S₂

1. What conditions can cause wide splitting of the S_2 as a result of a delay in pulmonary valve closure?

   ANS.: Delays of P_2 are caused by the following:

   a) Conditions that cause electrical delay of activation of the RV (e.g., right bundle branch block [RBBB]).

   * *Note:* a) The delay in P_2 with RBBB is due not only to delayed onset of right ventricular contraction but also to a slower rate of rise of right ventricular pressure [33].

   b) Type A atrioventricular preexcitation also causes a wide split (usually 50–70 msec) because the accessory bundle in type A enters the LV first and therefore acts like a RBBB [61].

   b) Conditions that cause an increased volume in the RV in comparison with the LV (e.g., at least a moderately sized ASD or a moderate amount of pulmonary regurgitation [PR], either congenital or as a result of pulmonary valve surgery).

   * *Note:* For some unknown reason the S_2, even in severe congenital PR, may occasionally be narrowly split.

   c) Conditions that cause a gradient across the pulmonary valve due to valvular or infundibular PS.

   d) Conditions that cause either acute or chronic RV failure, as in massive pulmonary embolism, or in the late stages of chronic pulmonary embolism or primary hypertension [16].

   e) Conditions that decrease the elastic recoil and increase the capacitance of the pulmonary artery (e.g., idiopathic dilatation of the pulmonary artery [53, 62]).

   * *Note:* The reason for the lack of wide splitting in some patients with idiopathic dilatation of the pulmonary artery may be a relatively smaller loss of elastic tissue. The exceptionally broad P_2 heard in some patients with idiopathic dilatation is unexplained.

   * f) Bilateral pulmonary artery branch stenosis [21, 32].

* 2. What has been shown to cause the delay of P_2 in patients with ASD or VSD besides the volume overload of the RV?

   ANS.: The $Q–P_2$ interval is lengthened because in VSDs there is a delay in the onset of RV contraction. The interval from Q to the onset of RV contraction (electromechanical interval) may be prolonged by as much as 60 msec more than the normal 40–60 msec. This interval has not been investigated in ASDs, but it is known that the preejection period (Q to carotid upstroke) is prolonged in ASDs [80].

   Note: a) The electromechanical interval (Q to onset of ventricular contraction) is relatively independent of heart rate. It is almost not measurable under the age of 1 year and is less than 5 msec by age 4. It reaches about 30 msec by puberty.

b) In uncomplicated ASDs the interval from Q to the end of the total ventricular systole (to the bottom of the ventricular pressure curves) is the same in both ventricles [39]. The P_2 occurs late in ASDs because the pulmonary incisura is late. The cause of the late incisura is thought to be due to
   1) The increased difficulty of halting the high velocity of flow into the pulmonary artery.
   2) The low impedance of the pulmonary vascular bed, which is partly due to dilatation of the main pulmonary artery (increased capacitance).
c) In more than 75 percent of postoperative ASD patients the wide splitting of the S_2 persists. This suggests that the theory that a dilated pulmonary artery causes delay of the incisura might be correct, because the pulmonary artery remains dilated after corrective surgery. This theory is further supported by the absence of a significant relationship between the width of the split in ASD patients and the size of the shunt [13].
d) If a VSD shunts into the right atrium, the S_2 split is often not wide. The reason is unknown.

3. Will a RBBB pattern (i.e., an S in lead 1 and an R' in V_1, with no prolongation of the QRS) cause a wide split of the S_2?

   ANS.: No. There must be terminal delay or slowing of conduction, as in incomplete or complete RBBB, in order to produce a widely split S_2.

4. When can a wide split occur owing to early closure of the A_2?

   ANS.: a) In **tamponade** the early occurrence of the A_2 is due to a markedly disproportionate decrease in the size of the LV in comparison with the RV on inspiration [28]. (The Q–P_2 does not change with inspiration in tamponade.) The Q–A_2, on the other hand, shortens due to a marked decrease in LV volume.

   *b) A wide split can occur in the presence of a left atrial tumor, usually a myxoma, due to underfilling of the LV [36].

   *Note: a) It has been assumed in the past that the widely split S_2 that occurs in severe MR is due to an early A_2 secondary to shortening of the ejection time because of the presence of two outlets for systole. This is unreasonable because
      1) There may be two outlets, but there is also more volume to be ejected.
      2) The S_2 is not widely split in mild to moderate MR.
      3) Left ventricular ejection times are normal in MR unless the output is decreased at rest.

   b) It is important to know that MR can produce a widely split S_2 because a wide split tells you not only that the MR is at least moderately severe but also that you must not assume that a widely split S_2 with MR is due to an A_2-opening snap. (How to tell the difference between an A_2–P_2 and an A_2-opening snap is discussed on pages 236–239.)

   c) It is surprising to find a widely split S_2 in MR because one study has shown a delayed Q-1 in most patients with ruptured chordae and in almost all patients with rheumatic mitral regurgitation. This correlates with the delay in electromechanical interval (i.e., MR seems to cause a delay in the onset of LV pressure). This should delay LV events enough to delay the A_2 also and cause either a single S_2 or even a reversed split of the S_2 [37].

5. In tamponade, why does the LV decrease in size so markedly in comparison with the RV during inspiration?

ANS.: The increase in RV volume during inspiration stretches the entire pericardium, which also covers the atria. This restricts the expansion of the left atrium, so that it cannot dilate with the blood it receives from the pulmonary veins. During inspiration the left atrial pressure may actually rise higher than the pulmonary venous pressure, and blood may flow backward into the pulmonary veins.

Another factor decreasing LV volume is an exaggerated shift of the ventricular septum toward the LV during inspiration.

Note: The extra-wide split that occurs during inspiration is usually manifest for only a few beats during the beginning of inspiration [6].

* 6. What is the *widest* normal split heard during held expiration?

ANS.: On held expiration or the end of normal expiration, the widest normal split is about 30 msec. This is rare over age 40. Roll the tongue as in the Spanish *tr* to imitate this.

Note: At all ages from 1 to 80, normal expiration produces a single S_2 in more than 85 percent of subjects. Over age 50, the S_2 closes in expiration in 95 percent of normal subjects in the recumbent position [2]. The greatest difference in the split of the S_2 between inspiration and expiration in normal subjects during quiet respiration is about 50 msec. Exceptionally wide splitting (80 msec on inspiration) is found in some normal children. The reason is unknown [23].

* 7. What should happen to the width of the split of the S_2 when both ventricles are volume-overloaded by a rupture of a sinus of Valsalva into the right atrium or RV?

ANS.: Such a rupture produces a volume overload of both ventricles, which widens the split S_2 no matter what the cause, except a VSD-to-right atrial shunt.

THE A_2–P_2 IN PULMONARY STENOSIS

1. Why will a stenotic RV outflow tract or valve cause a delay of the P_2?

ANS.: In PS, RV pressure is much higher than pulmonary artery pressure. Thus it takes an extra-long time for the RV pressure to drop to the closing pressure of the pulmonary artery valve. (See figure on page 217.) Also, the stiff pulmonic valve will require a greater fall in RV pressure below the pulmonary artery pressure before it can move the rigid valve into the closed position. Furthermore, if there is poststenotic dilatation, the increased pulmonary capacitance plus the poor elastic recoil will increase the delay in P_2.

*Note: There is less delay in RV emptying in supravalvular PS than in valvular PS because in the former there is a high pressure between the valve and the supravalvular obstruction. In supravalvular PS or in unilateral pulmonary artery stenosis, the A_2–P_2 split is usually normal or narrow [21, 51].

*2. Does the PS seen in severe tetralogy of Fallot produce a wide split of the S_2?

ANS.: In actual practice, the P_2 is audible in only about one-third of cyanotic adults with tetralogy of Fallot [31]. Intracardiac phonocardiography with the microphone in the pulmonary artery, however, has always shown the delayed P_2 [24]. Also, after shunt operations that increase pulmonary flow, the P_2 has been seen to be very delayed.

Note: A long systolic murmur that continues into or through the A_2 along the left sternal border can obscure the widely split S_2. This occurs with the murmur of VSD or with severe PS.

You can easily tell if the murmur is obscuring an A_2 by exploring the split S_2 away from the maximal murmur area and by comparing simultaneous phonocardiograms at the apex, where the aortic component will be seen, with the left sternal border, where only the P_2 may be seen.

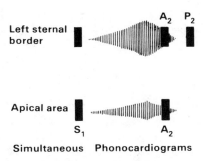

At the apex, the easily recorded A_2 may be heard despite the murmur, which is much softer in that area.

3. How can the A_2–P_2 interval tell you the probable RV pressure in PS?

ANS.: In general, the more severe the obstruction and the higher the RV pressure, the longer the A_2–P_2 interval.

*Note: a) If the A_2–P_2 interval is 40 msec or less, the RV pressure will range from normal to about 45 mm Hg. If the A_2–P_2 is 50 msec, the RV pressure will range widely from normal to about 55 mm Hg. If the A_2–P_2 is 60 msec, the RV pressure is no longer likely to be normal but ranges from about 45 mm Hg to about 80 mm Hg. If the A_2–P_2 is 80 msec, the range of RV pressure is from 60 mm Hg to about 120 mm Hg. If the A_2–P_2 is 100 msec, the range is from 70 mm Hg to 160 mm Hg [27]. If there is marked poststenotic dilatation of the pulmonary artery, the increase in capacitance of the

pulmonary artery may delay pulmonary valve closure so that the RV pressure will be thought to be higher than it really is. Therefore, the lower end of the range of RV pressure is more likely to be the correct one if pulmonary artery dilatation is marked [65].
  b) If the infundibulum is hypertrophied (usually secondary to valvular PS), contraction of the infundibulum may occur considerably later than that of the body of the RV even with only moderate gradients.
  c) The wide split of S_2 in PS is relatively fixed, either with mild PS and marked dilatation of the pulmonary artery or with severe PS and marked RV hypertrophy (RVH) [67].

THE FIXED SPLIT OF THE S_2

1. What is meant by a fixed or relatively fixed split of the S_2?
   ANS.: If the split changes less than 20 msec (0.02 sec) with quiet respiration, it is called a fixed or relatively fixed split.
2. What can cause a fixed or relatively fixed split of the S_2?
   ANS.: a) ASDs.
       b) Heart failure, because
           1) It prevents the ventricles from responding to changes in volume and pressure [50]. The heart in failure is relatively insensitive to changes in filling pressure; for example, a rise in LV end–diastolic pressure of a few millimeters of mercury in the normal ventricle can almost double cardiac output. In the failing ventricle the output rises only slightly or not at all.
           2) It does not permit much change in the volume of the ventricle with respiration because breathing with congested lungs is shallow.
            * Note: In patients with chronic cor pulmonale and failure, the fixed split moves normally after compensation is attained with medical treatment [9].
     * c) Moderate to large VSDs [8]. An obviously moving split on the phonocardiogram of a patient with a VSD usually implies a small shunt (with a pulmonary-systemic flow ratio of less than 2:1) and a pulmonary artery systolic pressure of less than 50 mm Hg [34].
       d) Pulmonary stenosis in some patients.
     * e) Pulmonary embolism (massive pulmonary embolism or with the late sequelae of chronic pulmonary embolism, when the pulmonary artery pressure is at least two-thirds of the systemic pressure [17]).
       f) Idiopathic dilatation of the pulmonary artery. In 6 of 8 patients with idiopathic dilatation of the pulmonary artery in one series, the split was relatively fixed [35].
       Note: A relatively fixed split is a variation of normal in children and young men, especially in the supine position. The reason is unknown. If the split is fixed when the patient is supine, it will not be fixed in the sitting position, and vice versa [11, 44].
3. Does complete RBBB produce a fixed split?
   ANS.: No [63].

The Fixed Split of the S_2 in ASD

1. Why is the S_2 split in ASD relatively fixed?

   ANS.: In ASD the LV does not become smaller on inspiration and may even become larger. This occurs because on inspiration vena caval blood is drawn into the right atrium, where pressure then rises and thereby the left–to–right shunt through the ASD is decreased. This nonshunted left atrial blood passes instead through the mitral valve into the LV and thus tends to keep LV volume constant during inspiration [7].

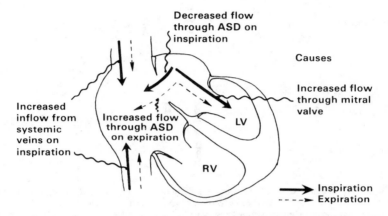

The increased inflow into the right atrium on inspiration (vertical solid arrows) causes a decreased flow through the ASD and thus increased flow through the mitral valve.

   * *Note:* a) If the left–to–right shunt is *markedly* decreased on inspiration due to a poorly compliant RV, the LV volume may even *increase* with the large inflow of blood from the left atrium during inspiration.

   b) There is physiological proof that the shunt from the left to the right atrium in ASD is decreased by inspiration. Oxygen saturation in the pulmonary artery has been shown to be less during inspiration in subjects with ASD [5]. It has been found that a 50 percent decrease in left–to–right shunt can occur with inspiration.

* 2. Does the P_2 move normally with respiration in the presence of an ASD?

   ANS.: With normal respiration the P_2 moves only slightly or not at all. The $Q–P_2$ interval moves less than 20 msec in ASDs during quiet inspiration [5]. (In normal subjects the $Q–P_2$ is almost always lengthened on quiet inspiration by at least 20 msec and in most cases by about 40 msec.) With deep inspiration, however, the P_2 in patients with ASD can move almost normally, as shown by the following evidence that deep inspiration can increase the flow into the RV.

   a) A tricuspid diastolic flow murmur due to torrential flow through the valve is often heard only on deep inspiration.

   b) The P_2 may become louder on deep inspiration on both external and intracardiac phonocardiograms [25].

* 3. How does the A_2 move in ASDs?

   ANS.: Either not at all or slightly toward the P_2 on inspiration.

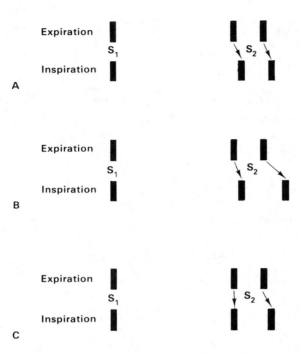

If, as in A, the A_2 moves forward on inspiration exactly the same amount as the P_2, the split will be absolutely fixed on respiration. This is uncommon. Usually, even when the A_2 moves forward with inspiration, it does not move as much as does the P_2 as in B and C.

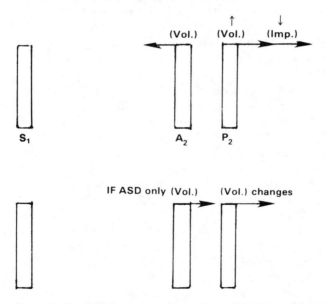

On inspiration the P_2 is shown to be moving to the right away from the S_1 by two mechanisms, the increased volume in the RV and the decreased impedance of the pulmonary circuit. The A_2 is shown moving to the left (toward the S_1) by only one mechanism, the decreased volume in the LV. In ASDs the P_2 moves with inspiration due only to its increased volume, because there is no significant impedance effect when the lung vessels are overfilled because of the shunt flow. The A_2 may either not move at all with inspiration or actually move in the same direction as the P_2.

ASDs WITH NARROW SPLITS

1. How common is a narrow split of the S_2 with ASDs?

    ANS.: Although ASDs are noted for their wide splits, the majority of adults with ASDs do not have a split of more than 60 msec [24]. Some normal young subjects have wider inspiratory splits than this.

*2. How is a narrow split of the S_2 in ASDs related to the size of the shunt?

    ANS.: In subjects with an ASD a narrow split of the S_2 is unrelated to the size of the shunt. The duration of RV ejection is not necessarily proportional to the stroke volume of the RV because the larger the stroke volume, the faster the RV contracts [20].

    *Note: a) A narrow split on inspiration that remains split on expiration, especially during sitting or standing, is an excellent sign of a relatively fixed split, because if a split is narrow on inspiration, it should *close* on expiration especially in the sitting or standing position.

    b) It is not surprising that in ASD patients even a narrow split of the S_2 remains open in the sitting position because it has been shown that in uncomplicated left-to-right shunts the shunt flow increases in the upright position [12].

    c) In ASD patients there is often more variation of the split S_2 with respiration in the sitting position; the longer the subject sits, the more variation there may be.

    d) Tachycardias also narrow the S_2 split in patients with ASDs [13].

    e) In infants with ASDs and congestive failure wide splitting is the rule [13].

    f) Marked dilatation of the pulmonary artery, which is common with ASDs, perhaps as an associated anomaly, can increase the capacitance of the pulmonary vascular tree and so delay closure of the P_2. It may be that with a narrow split in patients with an ASD one should suspect that the pulmonary artery is only minimally dilated [65].

*3. If a split is narrow, how can a long pause after a premature ventricular contraction or in atrial fibrillation suggest the presence of a fixed split in a patient with an ASD?

    ANS.: After a long pause, the split widens markedly (as much as 40 msec) [75]. This widening may be due to an increase in the left-to-right shunt during long diastoles. In the normal heart the split S_2 is also widened after long diastoles but not as much as in the presence of an ASD [49].

    Note: The left-to-right shunt in diastole is controlled largely by the relative resistance to expansion of the RV and the LV. It may be that the difference in distensibility between the RV and the LV is exaggerated by a long diastole.

DIFFERENTIAL DIAGNOSIS OF THE FIXED SPLIT

*1. Why is the split S_2 of some patients with PS relatively fixed?

    ANS.: There are at least three possibilities:

a) Because the split is usually fixed only when there is marked poststenotic dilatation of the pulmonary artery, the loss of elastic recoil may somehow be responsible. (The dilated segment has been shown to be more distensible than normal.) [53]

b) The markedly hypertrophied RV often has much fibrosis and may not be able to respond as well as a more normal RV to the increased blood volume brought to it by inspiration.

c) Shortening of the RV isovolumic contraction time as a result of the more powerful right atrial contraction that occurs during inspiration may also contribute to the poor movement of the P_2.

Note: If an ASD is diagnosed, suspect the presence of PS in addition when the split on expiration is 60 msec or more and the P_2/A_2 loudness ratio is less than one-half at the left sternal border in a high-frequency phonocardiogram.

2. What may mimic a wide fixed split of the S_2?

ANS.: a) A paradoxical split in complete LBBB, especially with some heart failure. (The paradoxical split is explained on page 220.)

b) The A_2 followed by an opening snap. (The six ways of distinguishing an A_2–P_2 from an A_2–opening snap are detailed on pages 236–239.)

c) A very wide split in which normal movements of the A_2–P_2 are difficult to perceive by auscultation. It is much easier to perceive movement of two sounds when they are close together than when they are very far apart. The solution to this dilemma is to make the two sounds approach one another by causing less blood to return to the heart, as with sitting or standing.

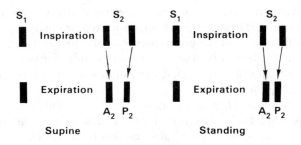

It would be difficult to perceive movement of the split in the supine position shown in the S_2 on the left, and you might call it a relatively fixed split until the patient sits or stands up.

3. Why does the split S_2 in the normal subject tend to narrow on sitting or standing?

ANS.: This happens because when both ventricles receive less blood (due to pooling in the abdomen and the legs), the RV responds by ejecting its blood relatively faster than does the LV [46]. The RV responds more to changes in filling pressure than does the LV [58]. Some normal subjects have a relatively fixed split in the supine position.

4. How can placing a patient in the sitting position help to distinguish the supine expiratory splitting of the S_2 in a normal young patient from the relatively fixed split of a patient with an ASD?

ANS.: The normal patient usually shows increased respiratory variation on sitting or standing, and the split will close on expiration [2, 14, 44]. The ASD patient on sitting or standing will maintain the split on expiration, even though respiratory variation may also increase in these positions.

Note: To complicate matters, however, about 15 percent of normal children may have splits that appear to be fixed in the sitting but not in the supine position [14].

*5. What happens to the splitting of the S_2 after a Valsalva maneuver during the period immediately following release and then a few seconds afterward? How can you use this maneuver to detect the presence of an ASD?

ANS.: In normal subjects the split widens by more than 20 msec immediately on release [5]. This occurs because the Valsalva maneuver dams up venous blood behind the RV. On release of this dammed-up blood, there is extra filling in the RV for a few beats, in contrast to the LV, which actually contains less blood for a few beats because the lungs have been partially emptied.

A few seconds after the release of the strain, the split S_2 becomes very narrow or single because the dammed-up blood now reaches the LV after a few beats, pushing a comparatively greater volume into the LV than into the RV for a few beats.

In patients with ASDs, however, the atria act almost as a single chamber, so that any rise in right atrial pressure is also reflected in a rise in left atrial pressure. Thus, on release of the Valsalva, any increased venous blood that rushes into the RV will also cause more blood to enter the LV, and there will be only slight immediate widening (not more than 20 msec) and no delayed narrowing of the S_2 [5].

After surgery on an ASD, the wide and relatively fixed split may persist for at least a year. The post-Valsalva effect will, however, indicate the true situation [79].

Note: You can overcome difficulties in a patient's understanding of how to perform a Valsalva maneuver by asking him to push against your hand pressed against his abdomen. He will inadvertently perform a Valsalva maneuver in the process of doing this [29]. Blowing a manometer up to 40 mm Hg is the ideal method of performing a Valsalva.

6. Which abnormalities besides an ASD may produce not only a relatively fixed split of the S_2 but also a *wide* split?

ANS.: a) Right bundle branch block plus heart failure. The RBBB makes the split wide, and the heart failure fixes it.

b) **Right ventricular failure** secondary to pulmonary hypertension. The wide split is probably due to a prolonged isovolumic contraction time in the failing RV.

Note: Normally, a prolonged isovolumic contraction time is usually associated with a shortened ejection time, and this will prevent late closure of the pulmonary valve [19]. We must assume, therefore, that high pressure during ejection is interpreted by the RV as if it were still isovolumically contracting, and ejection therefore takes longer than expected [16].

*   c) Some moderately large VSDs have wide and relatively fixed splits. The widening here is partly due to a delayed P_2 [8].
* d) Some patients with partial anomalous pulmonary venous drainage into the right atrium have relatively fixed, wide splits.
  * *Note:* Although this anomaly may cause the same physical, ECG, and x-ray signs as an ASD, the effect of respiration on the split of the S_2 often enables you to distinguish the two lesions. If the splitting is normal, the differentiation is easy [26]. Some subjects with partial anomalous pulmonary venous drainage, however, have relatively fixed splits due to a prolongation of the P_2 on expiration. A phonocardiogram showing a prolongation of the $Q-P_2$ interval on expiration can help in differentiating the lesions. This should be done during prolonged expiration to allow maximum filling of the right atrium by way of the anomalous pathway [38].

* 7. How can you distinguish the wide, fixed split and loud P_2 of RV failure due to pulmonary hypertension from that of ASD with pulmonary hypertension?

ANS.: a) Exercise will widen the split still further only in RV failure because it delays the P_2, probably because the rise in pulmonary artery pressure with exercise will increase the isovolumic contraction time of the failing RV and leave the isovolumic contraction of the normal LV relatively unchanged.

   b) Phonocardiograms taken at rest can show that in RV failure due to pulmonary hypertension inspiration causes the $Q-P_2$ either to remain the same or to be prolonged without any change in the $Q-A_2$. In ASDs, deep inspiration will cause prolongation not only of the $Q-P_2$ but also of the $Q-A_2$, even when there is severe pulmonary hypertension as in the Eisenmenger reaction.

THE NARROWLY SPLIT S_2

1. List the usual causes of a narrowly split S_2 due to a delayed A_2.

ANS.: 1) Conditions that cause electrical delay of LV conduction: LBBB and some types of **Wolff-Parkinson-White** (W-P-W) **preexcitation** that imitate LBBB by causing premature depolarization of the RV.

   2) Conditions that increase the volume of the LV but without an extra outlet (a VSD or MR is an extra outlet)—e.g., **persistent ductus arteriosus** (PDA) and AR.

   * *Note:* a) Hypertension can prolong the $Q-A_2$ more than the $Q-P_2$, probably by delaying the *onset* of LV contraction (electromechanical interval) and also by slightly prolonging the ejection time. If myocardial damage is superimposed on the hypertension, the isovolumic contraction time is prolonged as well, and a paradoxical or reversed split (P_2, A_2) may result.

      b) Aging not only prolongs the LV ejection time, thus delaying the A_2, but also causes a shortening of the $Q-P_2$ interval, thus bringing the P_2 earlier. The A_2 in the elderly often does not move at all.

Conditions that cause a significant gradient across the outflow of the LV (e.g., AS), so that there is a delay in LV pressure dropping below aortic pressure.

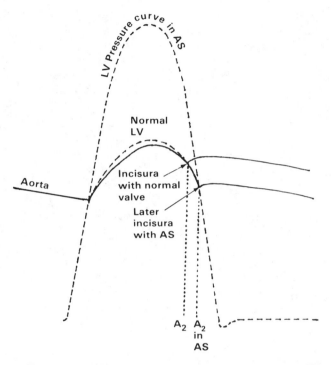

In AS the LV pressure rises high above aortic pressure during systole. It then takes so long to drop down to aortic diastolic pressure and close the valve that the incisura is low and late on the aortic pressure curve. The A_2 is also late because it is simultaneous with the incisura.

Note: *a) The delay in the A_2 in AS is not due to prolonged LV contraction. The time from the Q wave to the end of LV systole (i.e., from the Q to the beginning of the fall in LV pressure [end of LV systole] on an LV pressure curve) is *shorter* than the time from the Q wave to the end of RV systole in all degrees of AS [39A].

*b) Marked poststenotic dilatation may further delay the A_2 by decreasing the impedance beyond the valve [53].

2. List the causes of a narrowly split S_2 due to an early P_2.

ANS.: 1. Conditions that increase impedance of the pulmonary vasculature, e.g., pulmonary hypertension. (In the late stages the split widens owing to RV failure.)

Note: Although as a person grows older, the isovolumic contraction time of the LV becomes slightly longer [68], there is also some indication that the P_2 occurs slightly earlier (i.e., the Q–P_2 interval shortens [64] owing to the increase in impedance in the pulmonary circuit with aging [20]).

*2. Shortening of RV systole due to underfilling of the RV secondary to a right atrial tumor, usually an atrial myxoma [36].

3. In about what percentage of normal subjects is the S_2 single on quiet inspiration (a) under age 50, and (b) over age 50?

ANS.: The S_2 is single
    a) In about 30 percent of subjects under age 50.
    b) In about 60 percent of subjects over age 50 [2].

4. What causes a split second sound on auscultation to seem to be single as well as too narrow, that is, less than 30 msec (0.03 sec)?

ANS.: a) Too deep an inspiration may interpose too much lung between the stethoscope and the heart, causing one of the S_2 components (usually the P_2) to disappear.
    b) One component of the split may be so loud that it masks a soft component before or after it. This is known as masking, which may be due to the auditory fatigue effect produced by a loud sound (analogous to the momentary blindness caused by the flash of a bright light).

5. How can you tell that an S_2 is split on inspiration even if you do not hear two distinct components?

ANS.: If the S_2 is clean and sharp on expiration and becomes impure or rough on inspiration, then it probably has opened up slightly on inspiration (to about 20 msec [0.02 sec]).

6. What kinds of respiration will obscure awareness of whether the split moves?

ANS.: a) Too deep an inspiration will interpose too much lung between the stethoscope and the heart, causing one or both of the S_2 components to disappear.
    b) Too shallow an inspiration may not open the S_2 at all.
    c) Rapid respiration will not allow time for the hemodynamic changes that produce splitting on inspiration and narrowing on expiration.

7. How can you control the respiration of a patient so that there are enough cardiac cycles on inspiration and expiration for you to distinguish normal from abnormal splitting?

ANS.: Ask the patient to follow your arm, raising it for inspiration and lowering it for expiration; you may "conduct" his respiration so that there are at least two or three cycles during each phase of respiration. Be certain that the patient does not breathe too deeply, or he will make too much chest noise or even close his glottis at the end of inspiration, producing either a Valsalva maneuver or a **Müller maneuver**.

THE S_2 SPLIT IN PULMONARY HYPERTENSION

1. What are the three general types of pulmonary hypertension?

ANS.: a) Hyperkinetic pulmonary hypertension, i.e., that due to excess volume flow, as in large left-to-right shunts. The pulmonary arterioles can dilate to accommodate up to three times the normal cardiac output before the pulmonary artery pressure must rise. When the excess flow causes the pulmonary artery pressure to rise, vasoconstriction probably also occurs.

b) Vasoactive pulmonary hypertension, i.e., that due primarily to pulmonary arteriolar constriction, as in response either to hypoxia or to a high left atrial pressure, as in patients with MS.

c) Obstructive pulmonary hypertension, i.e., that due to fixed lumen obliteration, as with pulmonary emboli, or to narrowing, as with the endothelial and medial hypertrophy seen in some ASDs, PDAs, and VSDs with bidirectional shunting (Eisenmenger reaction), or with primary pulmonary hypertension.

*2. In which of the preceding causes of pulmonary hypertension do you expect (a) normal or narrow splitting, (b) wide splitting, or (c) no splitting?

ANS.: 1) Normal or narrow splitting is expected in the early stages of primary pulmonary hypertension in some subjects and with the pulmonary hypertension of most subjects with PDA or MS [74]. The increased impedance due to the high resistance and tense pulmonary artery ordinarily causes an early P_2, making the S_2 single. However, the dilated pulmonary artery, so often found in patients with pulmonary hypertension, decreases the impedance to pulmonary flow and may cause separation of the S_2 to normal degrees on inspiration.

Note: a) The level of pulmonary hypertension does not correlate with the width of splitting in MS (range, 20–60 msec) or in MR (range, 40–70 msec) [74].

b) After pulmonary artery banding an A_2–P_2 interval of less than 40 msec has been found in one study to imply persistent pulmonary hypertension and increased pulmonary vascular resistance [18].

2) Wide splitting is expected in ASDs, in massive pulmonary embolism, and in some patients with severe primary pulmonary hypertension with a prolonged RV isovolumic contraction time.

3) No splitting is expected in VSDs with an Eisenmenger reaction, but in VSDs with hyperkinetic pulmonary hypertension, the S_2 may be either single or split normally [74].

*Note: Although a single S_2 in VSDs does not indicate whether or not the pulmonary hypertension is too fixed to be operable, a split S_2 usually implies that an operation is feasible.

3. How much obstruction is necessary before an acute pulmonary embolism can produce wide, relatively fixed splitting of the S_2?

ANS.: Almost the entire pulmonary tree on both sides must be obstructed. If, however, pulmonary hypertension is already present due to previous disease, a further embolus to one branch may cause wide, fixed splitting.

*Note: a) Moderate exercise can bring out the wide splitting in borderline cases and exaggerate it still more in advanced obstruction. In severe obstruction, the split may be almost 80 msec. Because it is relatively fixed, it may be mistaken for an opening snap. This wide split often narrows with lysis of the embolus during 3 to 6 days.

b) The cause of the wide split in acute pulmonary embolism is due to a shortened Q–A_2 and a normal Q–P_2. The early A_2 is probably due to shortening of the LV systole, partly by catecholamines and partly by a reduced LV stroke volume.

4. What is an ASD, VSD, or PDA with bidirectional shunting called?

ANS.: An Eisenmenger situation, syndrome, or reaction. The pulmonary hypertension may be so severe that only right-to-left shunting occurs.

Note: When a VSD is the cause of the pulmonary hypertension, it is often called an Eisenmenger *complex* because this is the original lesion described by Eisenmenger in 1897.

5. Why does the S_2 of a VSD with an Eisenmenger reaction become single on both phases of respiration?

ANS.: This occurs because only a large VSD could produce an Eisenmenger reaction, and such a large communication between the ventricles tends to make them function as a single chamber.

6. How does the S_2 differ among the three different levels of Eisenmenger syndromes, i.e., VSD, ASD, and PDA?

ANS.: In VSDs the S_2 is single; in ASDs it is split and fixed (often widely split); in PDAs it is normally or narrowly split, and when split, it moves normally [74].

Note: a) Early in the course of development of an ASD Eisenmenger reaction, the high resistance beyond the pulmonary valve may narrow the split S_2. As the RV begins to fail, its isovolumic contraction time is prolonged, and the split becomes wide again.

b) The A_2/P_2 loudness ratio at the second left interspace can be used to suggest the presence of hyperkinetic pulmonary hypertension in a subject with a VSD. In a VSD with normal pulmonary artery pressure, the A_2 is generally louder than the P_2. Therefore, if the P_2 is louder, pulmonary hypertension is probably present.

*7. What auscultatory signs suggest that the pulmonary hypertension is primary?

ANS.: Primary pulmonary hypertension tends to have a vibratory S_1, which is thought to be due to loud tricuspid valve closure [75].

THE REVERSED OR PARADOXICALLY SPLIT S₂

Physiology and Etiologies

1. What is meant by a reversed or paradoxical split of the S_2?

ANS.: This is a split in which the order of components is P_2A_2 instead of the normal A_2P_2.

2. Can too early a P_2 cause a reversed split?

ANS.: A reversed split caused by such a phenomenon is very rare. A reversed split is nearly always caused by a delayed A_2.

3. What can delay the A_2 enough to cause paradoxical splitting?

ANS.: a) Conduction defects that delay depolarization of the LV, such as complete LBBB and some types of Wolff-Parkinson-White preexcitation that imitate LBBB [54, 61, 83].

Note: The type of W-P-W preexcitation that acts like LBBB is one in which the initial conduction passes to the RV muscle first. This is known as type B, in which the QRS and delta wave in V_1 point predominantly posteriorly (i.e., they are predominantly negative).

b) A marked systolic gradient across the aortic valve, causing a delay in the fall of LV pressure to below aortic pressure, as in severe AS (see p. 217).

  Note: Poststenotic dilatation can contribute to the delay in A_2 by producing a loss of elastic recoil as well as by increasing the capacitance of the aorta [39A].

*c) Marked volume loads on the LV with only one outlet for systole (e.g., a large PDA).

*d) Rarely, acute ventricular dysfunction, as in acute myocardial infarction or acute myocarditis or during angina pectoris.

*e) Hypertension plus myocardial damage, especially if the increase in blood pressure is transiently higher than average for that patient. (See page 414 for the effect of increased blood pressure on the ejection time.)

4. What causes the widest reversed split?

  ANS.: Complete LBBB (i.e., with a QRS of 120 msec [0.12 sec] or longer). This is also the commonest cause of a reversed split and the only one that is easily recognized by the noncardiologist.

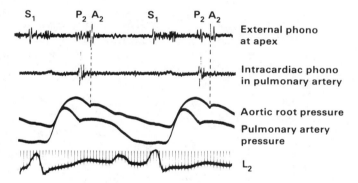

These simultaneous intra-arterial and phonocardiogram tracings are from a 59-year-old man in heart failure due to an idiopathic cardiomyopathy. Because of LBBB, the incisura of the pulmonary artery and its simultaneous P_2 comes before the aortic incisura and its simultaneous A_2. (His pulmonary artery systolic pressure was 35 mm Hg; his LV pressure, 120 mm Hg; and his cardiac index, 2.4.) These are catheter-tip electromanometer tracings, so that there are no tubing delays.

*5. What produces the delayed A_2 in LBBB?

  ANS.: The delay is usually due to prolongation of isovolumic contraction time. This has been shown in subjects with intermittent LBBB [10, 59]. Prolongation of the electromechanical interval (i.e., Q to onset of ventricular contraction [Q–C]), is prolonged in some patients but not in others. When the main left bundle is cut in dogs, the Q–C is always prolonged [82].

  Note: In transposition of the great vessels, the RV is the systemic ventricle. Therefore, a RBBB acts the same as a LBBB without a transposition and can cause a reversed split [84].

6. What is the significance of a reversed split in AS?

  ANS.: It implies that the gradient is at least 60 mm Hg or more. This is more reliable in congenital than in rheumatic stenosis because in the latter, myocardial damage may add extra delays to the A_2 by delaying the onset of the

aortic valve opening (i.e., the isovolumic contraction time may be prolonged).

> *Note:* In hypertrophic subaortic stenosis (HSS) there may be day-to-day
> variation in S_2 splitting, so that splitting may change from normal to
> single to reversed. The highest incidence of audible reversed splits
> apparently occurs in severe HSS, probably because there is no
> calcification of the valve to cause the A_2 to disappear [76].

* 7. When do reversed splits occur in patients with ischemic heart disease in the absence
   of LBBB?

   ANS.: It is rare to observe reversed splitting in chronic coronary disease [15]. It
   does, however, occur in the following situations:

   a) During acute angina or after exercise in the presence of significant coronary obstruction [22].

   b) During the first three days of acute myocardial infarction in about 15
   percent of patients [73].

   c) In patients over 70 years old with coronary disease and usually enough
   heart damage to produce an S_3 [3].

   d) In such patients who are hypertensive.

   > *Note:* a) Reversed splits occur in chronically hypertensive patients only
   > if they have myocardial damage as well. Proof of this is the
   > appearance of the reversed split with the development of early
   > failure and its disappearance after digitalis is given [1].
   >
   > b) A reversed split may also be detected during an acute hyperten-
   > sive crisis.
   >
   > c) The reversed split is so narrow in coronary disease problems
   > that the only sign of reversal may be a pure S_2 on inspiration
   > and an impure sound on expiration.
   >
   > d) The delay of the S_2 in patients with coronary disease is usually
   > due to a prolonged isovolumic contraction time.

8. What is the significance of expiratory splitting of the S_2?

   ANS.: Expiratory splitting indicates either a wide split, a fixed split, or a paradoxical split.

   > *Note:* Of normal subjects over age 50, only about 5 percent have expiratory
   > splitting of the S_2. Therefore, when expiratory splitting is found in
   > this age group, it may be abnormal and should be accounted for.

9. What can be confused with paradoxical splitting of the S_2?

   ANS.: a) An S_2-opening snap. (This is discussed in detail on page 237.)

   * b) A widely split A_2–P_2 in atrial fibrillation. After short diastoles there is
   narrow splitting. Inspiration, because of its vagolytic effect on the AV
   node, may cause a faster rate. Therefore, the split may narrow on inspiration because of the shorter R–R intervals. The widening on expiration
   and narrowing on inspiration will sound like a reversed split [41].

* 10. When will an electronic pacemaker in the RV in a patient with complete AV block
   not produce a reversed split? Why?

   ANS.: A reversed split will not occur when a P wave precedes the QRS. This is true
   because the booster pump action of the atrial kick affects the RV ejection
   time more than the LV ejection time, prolonging the RV ejection time more
   than that of the LV [58].

Eliciting and Recognizing Reversed Splits

1. What should make you suspect paradoxical or reversed splitting?
   ANS.: A split that widens on expiration and narrows on inspiration implies that the P_2 comes first.

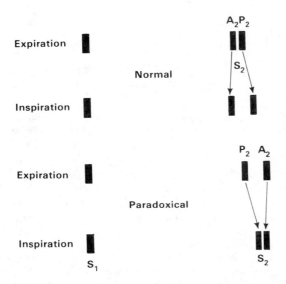

If the split narrows on inspiration, the P_2 must come first, and the split S_2 is reversed.

2. How can you confirm by auscultation that a wide split is reversed when the respiratory movements are so erratic that the respiratory changes cannot be recognized?
   ANS.: a) At the apex the A_2 is either the only sound heard, or it is the loudest component of the S_2 if both are heard there. Therefore, you should gradually move your stethoscope from the left sternal border toward the apex as you listen to the split second sound. The S_2 component that either disappears or becomes softer at the apex will be the P_2. If it is the second component that disappears or becomes softer, then you know that the order of components is A_2P_2. If, on the other hand, you hear the first component becoming softer or disappearing in relation to the second component, then the order is P_2A_2. Since the A_2 is usually the only component of S_2 heard at the second right interspace, the same maneuver can be used by gradually shifting your chest piece toward the second left interspace.
   b) The component that increases in loudness with inspiration is the P_2.

If the split is fixed at the left sternal border, it may be difficult to tell whether it has a normal or paradoxical sequence. Toward the apex, the component that becomes relatively softer must be the P_2.

c) Have the patient perform a Valsalva maneuver for about 10 seconds. During the strain, while blood is being withheld from both ventricles, the P_2 will come relatively early, and the reversed split will widen. In normal subjects, the S_2 split usually becomes narrower during a Valsalva strain.

Immediately on release of the Valsalva maneuver, more blood comes back to the right side, and the P_2 occurs later. If the split S_2 narrows, the order is P_2A_2. In normal subjects, the sudden return of blood into the RV causes an immediate widening of the S_2 split.

A few beats after the release of the Valsalva, the reversed split widens again markedly. In normal subjects, on the contrary, the split narrows as the excess pulmonary blood reaches the LV after traversing the lungs.

* 3. How can you confirm by phonocardiogram alone that a reversed split is present?
   ANS.: a) Simultaneous phonocardiograms at the second left interspace and apex will show the louder component or even the only component of the S_2 at the apex to be simultaneous with the second component at the sternal border.

       b) You can confirm by recording a phonocardiogram and carotid pulse tracing simultaneously that the split is reversed by timing the split with the carotid tracing. We know that the aortic component of the S_2 is almost simultaneous with the dicrotic notch (except for a slight delay in the carotid tracing). Therefore, any component that occurs before the aortic component is likely to be a P_2.

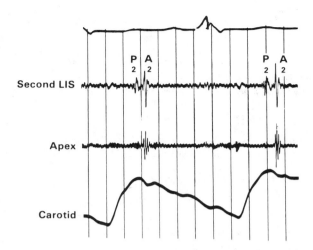

Note that (1) the two components of S$_2$ come before the carotid dicrotic notch, and (2) the second component of the S$_2$ is coincident with the only sound at the apex, which is always the A$_2$.

*4. What is meant by nonparadoxical reversed splitting?

ANS.: The order is P$_2$A$_2$, but the S$_2$ splits more widely on inspiration than on expiration. It can occur in the presence of LBBB in a patient with a cardiomyopathy or acute myocardial infarction. It is apparently due to an excessively early P$_2$ on inspiration and can be diagnosed only by simultaneous phonocardiograms or pulse tracings, but it can be suspected if a patient with a known LBBB has an apparently normal movement with a widely split S$_2$ [60].

REFERENCES

1. Abbott, J. A., and Whipple, G. H. Paradoxic splitting of the second heart sound in systemic hypertension. *Dis. Chest* 46:304, 1964.
2. Adolph, R. J., and Fowler, N. O. The second heart sound: A screening test for heart disease. *Mod. Concepts Cardiovasc. Dis.* 39:91, 1970.
3. Agnew T., et al. Delayed closure of the aortic valve in ischaemic heart disease. *Br. Heart J.* 29:775, 1967.
4. Anastassiades, P. C., et al. Aortic valve closure: Echocardiographic, phonocardiographic and hemodynamic assessment. *Am. Heart J.* 91:228, 1976.
5. Aygen, M. M., and Braunwald, E. The splitting of the second heart sound in normal subjects and in patients with congenital heart disease. *Circulation* 25:328, 1962.
6. Beck, W., Schrire, V., and Vogelpoel, L. Splitting of the second heart sound in constrictive pericarditis with observations on the mechanism of pulsus paradoxus. Am. Heart J. 64:765, 1962.
7. Berry, W. B., and Austen, W. G. Respiratory variations in the magnitude of the left to right shunt in experimental interatrial communications. *Am. J. Cardiol.* 14:201, 1964.
8. Blazek, W. V., and Bliss, H. A. The second sound in uncomplicated ventricular septal defect. *Med. Clin. North Am.* 50:111, 1966.
9. Bose, H. K., and Das, P. C. Importance of auscultation of the second heart sound in chronic cor pulmonale. *Indian Heart J.* 18:30, 1966.
10. Bourassa, M. G., Boiteau, G. M., and Allenstein, B. J. Hemodynamic studies during intermittent left bundle branch block. *Am. J. Cardiol.* 10:792, 1962.

11. Breen, W. J., and Rekate, A. C. Effect of posture on splitting of the second heart sound. *J.A.M.A.* 173:106, 1960.
12. Bruce, R. A., and John, G. G. Effect of upright posture and exercise on pulmonary hemodynamics in patients with central cardiovascular shunts. *Circulation* 16:776, 1957.
13. Castle, R. F. Variables affecting the splitting of the second heart sound in atrial septal defect. *Am. Heart J.* 73:468, 1967.
14. Castle, R. F., Hedden, C. A., and Davis, N. P., II. Variables affecting splitting of the second heart sound in normal children. *Pediatrics* 43:183, 1969.
15. Caulfield, W. H., Jr., Smith, R. H., and Franklin, R. B. The second heart sound in coronary artery disease. A phonocardiographic assessment. *Am. Heart J.* 77:197, 1969.
16. Cobbs, B. W., Jr. The second heart sound in pulmonary embolism and pulmonary hypertension. *Am. Heart J.* 71:843, 1966.
17. Cobbs, B. W., Jr. The second heart sound in pulmonary embolism and pulmonary hypertension. *Am. Heart J.* 71:843, 1966.
18. Cumming, G. R. Second heart sound after pulmonary arterial banding operation. *Br. Heart J.* 38:497, 1976.
19. Curtiss, E. I., et al. Alterations of right ventricular systolic time intervals by chronic pressure and volume overloading. *Circulation* 53:007, 1976.
20. Curtiss, E. I., et al. New concepts in physiologic splitting of the second heart sound. *Physiologic Principles of Heart Sounds and Murmurs*. Am. Heart Assoc. Monograph 46, 1975.
21. D'Cruz, I. A., et al. Stenotic lesions of the pulmonary arteries. *Am. J. Cardiol.* 13:441, 1964.
22. Dickerson, R. B., and Nelson, W. P. Paradoxical splitting of the second heart sound. *Am. Heart J.* 67:410, 1964.
23. Ehlers, K. H., et al. Wide splitting of the second heart sound without demonstrable heart disease. *Am. J. Cardiol.* 23:690, 1969.
24. Feruglio, G. A., and Gunton, R. W. Intracardiac phonocardiography in ventricular septal defect. *Circulation* 21:49, 1960.
25. Feruglio, G. A., and Sreenivasan, A. Intracardiac phonocardiogram in thirty cases of atrial septal defect. *Circulation* 22:1087, 1959.
26. Frye, R. L., et al. Anomalous pulmonary venous drainage of the right lung into the inferior vena cava. *Br. Heart J.* 24:969, 1962.
27. Gamboa, R., Hugenholtz, P. G., and Nadas, A. S. Accuracy of the phonocardiogram in assessing severity of aortic and pulmonic stenosis. *Circulation* 30:35, 1964.
28. Golinko, R. J., Kaplan, N., and Rudolph, A. M. The mechanism of pulsus paradoxus during acute pericardial tamponade. *J. Clin. Invest.* 42:249, 1963.
29. Hamby, R. I., Meron, J. M., and Roberts, G. S. Valsalva maneuver made easy. *Am. Heart J.* 82:838, 1971.
30. Harris, A., and Sutton, G. Second heart sound in normal subjects. *Br. Heart J.* 30:739, 1968.
31. Higgins, C. B., and Mulder, D. G. Tetralogy of Fallot in the adult. *Am. J. Cardiol.* 29:837, 1972.
32. Honey, M. Delayed closure of the pulmonary valve. *Lancet* 5:318, 1966.
33. Johnston, R. R., et al. Effect of intermittent right bundle branch block on right ventricular contractility. *Am. J. Cardiol.* 1:813, 1966.
34. Kardalinos, A. The second heart sound. *Am. Heart J.* 64:610, 1962.
35. Karnegis, J. N., and Wang, Y. The phonocardiogram in idiopathic dilatation of the pulmonary artery. *Am. J. Cardiol.* 14:75, 1964.
36. Kaufmann, G., Rutishauser, W., and Hegglin, R. Heart sounds in atrial tumors. *Am. J. Cardiol.* 8:350, 1951.
37. Kinoshita, M., et al. Phonocardiographic findings of mitral insufficiency due to ruptures chordae tendineae. *CV Sound Bull.* 5:263, 1975.
38. Kraus, Y., et al. Splitting of the second heart sound in partial anomalous pulmonary venous connection with intact interatrial septum. In *Proceedings of Fourth Asian-Pacific Congress of Cardiologists*. New York: Academic, 1969. P. 147.
39. Kumar, S., and Luisada, A. A. Second heart sound in atrial septal defect. *Am. J. Cardiol.* 28:168, 1971.
40. Laniado, S., et al. Hemodynamic correlates of the normal aortic valve echogram. A study of sound, flow, and motion. *Circulation* 54:729, 1976.

41. Leacham, R. D., Talat, A., and Cokkinos, V. P. Narrowed splitting of the second heart sound on inspiration in patients with giant left atrium. *Chest* 60:151, 1971.
42. Leatham, A., and Gray, I. Auscultatory and phonocardiographic signs of atrial septal defect. *Br. Heart J.* 18:193, 1956.
42A. Leighton, R. F., et al. Right and left ventricular systolic time intervals: Effects of heart rate, respiration and atrial pacing. *Am. J. Cardiol.* 27:66, 1971.
43. Macieira-Coelho, E., and Guimaraes, C. Phonocardiography in atrial septal defects of the ostium secundum type. *Cardiologia* 44:78, 1964.
44. MacKenzie, J. C., et al. Postural variation in second sound splitting. *Chest* 63:56, 1973.
45. Mills, P., et al. Non-invasive diagnosis of subpulmonary outflow tract obstruction. *Br. Heart J.* 43:276, 1980.
46. Moss, W. G., and Johnson, V. Differential effects of stretch upon the stroke volumes of the right and left ventricles. *Am. J. Physiol.* 139:52, 1943.
47. Nandi, P. S., Pigott, V. M., and Spodick, D. H. Sequential cardiac responses during the respiratory cycle: Patterns of change in systolic intervals. *Chest* 63:380, 1973.
48. Nelson, W. P., and North, R. L. Splitting of the second heart sound in adults forty years and older. *Am. J. Med. Sci.* 56:805, 1967.
49. O'Toole, J. D., et al. The mechanism of splitting of the second heart sound in atrial septal defect. *Circulation* 56:1047, 1977.
50. Perloff, J. K., and Harvey, W. P. Mechanisms of fixed splitting of the second heart sound. *Circulation* 18:998, 1958.
51. Perloff, J. K., and Lebauer, E. J. Auscultatory and phonocardiographic manifestations of isolated stenosis of the pulmonary artery and its branches. *Br. Heart J.* 31:314, 1969.
52. Piemme, T. E., Barnett, O., and Dexter, L. Relationship of heart sounds to acceleration of blood flow. *Circ. Res.* 18:303, 1966.
53. Roach, M. R. Changes in arterial distensibility as a cause of poststenotic dilatation. *Am. J. Cardiol.* 12:802, 1963.
54. Rodriguez-Torres, R., Yao, A. C., and Lynfield, J. Significance of split heart sounds in children with Wolff-Parkinson-White syndrone. *Bull. N.Y. Acad. Med.* 44:511, 1968.
55. Ruskin, J., et al. Pressure-flow studies in man: Effect of respiration on left ventricular stroke volume. *Circulation* 48:79, 1973.
56. Sabbah, H. N., et al. The aortic closure sound in pure aortic insufficiency. *Circulation* 56:859, 1977.
57. Sainani, G. S., and Luisada, A. A. "Mapping" the precordium. *Am. J. Cardiol.* 19:788, 1967.
58. Sakai, H., et al. Influence of the atrial contraction on the left ventricular systolic time intervals (LVSTI) and the modes of the splitting of the second heart sound in patients with right ventricular pacemakers. *J. Cardiography* 9:363, 1979.
59. Sakamoto, T., et al. QRS dependence of the split interval of the second heart sound in complete right and left bundle branch block. *Jap. Heart J.* 8:459, 1967.
60. Sakamoto, T., et al. Methoxamine induced "non-paradoxical" reversed splitting. *Jap. Heart J.* 8:642, 1967.
61. Sato, H., et al. Second heart sound in WPW syndrome with special reference to the accessory pathway. *J. Cardiography* 7:225, 1977.
62. Schrire, V., and Vogelpoel, L. The role of the dilated pulmonary artery in abnormal splitting of the second heart sound. *Am. Heart J.* 63:501, 1962.
63. Shafter, H. A. Splitting of the second heart sound. *Am. J. Cardiol.* 6:1013, 1960.
64. Shah, P. M., and Slodki, S. J. The Q-II interval. *Circulation* 29:551, 1964.
65. Shaver, J. A., et al. Sound pressure correlates of the second heart sound. *Circulation* 49:316, 1974.
66. Shuler, R. H., et al. The differential effects of respiration on the left and right ventricles. *Am. J. Physiol.* 137:620, 1942.
67. Singh, S. P. Unusual splitting of the second heart sound in pulmonary stenosis. *Am. J. Cardiol.* 25:28, 1970.
68. Slodki, S. J., Hussain, A. T., and Luisada, A. A. The Q-II interval. III. A study of the second heart sound in old age. *J. Am. Geriatr. Soc.* 17:673, 1969.
69. Stein, P. D., Sabbah, H. N., and Blick, E. F. Dependence of the intensity of the aortic closure sound upon the rate of ventricular diastolic relaxation and ventricular performance. *Am. J. Cardiol.* 39:287, 1977.

70. Stein, P. D., et al. Hemodynamic and anatomic determinants of relative differences in amplitude of the aortic and pulmonary components of the second heart sound. *Am. J. Cardiol.* 42:539, 1978.

71. Stein, P. D., et al. Frequency spectrum of the aortic component of the second heart sound in patients with normal valves, aortic stenosis and aortic porcine zenografts. *Am. J. Cardiol.* 46:48, 1980.

72. Stein, P. D., et al. Exploration of cause of low-intensity aortic component of second sound in nonhypotensive patients with poor ventricular performance. *Circulation* 57:590, 1978.

73. Stock, E. Auscultation and phonocardiography in acute myocardial infarction. *Med. J. Aust.* 1:1060, 1966.

74. Sutton, G., Harris, A., and Leatham, A. Second heart sound in pulmonary hypertension. *Br. Heart J.* 30:743, 1968.

75. Tanaka, C., et al. Phonocardiographic findings in adult ASD. *CV Sound Bull.* 5:107, 1975.

76. Tavel, M. E. Clinical phonocardiography. *J.A.M.A.* 203:123, 1968.

77. VanBogaert, A. Role of the valves in the genesis of normal heart sounds. *Cardiologia* 52:330, 1968.

78. Victorica, B. E., Gessner, I. H., and Schiebler, G. L. Phonocardiographic findings in persistent truncus arteriosus. *Br. Heart J.* 30:812, 1968.

79. Wang, Y. Wide fixed splitting of the second heart sound and right ventricular diastolic overload. *Circulation* 36 (Suppl.):11, 1967.

80. Weinstein, P. B., et al. Mechanism for splitting of the second heart sound in atrial septal defects. *Circulation* 36 (Suppl.):11, 1967.

81. Weisse, A. B., et al. Intensity of the normal second heart sound components in their traditional auscultatory areas. *Am. J. Med.* 43:171, 1967.

82. Wennemark, J. R., Blake, D. F., and Keydie, P. Cardiodynamic effects of experimental bundle branch block in the dog. *Circ. Res.* 10:280, 1962.

83. Zuberbuhler, J. R., and Bauersfeld, S. R. Paradoxical splitting of the second heart sound in the Wolff-Parkinson-White syndrome. *Am. Heart J.* 70:595, 1965.

84. Zuberbuhler, J. R., Bauersfeld, S. R., and Pontius, R. G. Paradoxic splitting of the second sound with transposition of the great vessels. *Am. Heart J.* 74:816, 1967.

10. *The Opening Snap*

MECHANISM AND TIMING

1. Draw a simultaneous normal (left ventricular) (LV) and left atrial (LA) pressure curve. At what point on the curve does the mitral valve open?

    ANS.: The mitral valve opens when LV pressure drops below LA pressure. The normal peak LA pressure is about 10 mm Hg. Therefore, when LV pressure drops to about 9 mm Hg, the mitral valve should open.

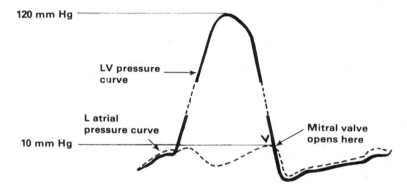

Note that the left atrial V wave rise is abruptly interrupted by LV pressure's falling below left atrial pressure and opening the mitral valve.

2. Draw a LV, LA, and simultaneous aortic pressure curve. Which left-sided event produces a sound just before the mitral valve opens?

    ANS.: Closure of the aortic valve produces the A_2 about 100 msec (0.10 sec) before the mitral valve opens. This 100-msec interval takes about as long as it takes to say "pa-pa" as quickly as possible.

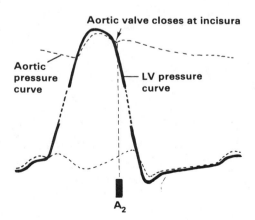

The A_2 is simultaneous with the aortic valve incisura and occurs shortly before the LV pressure drops below left atrial pressure, to open the mitral valve. The interval between the aortic valve closure (A_2) and the opening of the mitral valve is the isovolumic relaxation time.

3. What is usually necessary before the opening of the mitral valve becomes audible?
   ANS.: At least some mitral stenosis (MS). MS is due primarily to fibrous thickening and often to calcification of the margins of the mitral leaflets, especially
   the large anterior leaflet. The commissures are also fused by fibrosis or
   calcium. The mitral valve belly may act like a sail that billows downward
   into a dome in diastole as the LV attempts to "suck" left atrial blood into the
   LV cavity. This sudden diastolic doming causes the anterior leaflet to bulge
   downward with a snap [6].

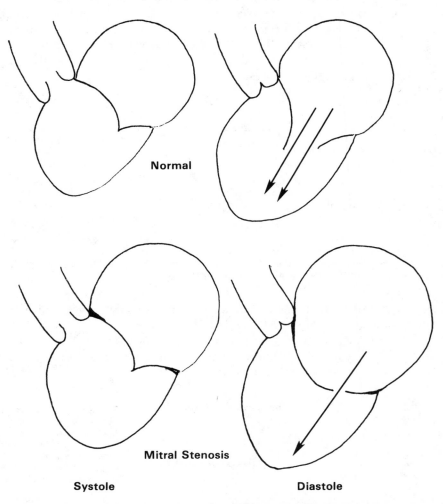

Normal

Mitral Stenosis

Systole   **Diastole**

The opening snap is produced by the belly of the stenotic anterior leaflet bulging or doming
downward with a jerk to produce a clicking or snapping sound. The anterior leaflet, therefore,
must also close with a snap as it domes upward. The posterior leaflet has too short a ring-to-
free edge distance to produce a "belly snap."

*Note: a) Torrential flow through the mitral valve may on rare occasions produce an opening snap (OS) in the absence of MS. It has been recorded on rare occasions in ventricular septal defect (VSD), persistent ductus arteriosus, tricuspid atresia, thyrotoxicosis, and after a Blalock-Taussig operation for tetralogy of Fallot.

b) In congenital MS in infants there is rarely an OS because congenitally abnormal leaflets usually do not have pliable bellies.

c) An OS-like sound has been heard in patients who have a prolapsed mitral valve either with a click or with both a click and a systolic murmur [1, 7, 18, 35]. Because the sound may be simultaneous with the D point on an echocardiogram, it is probably due to recoaptation of a prolapsed posterior leaflet with the anterior leaflet when the LV pressure falls below the LA pressure [1, 7, 35]. When, however, it is associated with a "floppy valve," i.e., marked anterior leaflet prolapse and a severe pansystolic mitral regurgitation (MR) murmur, the OS is synchronous with the E point of the mitral echocardiogram and is due to marked anterior leaflet prolapse [18]. These sounds are best heard at the apex.

d) An OS-like sound has also been heard about 70 msec after the A_2 in patients with massive ascites. It occurs simultaneously with the onset of opening of the mitral valve on echophonocardiograms and is thought to be due to the heart striking against the high diaphragm because it disappears on inspiration and when the ascites is gone [13].

e) The early S_3 of a left atrial myxoma called the "tumor plop" often occurs only 0.07 to 0.11 sec after the A_2, which is the same range as the OS from the A_2 [3].

4. Why is the audible opening of the mitral valve called an opening snap?

ANS.: Because most of the time the sound is a short, high-frequency (see **frequency**), crisp crack, click, or snap.

5. Why must it be the anterior leaflet that is responsible for the OS of MS?

ANS.: Not only is the anterior leaflet three times broader than the posterior leaflet, but also the surface chordae tendineae of the anterior leaflet are attached to the peripheral zone of the valve, leaving the bellies intact, whereas the surface chordae of the posterior leaflets are attached to its entire ventricular surface [34]. Therefore, even though MS tends to convert the two semi-independent leaflets into a continuous funnel-like sleeve with a fish-mouth opening, the belly of the anterior leaflet contributes most to the valve sounds, i.e., the loud S_1 and the OS.

*Note: An OS can occur with dominant MR if the regurgitation is due to a thickened, rolled, immobile posterior (mural) leaflet and if the anterior (septal) leaflet still has a mobile belly [20].

6. What do we call the interval between the closing of the aortic valve and the opening of the mitral valve?

ANS.: The **isovolumic relaxation** period.

---

*Material marked with an asterisk is for reference and for advanced students in cardiology.
Boldface type indicates that the term is explained in the Glossary.

7. What do cardiologists call the isovolumic relaxation interval between the aortic closure sound and the OS sound?

ANS.: The A_2–OS interval or, simply, the 2–OS interval.

> *Note:* When referring to a tricuspid OS, it is necessary to say the "P_2 to the tricuspid OS interval." When no specific mention of which side of the heart is meant, the 2–OS interval refers to the A_2 to mitral OS interval because a tricuspid OS is relatively rare.

RELATION BETWEEN THE 2–OS AND THE SEVERITY OF MITRAL STENOSIS

1. What controls the duration of isovolumic relaxation, or the 2–OS interval?

ANS.: a) The pressure in the LA at the time the mitral valve opens.

    b) The heart rate. The more rapid the heart rate, the shorter the 2–OS interval because
       1) Isovolumic relaxation is faster under the influence of the increased sympathetic tone or catecholamines that cause the faster rate, and
       2) Left atrial pressure is higher owing to the reduced atrial emptying time with the short diastoles.

    c) The stiffness of the mitral valve (due mostly to calcium) [23]. (See Question 5 below.)

    d) The rate and strength of relaxation of the myocardium, i.e., the state of myocardial function or inotropic state (contractility) of the myocardium.

    e) The pressure at which the aortic valve closes (near systolic pressure).

2. What is the relationship between the degree of MS and the height of the V wave in the left atrium?

ANS.: The greater the stenosis, the greater the obstruction to flow and thus the slower and more incomplete the emptying of the left atrium. Therefore, the greater the MS, the higher the V wave.

> *Note:* This will be clear only if you recall that the V wave is built up during ventricular systole when the mitral valve is closed. If the V wave begins to build up from a high pressure, that wave will rise even higher. If the left atrium did not empty well in diastole due to MS, the V wave will start to build up from an already high pressure.

3. Does a high left atrial pressure make the 2–OS interval shorter or longer? Why?

ANS.: Shorter, because the LV pressure does not have to fall so far to open the mitral valve after closure of the aortic valve or A_2.

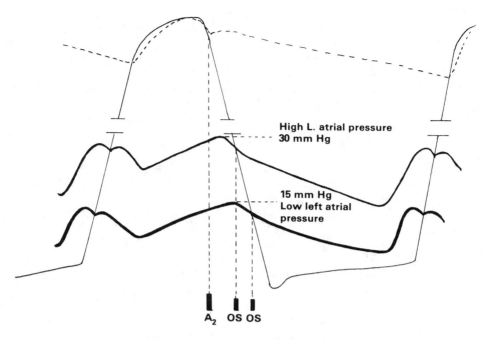

High L. atrial pressure
30 mm Hg

15 mm Hg
Low left atrial
pressure

A₂ OS OS

Note that the distance between the A_2 and the OS is shorter with the higher left atrial pressure.

*Note: The high V wave caused by concomitant MR does not necessarily cause an early OS, probably because the OS in MS occurs not at the peak but early on the Y descent, and if MR is also present, the OS may occur farther down on the Y descent [26]. Even though the descent of the mitral leaflets begins at the crossover of left ventricular and left atrial pressures, maximum excursion of the leaflets may take another 25–70 msec. The OS occurs at the moment of maximum excursion. It is probably this valvular descent before the OS that expands the left atrial capacity and allows the beginning of the Y descent to occur before the OS. With prosthetic mitral valves, the prosthetic descent may be so rapid that MR and a high V wave do cause an early opening click.

4. Will the beat that follows a long diastole in atrial fibrillation produce a long or a short 2–OS? Why?

ANS.: It produces a long 2–OS because a long diastole gives more time to empty the left atrium, allowing its pressure to drop. The next systole will begin and end with a lower left atrial pressure, thus making a long 2–OS.

5. Will a very stiff mitral valve make the OS earlier or later, i.e., will the 2–OS interval be shortened or lengthened? Why?

ANS.: The 2–OS interval will be lengthened, because the stiffer the valve, the lower the LV pressure will have to fall below atrial pressure before it can "suck" the valve open [23]. Stiffness refers not to the degree of stenosis but to the degree of *mobility* of the belly of the anterior leaflet.

*Note: Calcification also has been shown to slow the velocity of mitral valve opening. The 2–OS interval is the sum of the true isovolumic relaxation period (A_2 to the beginning of the opening of the mitral valve) plus mitral valve excursion. Therefore, a high left atrial pressure will shorten the true isovolumic relaxation time, whereas valve calcification and stiffness will lengthen the mitral valve excursion period. The result will be a longer than expected 2–OS for the degree of MS [14, 15]. (Echophonocardiographic correlations have shown that the true isovolumic relaxation period [A_2 to the onset of mitral valve opening] correlates better with MS severity than does the 2–OS interval.)

6. List the causes of a late OS aside from a mild degree of MS or a heavily calcified mitral valve.

ANS.: a) Bradycardia. This prolongs the isovolumic relaxation time mainly because long diastoles also allow more left atrial emptying and lower left atrial pressure. (Bradycardia may also decrease the slope of fall of LV pressure.)

b) Poor myocardial function due to either damage or aging. This causes prolongation of the isovolumic relaxation time. (Isovolumic relaxation time increases strikingly with age [12].)

c) Aortic regurgitation (AR). This is presumably due to the aortic regurgitation jet striking the underbelly of the anterior mitral leaflet and preventing rapid downward excursion. (AR may even eliminate an OS.)

d) A low left atrial pressure due to a large left atrium and severe failure with low flow.

e) High aortic pressure. If the aortic valve closes at a high pressure, more time will be required for the LV pressure to drop below left atrial pressure, to open the mitral valve and create the OS.

Note: At an aortic systolic pressure of more than 130 mm Hg, the 2–OS interval will be unreliable in indicating the degree of MS [5]. (Remember that aortic valve closure and the A_2 occur at near aortic systolic pressure.)

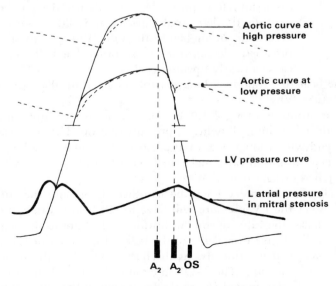

Note that the higher the aortic pressure, the longer the A_2–OS interval.

7. Which is more reliable in predicting the degree of MS, a narrow 2–OS or a wide one? Why?

ANS.: A narrow 2–OS is more reliable because there is not much besides a tight MS or a tachycardia that can narrow a 2–OS interval, whereas there are at least five causes besides mild MS for a wide 2–OS.

*Note: a) Unequivocally tight MS is suggested by a resting 2–OS of 50 msec or less [32].

The lowest normal isovolumic relaxation time (measured from the aortic incisura to the LV–left atrial pressure curve crossover) is 55 msec [2]. Because the mitral OS is later than the crossover of pressure by about 40 msec, the shortest 2–OS interval with almost normal left atrial pressures would be about 95 msec.

b) A supine post-exercise 2–OS of 80 msec or more suggests mild MS (mean left atrial pressure of not more than 12 mm Hg). If the 2–OS after exercise is 50 msec or less, the stenosis is severe (mean left atrial pressure of at least 25 mm Hg [10]).

8. Without a phonocardiograph, how can you estimate the width of the 2–OS interval?

ANS.: a) If you say "pa-pa" as quickly as possible, you will be separating the sounds by about 100 msec (0.01 sec). This is a wide 2–OS interval.

b) If you say "pa-da" as quickly as possible, you should be able to separate the sounds by about 50–70 msec (0.05–0.07 sec). This is a narrow 2–OS and suggests moderate to tight MS.

Note: You should time yourself on a phonocardiogram. Some physicians say "pa-pa" so slowly that the syllables are really 120 msec apart, which is the distance of an S_2 to an S_3. (See page 205 for imitations of intervals between 30 and 100 msec.)

THE LOUDNESS OF THE OPENING SNAP

1. Other than an obese or emphysematous chest, what can cause a soft or absent OS despite significant MS?

ANS.: 1. The mitral valve may be too calcified for the bellies to snap into their maximal open position.

* Note: a) Fibrosis alone is rarely responsible for a soft OS.

b) A calcified mitral valve tends to cause a loss of high frequencies [4]. This is the opposite to degeneration of a bioprosthesis, which loses low frequencies when it becomes fibrotic.

2. Extremely low flow due to
   a) Exceptional severity of the stenosis.
   b) Secondary pulmonary hypertension.
   c) Concomitant aortic or tricuspid valve disease.
   d) Myocardial failure.

3. A large RV (usually due to pulmonary hypertension or tricuspid regurgitation) that pushes the LV away from the chest wall.

4. Moderate to severe AR that can "cushion" the mitral valve anterior leaflet as it domes downward.

        * *Note:* When a patient with AR and MS sits up, you may hear a soft OS for the first time, probably because the decreased venous return of the sitting position reduces the amount of AR.

2. Why will severe pulmonary hypertension in a patient with MS produce a low flow and therefore a soft OS?

    ANS.: Because there are then two causes of a low flow: the obstruction at the mitral valve and obstruction at the pulmonary arterioles.

        * *Note:* a) A reduced flow occurs with pulmonary hypertension, probably because elevation of the RV pressure does not completely compensate for the high resistance produced by the pulmonary arteriolar constriction. (It may be that compensatory mechanisms in biological systems are rarely if ever complete.)

            b) Further proof that low flow can prevent the appearance of an OS is the observation that standing can cause a soft OS to disappear, and raising the legs can make it louder.

3. How often does a mitral commissurotomy eliminate the OS?

    ANS.: Probably in not more than half the cases.

        Note: Normally, a porcine valve may produce a soft OS in two-thirds of patients. The presence or absence of an OS reveals nothing about porcine valve malfunction [24].

HOW TO TELL AN A_2–P_2 FROM AN A_2–OS

Similarities Between a P_2 and the OS

1. Where on the chest wall is the OS usually best heard? Why is it often confused with a P_2?

    ANS.: An OS is usually best heard between the apex and the left sternal border or at the left sternal border. This is not too surprising when one considers that the anterior leaflet of the mitral valve, which creates most of the sound, makes its opening motion in a line that points almost directly toward the left sternal border. A P_2 is also best heard at the left sternal border, and because the chest wall may keep the stethoscope farther away from the heart when one is listening at the upper left sternal border, the P_2 may be better heard at the third or fourth left interspace just as with an OS.

    Peculiarly, an OS can often be heard well at the second right interspace, even if it is only moderately loud at the left lower sternal border. This may be because the mitral valve is in fibrous continuity with the aortic root, which may be more anterior than usual due to the dilated left atrium. A louder than normal P_2, however, may also be heard at the second right interspace.

    Note: Like all sounds and murmurs, a loud OS can be heard anywhere on the chest wall. An OS may even be grade 6 in loudness.

  * 2. How does the range of a 2–OS interval differ from that of an A_2–P_2 interval?

    ANS.: They do not differ much. The 2–OS may range from 30–100 msec (0.03–0.10 sec). Although the A_2–P_2 may be as long as 100 msec, it is often as short as 20 msec, which would be unusual for a 2–OS.

3. How does the quality, frequency, and duration of an OS differ from that of a P_2?

ANS.: They do not differ much. Occasionally the OS may consist mostly of low frequencies, especially if the valve is heavily calcified.

Differences Between the A_2–P_2 and the 2–OS

1. Is a loud P_2 ever as loud at the apex as it is at the left sternal border?

   ANS.: No. However, an occasional chest shape may attenuate all sounds at the left sternal border, but if it allows the apex beat to fall between the ribs in the left lateral decubitus position a P_2 may be heard as loud at the apex as at the left sternal border.

2. When is an OS louder or as loud at the apex as it is at the left sternal border?

   ANS.: As a rule, this occurs only when the LV is dilated, or if a rib has been removed in previous heart surgery. These conditions place the stethoscope almost directly on the heart at the apex.

   OS VS P_2 RULE NO. 1: If the second component of a split S_2 is louder or as loud at the apex as elsewhere, it is probably an OS.

3. How does the effect of respiration affect the loudness of the P_2 and of the OS?

   ANS.: Inspiration makes the P_2 louder (more blood is drawn into the right side of the heart with inspiration) and the OS softer (blood is withheld from the left atrium on inspiration so that less blood flows through the mitral valve).

   Note: a) The P_2 can be expected to become louder on inspiration only at the left *lower* sternal border because all sounds tend to become softer on inspiration high on the chest.

   b) Lung expansion between the stethoscope and the heart adds to the hemodynamic effect of inspiration on the OS—i.e., it exaggerates the inspiratory decrease in the loudness of the OS.

   OS VS P_2 RULE NO. 2: If the second component of an S_2 split becomes softer on inspiration at the left lower sternal border (in the absence of LBBB), it is probably a mitral OS.

*4. When will a 2–OS sound like a reversed split?

   ANS.: A 2–OS interval sometimes appears to widen on expiration but actually does not, i.e., it is an illusion. The pulmonary component on expiration moves slightly toward the aortic component and, therefore, away from the OS. This gives the illusion of a wider splitting of the 2–OS interval on expiration.

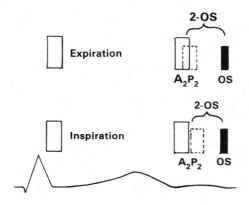

Note that the respiration will give the impression of a reversed split, because the P_2 moves away from the OS on expiration and toward the OS on inspiration.

Note: a) Sinus arrhythmia may contribute to the widening of the 2–OS on expiration by slowing the heart rate on expiration.

b) Even though the left atrial pressure rises on expiration and therefore should make the 2–OS shorter, the aortic pressure also rises on expiration, thereby keeping the 2–OS about the same.

OS VS P$_2$ RULE NO. 3. A widely split S$_2$ on inspiration that tends to become wider on expiration is an OS in the absence of LBBB.

5. How can you recognize an A$_2$, P$_2$, and OS as three distinct sounds in one place?

ANS.: A triple S$_2$ can often be recognized along the left sternal border in MS by listening for a snare-drum effect, a "trill," or a tongue-rolling Spanish R effect with the second sound. This snare-drum triple S$_2$ is most likely to be heard during inspiration, when the P$_2$ pulls away from the A$_2$. But occasionally the OS is so soft that it can be heard only on expiration, and if the split second sound A$_2$–P$_2$ happens to remain split on expiration, you will hear the snare-drum or trill effect only on expiration.

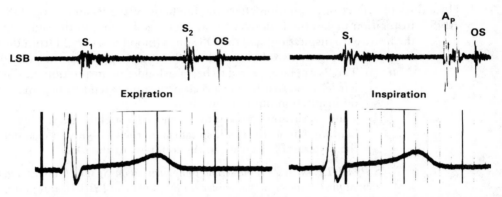

On inspiration, the S$_2$ split opened up into its A$_2$ and P$_2$ components. Together with the OS, a triple second sound is heard that produces a snare-drum effect.

OS VS P$_2$ RULE NO. 4: A triple second sound, in which the three sounds are close enough together to sound like a snare-drum, implies that an OS is present as the final component.

6. What effect does standing have on the 2–OS interval? Why?

ANS.: It widens it. The pooling of blood in the legs decreases venous return to the left atrium. This lowers the pressure behind the obstructed mitral valve. You have already learned why a low pressure in the left atrium makes a wide 2–OS interval.

7. What effect does standing have on the A$_2$–P$_2$ interval? Why?

ANS.: The A$_2$–P$_2$ interval either remains the same or narrows [28]. The reason for this is described on page 214. However, in brief, although there is a decrease in volume to both ventricles, the RV responds to the decrease more than does the LV.

Note: One proof that the RV responds to filling pressure changes to a greater extent than does the LV is seen in patients with RV pacemakers and complete AV block but without valvular disease. When the P wave falls before the QRS to give a good atrial kick, the P$_2$ occurs later than the A_2, i.e., reversed splits become narrower, single, or even normal [27].

> *OS VS P_2 RULE NO. 5: If a split second sound becomes wider on standing, its second component is an OS.*

8. Why should the presence of an OS imply that the first sound should have a snapping quality?

   ANS.: The stiffness and doming of the valve that produced the OS should also make a snapping S_1. In other words, a mitral valve that has an OS usually also has a "closing snap."

   > Note: A loud S_1 and closing snap may be present even with a completely immobile mitral valve that is too stiff to produce an OS. Therefore, a loud S_1 with a closing snap suggests the presence of an OS. A soft S_1 denies the presence of an OS.

   > *OS VS P_2 RULE NO. 6: If the S_1 is very soft or only a low-pitched thud, the second component of the S_2 is not likely to be an OS.*

Summary of Methods of Differentiating an A_2–P_2 from a 2–OS

1. If the second component of a split S_2 is as loud at the apex as at the left sternal border, it is probably an OS.
2. If the second component of an S_2 is only moderately loud and yet is heard at the second right interspace as well as at the apex, it is an OS (in the absence of LBBB).
3. If the second component decreases with inspiration, it is an OS (in the absence of LBBB).
4. If the split tends to narrow on inspiration, it is a 2–OS (in the absence of LBBB).
5. If there is a triple second sound at the left sternal border, an OS is present.
6. If the split widens on standing, the second component is an OS.
7. If the S_1 is soft or muffled, the second component of the split S_2 is probably not a mitral OS.

Differential Diagnosis of an Opening Snap

1. What can imitate a late OS?

   ANS.: a) The early S_3 of constrictive pericarditis (see p. 260). This is the "pericardial knock."

   b) The tumor plop of a left atrial myxoma (see p. 258).

   *c) A vegetation on the mitral valve that moves rapidly from the left atrium into the LV and strikes the base of the ventricular septum (very rare) [33].

---

*THE TRICUSPID OPENING SNAP

*1. When will a tricuspid OS be present in the absence of tricuspid stenosis (TS)?

   ANS.: a) When a large volume enters the RV by way of the tricuspid valve. With an ASD or anomalous pulmonary venous drainage into the right atrium, partial or complete, the torrential flow may cause a tricuspid OS along the left sternal border, 30–50 msec from the P_2. (It may be heard in more than three-quarters of patients over age 35 with ASD [30].)

Note: a) In one study a tricuspid OS was found only in patients with pulmonary-systemic flow ratios of 2:1 or more [25]. The left-to-right shunt in another study was 1½ to 2 times greater in patients with the tricuspid OS than in those without [11]. However, an OS can occur even with a reduced left-to-right shunt if the flow is reduced owing to pulmonary hypertension, provided that TR is present to add to the volume of blood flowing through the tricuspid valve in diastole. The dilated and hypertrophied RV may stretch the ring and stiffen the leaflets enough to cause an OS [11].

b) With a deformed tricuspid valve, as in Ebstein's anomaly, the second component of a widely split S_2 is synchronous with the echocardiographic maximum opening point of the tricuspid valve [9].

*2. How does the effect of respiration on the mitral and tricuspid opening snaps differ?

ANS.: A tricuspid OS becomes louder on inspiration because more blood flows through the tricuspid valve on inspiration. This fact is helpful because when a huge RV takes over the usual site of the apex beat, a tricuspid OS may be as loud at the apex area as at the left sternal border, thus mimicking a mitral OS.

*3. Which opens first, the tricuspid valve or the mitral valve?

ANS.: The tricuspid valve usually opens first when it is normal. However, in the presence of both MS and TS, the mitral OS usually occurs first because the MS is usually much more severe, making left atrial pressure higher than right atrial pressure [17].

Note: a) In the presence of mild MS, the tricuspid OS may occur prior to the mitral OS. This is expected in view of the fact that the isovolumic relaxation time of the RV is shorter than that of the LV by about 50–80 msec.

b) In Ebstein's anomaly, the tricuspid OS occurs late, presumably because the smaller than normal RV not only contracts poorly but also expands poorly.

*4. How can you distinguish a tricuspid OS from a widely split A_2–P_2?

ANS.: a) Listen for the snare-drum effect of a triple S_2 with the last sound becoming louder on inspiration.

b) Ask the patient to stand. An A_2–P_2 may remain the same or become narrower when the patient is standing, but an A_2–tricuspid OS interval either remains the same or becomes wider.

---

*THE Q–1 AND C–1 INTERVALS

*1. What is meant by the Q–1 interval?

ANS.: It is the time from the onset of the QRS complex to the first major component of the S_1, i.e., it is the Q–M_1 interval. It actually consists of two shorter intervals—namely, the Q–C and the C–1 intervals. The Q–C interval is the time between the onset of electrical activity and the onset of mechanical activity of the LV (electromechanical interval). This interval varies from person to person, ranging from 10–70 msec. The C–1 interval is the time between the onset of LV contraction and the closure of the mitral valves. This is the preisovolumic contraction period. It is also known as the deformation time.

> Note: a) The C–1 interval is better than the Q–1 interval for assessing the severity of MS because the C–1 eliminates the unknown factor of the electromechanical interval.
>
> b) Some factors that control the C–1 interval are
>   1) The ability of the LV to contract rapidly and strongly (inotropic state).
>   2) The difference between left atrial and LV pressure at the beginning of contraction.
>   3) The stiffness or resistance of the mitral valve.

*2. Why does MS prolong the Q–1 interval?

ANS.: The stiff mitral valve and the high left atrial to LV pressure gradient forces the LV to rise to a higher pressure and therefore to contract for a longer period of time before it can close the mitral valve.

> Note: a) A left atrial myxoma will also prolong the Q–1 interval because the tumor usually prolapses downward through the mitral valve in diastole, producing obstruction to flow and a high left atrial pressure [3].
>
> b) Some other factors known to prolong the Q–1 interval are hypertension, a poorly functioning myocardium, shunt flow through a VSD or patent ductus arteriosus, and conduction defects such as RBBB, LBBB, anterior divisional blocks, and Wolff-Parkinson-White preexcitation.

*3. In MS with atrial fibrillation, how does the Q–1 vary with various diastolic lengths, and how can this variation be used to determine the severity of the MS?

ANS.: The shorter the previous diastole, the longer the Q–1, because with short diastoles the left atrium cannot empty well through a stenotic valve. This results in a very high left atrial pressure at the beginning of the next ventricular contraction, and thus the ensuing Q–1 interval will be prolonged. (In patients without MS, atrial fibrillation does not cause significantly different Q–1 intervals.)

If the Q–1 does not become longer after 700–msec cycles, the MS is mild. If the Q–1 requires at least 1-sec cycles to stabilize, it is probably severe.

---

*The Q–1 Minus the 2–OS Interval

*1. How can the Q–1 and the 2–OS intervals be used together to estimate MS severity more accurately than either one alone?

ANS.: Because as MS increases in severity the Q–1 becomes longer and the 2–OS becomes shorter, the index (Q–1 minus 2–OS) becomes increasingly large as the MS worsens [36]. It has been found that with heart rates of between 70 and 80 a Q–1 minus 2–OS index of 20 msec or more always indicates severe MS [22, 29]. If the index is less than 20 msec, it may or may not be associated with severe MS, because the index may be made invalid by factors that prolong the 2–OS excessively [23].

Another way of using the Q–1 and 2–OS index is to correlate the Q–1/2–OS ratio with left atrial mean pressure. One study found the correlation coefficient to be 0.90 [38]. The calculated regression equation was

17.8 (Q–1)/(2–OS) + 1.33

To use the ratio, the systolic blood pressure should not be more than 150 mm Hg, and in patients with atrial fibrillation the ventricular rate should be between 70 and 90 per minute.

*2. In the presence of atrial fibrillation, how can the Q–1 and 2–OS tell you whether or not the mitral valve is pliable enough to permit a valvotomy?

ANS.: When the Q–1 changes inversely and the 2–OS changes directly with the previous cycle length, the valve will almost always be pliable enough for a successful valvotomy. If these intervals are fixed regardless of cycle length, the valve is likely to be rigid and will require replacement [8].

*USE OF THE APEX CARDIOGRAM IN ASSESSING THE SEVERITY OF MITRAL STENOSIS

*1. How can you use the C–1, i.e., the C–M$_1$ interval in helping to diagnose the presence or absence of MS if C represents the onset of LV contraction on an apex cardiogram?

ANS.: If the C–1 interval is less than 30 msec, MS is very unlikely. If, on the other hand, the C–1 interval is more than 50 msec, MS is probable [21].

*2. What is the O–F interval? How does MS affect this interval?

ANS.: The O–F is the interval from the O point on the apex cardiogram to the F point. It represents the early rapid filling movement of the LV, and it is either shortened or eliminated completely by MS. The more severe the MS, the shorter the O–F.

The C–1 and the O–F intervals can be used together to assess the severity of MS. If an index of C–1 minus O–F is used, the higher the number, the more severe the MS. (It is not necessary to correct for heart rate.) A value of − 1 or greater suggests severe MS. Even if MR is present, as long as the MS is dominant, a value of − 1 suggests that the diameter of the mitral orifice is 1.5 cm or less [22]. It must be realized, however, that the O point is highly dependent on the time constant of the transducer used to record the apex impulse. The longer the time constant, the later the O point after the OS. With an infinite time constant, the O point of the apex cardiogram is simultaneous with the nadir of the LV pressure curve [37]. The C–1 minus O–F criterion given here requires a pulse unit with a time constant of about 1.3 sec.

REFERENCES

1. Aintablian, A., et al. Opening snap in mitral valve prolapse-click syndrome. *N.Y. State J. Med.* 78:1764, 1978.

2. Arevalo, F., and Sakamoto, T. On the duration of the isovolumetric relaxation period (IVRP) in dog and man. *Am. Heart J.* 67:651, 1964.

3. Atsuchi, U., et al. Left atrial myxoma: Phonocardiographic, mechanocardiographic and echocardiographic features in 4 cases with special reference to comparison of mitral stenosis. *Cardiovasc. Sound Bull.* 5:329, 1975.

4. Battaglia, G., Fasoli, G., and Chioin, R. Revised phonocardiographic and polygraphic findings in calcified mitral stenosis. *Folia Cardiologica* 24:229, 1965.

5. Bayer, O., Loogen, R., and Wolter, H. H. The mitral opening snap in the quantitative diagnosis of mitral stenosis. *Am. Heart J.* 2:234, 1956.

6. Bjork, V. O., and Lodin, H. The evaluation of mitral stenosis with selective left ventricular angiocardiography. *J. Thorac. Cardiovasc. Surg.* 40:17, 1960.

7. Bonner, A. J., Jr., et al. Early diastolic sound associated with mitral valve prolapse. *Arch. Intern. Med.* 136:347, 1976.

8. Cheng, T. O. Phonocardiographic sign for pliability of a stenotic mitral valve. *N. Engl. J. Med.* 286:266, 1972.

9. Crews, T. L., et al. Auscultatory and phonocardiographic findings in Ebstein's anomaly. *Br. Heart J.* 34:681, 1972.

10. Delman, A. J., et al. The second sound–mitral opening snap (A_2–OS) interval during exercise in the evaluation of mitral stenosis. *Circulation* 33:399, 1966.

11. Funatsu, T., et al. The cause of tricuspid opening snap in atrial septal defect (especially about the aged patient). *Cardiovasc. Sound Bull.* 5:305, 1975.

12. Harrison, T. R., et al. The relation of age to the duration of contraction, ejection, and relaxation of the normal human heart. *Am. Heart J.* 67:189, 1964.

13. Ichiyasu, H., et al. Pseudo-knock sound in a patient with nephrotic syndrome and massive ascites. *Jpn. Heart J.* 23:137, 1982.

14. Kalmanson, D., et al. Opening snap and isovolumic relaxation period in relation to mitral valve flow in patients with mitral stenosis. Significance of A_2–OS interval. *Br. Heart J.* 38:135, 1976.

15. Kato, H., et al. A reassessment of the phonocardiogram in mitral stenosis. *J. Cardiography* 6:469, 1976.

16. Luisada, A. A., and Argano, B. Triplication and quadruplication of the second sound. *Chest* 59:316, 1971.

17. Luisada, A. A., Slodki, S. J., and Krol, B. Double (mitral and tricuspid) opening snap in patients with valvular lesions. *Am. J. Cardiol.* 16:800, 1965.

18. Matsue, T., et al. Anterior mitral leaflet prolapse with mitral opening snap: Report of a surgical case. *J. Cardiography* 7:243, 1977.

19. Millward, D. K., McLaurin, L. P., and Craige, E. Echocardiographic studies to explain opening snaps in presence of nonstenotic mitral valves. *Am. J. Cardiol.* 31:64, 1973.

20. Nixon, P. G. F., Wooler, G. H., and Radigan, L. R. The opening snap in mitral incompetence. *Br. Heart J.* 22:395, 1960.

21. Oreshkov, V. I. Q–1 or C–1 interval in the diagnosis of mitral stenosis. *Br. Heart J.* 29:778, 1967.

22. Oreshkov, V. I. A new mechanocardiographic index in evaluation of the severity of mitral stenosis: An apexcardiographic study. *Am. Heart J.* 79:789, 1970.

23. Rackley, C. E., et al. Phonocardiographic discrepancies in the assessment of mitral stenosis. *Arch. Intern. Med.* 121:50, 1968.

24. Raizada, V., et al. Non-invasive evaluation of normally functioning mitral bioprosthesis. Abstracts, World Congress Cardiology, Tokyo, p. 1330, 1978.

25. Rees, A., Farru, O., and Rodriguez, R. Phonocardiographic, radiological, and haemodynamic correlation in atrial septal defect. *Br. Heart J.* 34:781, 1972.

26. Ross, R. S., and Criley, J. M. Cineangiocardiographic studies of the origin of cardiovascular physical signs. *Circulation* 30:255, 1964.

27. Sakai, H., et al. Relation between the atrial contraction and the patterns of the splitting of the second heart sound in patients with right ventricular pacemakers. *J. Cardiography* 8:755, 1978.

28. Surawicz, B. Effect of respiration and upright position on the interval between the two components of the second sound and between the second sound and opening snap. *Circulation* 16:422, 1957.

29. Surawicz, B., et al. Role of the phonocardiogram in evaluation of the severity of mitral stenosis and detection of associated valvular lesions. *Circulation* 34:795, 1966.
30. Tanaka, C., et al. Phonocardiographic findings in adult ASD. *Cardiovasc. Sound Bull.* 5:107, 1975.
31. Tavel, M. E., Frazier, W. J., and Fisch, C. Use of phenylephrine in the detection of the opening snap in mitral stenosis. *Am. Heart J.* 77:274, 1969.
32. Uyttenhove, P., VanLoo, A., and Haerens, R. Phonocardiography in mitral stenosis. *Acta Cardiol.* 18:24, 1963.
33. Valois, R., and Charuzi, Y. Vegetation diastolic sound in mitral valve endocarditis. *Am. Heart J.* 103:432, 1982.
34. Van Der Spuy, J. C. The functional and clinical anatomy of the mitral valve. *Br. Heart J.* 20:471, 1958.
35. Wei, J. Y., and Fortuin, N. J. Diastolic sounds and murmurs associated with mitral valve prolapse. *Circulation* 63:559, 1981.
36. Wells, B. The assessment of mitral stenosis by phonocardiography. *Br. Heart J.* 16:261, 1954.
37. Willems, J. L., DeGeest, H., and Kesteloot, H. On the value of apex cardiography for timing intracardiac events. *Am. J. Cardiol.* 28:59, 1971.
38. Yigitbasi, O., et al. Q–1/IIA–OS formula for predicting left atrial pressure in mitral stenosis. *Br. Heart J.* 32:547, 1970.

11. *The Third Heart Sound (S₃)*

NOMENCLATURE

1. What are other names for the S₃?
    ANS.: The third heart sound, protodiastolic gallop sound, ventricular gallop, early filling gallop sound, and early or rapid filling sound.
2. What is the difference between *a* third heart sound and *the* third heart sound?
    ANS.: Any sound after a second sound (S₂) may be *a* third sound, e.g., an OS or a presystolic sound such as the S₄. What is meant by *the* third sound, however, is the specific sound that occurs just after the S₂ near the end of the rapid filling phase of a ventricle (about 120–180 msec [0.12–0.18 sec] after the S₂). (The term *S₃* is preferred because it has a specific meaning.)
    Note: 120 msec (0.12 sec) is about the length of time it takes to say "two–three" or "tu–huh" at a leisurely speed.
3. What is misleading about the word *protodiastolic* in describing the S₃?
    ANS.: a) It was originally coined by Wiggers [27] to represent the time on the aortic pressure pulse between the peak pressure and the closure of the aortic valve. This interval or period of reduced ejection was assumed to represent the beginning of ventricular relaxation or diastole. However, the auscultator defines *diastole* as the period beginning with aortic valve closure as signaled by the S₂.

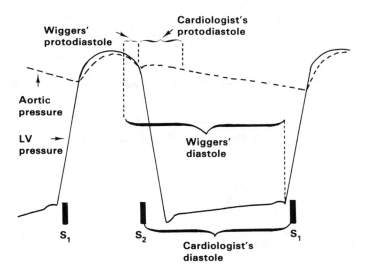

The physiologist considers diastole to begin with the earliest point suggestive of ventricular relaxation or where ejection begins to slacken off. This is not so precise or useful a point as the cardiologist would like, so he considers that diastole begins with the S₂ or the incisura of the arterial pulse.

b) *Protodiastolic* is used as a synonym for *early diastolic*, yet the prefix *protos* does not mean "early" but "first." Therefore, the S₄ should be called *hystidiastolic,* from the Greek *hystidos,* which means "last." Since we do not use such a word for the S₄, it is inconsistent to use Greek nomenclature only for the S₃.

4. What factors besides brevity make the term *S₃* preferable to the term *rapid filling sound?*
   ANS.: a) The S₄ is also due to rapid filling of the LV, but this is secondary to atrial contraction.
   b) Only *S₃* relates the sound and timing to the S₂.
   c) The S₃ has been produced in a vigorously contracting dog heart with no blood in it at all [26].

5. What is the difference between an S₃ and a ventricular gallop sound?
   ANS.: A gallop cannot be one sound. The word *gallop* must refer to a rhythm or cadence made by at least three sounds in succession. A ventricular gallop is the triple rhythm made by the sequence of the S₁, S₂, and S₃. Therefore, the term *S₃* is preferable.

6. How has the meaning of the term *gallop rhythm* changed over the decades?
   ANS.: This term was originally used to describe any rapid series of three or more sounds in the presence of a tachycardia and heart failure. It included any extra sounds in systole (systolic gallop) as well as diastole. It also eliminated any S₃ with a normal heart rate or without heart failure. Therefore, the term *gallop rhythm* has changed its meaning because it now refers to any series of three or more sounds in which the extra sounds occur *only in diastole* and are due to an S₃, an S₄, or both. Because most physicians cannot distinguish a gallop from a canter or a trot, some cardiologists prefer the term *triple or quadruple rhythm* to describe a series of sounds with an S₃ or an S₄. The term *S₃ or S₄ gallop,* however, is universally understood when referring to the rhythm of the usual heart sounds plus a specific extra diastolic sound.

TIMING

1. Which LV hemodynamic events occur in diastole after the S₂ but before the S₃?
   ANS.: **Isovolumic relaxation,** and after opening of the mitral valve, early rapid filling of the LV.
   *Note: This isovolumic period is an active metabolic process and should really be called isovolumic *expansion.* Usage forces us to continue using the term *relaxation.*

2. When does isovolumic relaxation begin and end in the LV?
   ANS.: It begins with aortic valve closure and ends with mitral valve opening. As soon as isovolumic relaxation ends and the mitral valve opens, the LV fills rapidly from the left atrium.

Boldface type indicates that the term is explained in the Glossary.
*Material marked with an asterisk is for reference and for advanced students in cardiology.

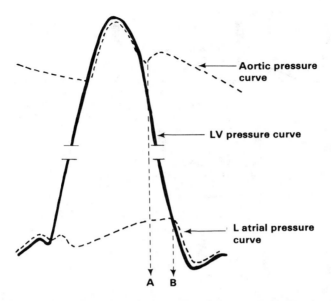

Aortic pressure curve

LV pressure curve

L atrial pressure curve

A   B

Between point A (aortic valve closure) and point B (mitral valve opening) the volume in the LV is unchanged. This is therefore the isovolumic relaxation period.

* *Note:* Normally, the duration of isovolumic relaxation ranges from about 60–100 msec in the LV, and from 30–120 msec in the RV [3].

3. Does the ventricle fill most rapidly in early, middle, or late diastole?

ANS.: In early diastole. The ventricle has two rates of expansion: an early rapid one and a later slow one. Once the aortic valve closes, the LV expands very rapidly. During this expansion it first goes through the stage of isovolumic expansion in about 100 msec, the time it takes to say "pa-pa" as quickly as possible, and then, when the mitral valve opens, through the stage of rapid filling while the ventricle continues its rapid expansion phase for about another 60 msec (0.06 sec). At the end of the rapid filling phase it is suddenly checked by unknown forces, and the slow expansion phase takes over.

4. What percentage of ventricular filling occurs in the early rapid filling phase of diastole in comparison with the later slow filling phase of diastole?

ANS.: About 80 percent. After the initial rapid filling, the volume of the ventricle changes very little until atrial contraction squeezes the last 20 percent of blood into the ventricle.

5. At what point during the rapid filling phase of the LV pressure curve does the S_3 occur?

ANS.: Near the end of the rapid pressure drop in the LV, i.e., near the point at which rapid expansion changes to the slow expansion phase.

* *Note:* Some rapid filling continues to occur after the S_3.

6. In what part of diastole does the S_3 usually fall?

ANS.: In the first third in patients with normal heart rates and in the middle third in those with tachycardias.

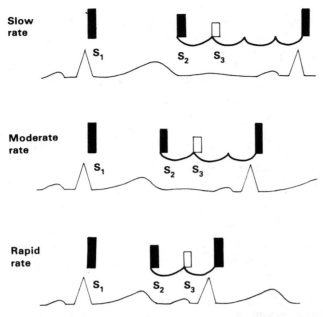

At slow rates (top line) the S₃ is much closer to the S₂ than to the following S₁; i.e., it falls in the first quarter of diastole. At fast rates (bottom line) it may occur in mid-diastole.

*7. Which conditions shorten the A_2–S_3 interval?

ANS.: Anything that shortens isovolumic relaxation time such as

   a) Restrictive cardiomyopathies or constrictive pericarditis, both of which limit the extent of early expansion.

   b) Heart rates of more than 100 beats per minute. Presumably sympathetic stimulation causes ventricular expansion to complete its early rapid filling phase more rapidly.

   Note: The time between the opening of the mitral valve and the S_3 remains relatively constant for all heart rates under 100 beats per minute.

MECHANISM OF PRODUCTION

1. How is the S_3 produced?

ANS.: There are two theories: an external theory and an internal production theory. In the internal production theory the S_3 is due to a sudden "pulling short" of the rapidly expanding ventricle by unknown myocardial forces at the end of the rapid expansion phase in early diastole [19]. At the moment of the S_3, the ventricle has stopped rapid expansion, and pressure in the ventricle is no longer falling but is relatively stable for about 40 msec, despite continued rapid filling due to the inertia of the blood mass. The S_3 seems to occur at the transition between rapid active and rapid passive ventricular filling [2]. The continued rapid increase in blood volume in the ventricle at the time of the sudden transition may act as a sudden distending force that causes the sound.

Note: A sudden change of slope from rapid to slow expansion of the LV septum and posterior wall at the time of the S_3 has been observed in echocardiograms. This is best seen near the apex [23].

*2. Can a sudden stretch of ventricular muscle or papillary muscle and chordae tendineae produce a heart sound?

ANS.: No sound was produced when one end of a piece of ventricle was fixed and the other end was suddenly pulled by various amounts of sudden force [6]. (Perhaps if the piece of muscle had been coupled to another structure with different acoustical properties, the inaudible vibrations would have been converted to audible ones.)

Note: The following facts are evidence that the S_3 is not caused by a sudden stretch of the papillary muscles and chordae attached to mitral leaflets.

a) An S_3 can occur with homograft (human cadaver) or heterograft (porcine) replacement of the mitral valve. This implies that chordae tendineae attachments to the valves are absent [7, 9, 20]. Even with a prosthetic ball valve, an S_3 occurs when the flow into the LV is increased by a severe paravalvular leak [5].

b) On an echocardiogram the S_3 occurs when the anterior mitral leaflet is between its maximum opening position and the nadir of its early partial closure position (see illustration below). There is no evidence here that the mitral valve apparatus plays any important role in the production of the S_3.

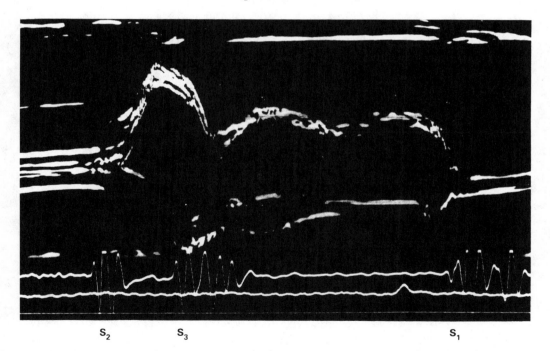

S_2 S_3 S_1

This simultaneous mitral valve echo and low-frequency phonocardiogram was taken at very fast film speed from a 20-year-old man with heart failure and atrial fibrillation due to a severe idiopathic cardiomyopathy. The apical phonocardiogram shows the loud S_3 beginning just before the change of slope in the first closing movement of mitral valve. This man had at times a double S_3 (very rare). However, on the day of this tracing the S_3 was more like a prolonged S_3 or an S_3 followed by a short rumble. (The cause of a split S_3 is unknown, but the split S_3 has been attributed to a transient opening and closing movement of the mitral valve.)

The External Production Theory of the S_3

1. Why is an external production theory necessary to account for the S_3?

    ANS.: a) An S_3 can often not be recorded inside the LV in a patient in whom it can be recorded externally on the chest wall [21].

    b) There is no feature of the LV pressure curve that consistently corresponds to the S_3.

    * c) Except for some change of motion near the apex, echocardiograms do not show any features elsewhere in the ventricular walls that are simultaneous with the S_3.

    * d) A sound is produced by the heart striking the chest wall in rare instances of pericardial effusion when a systolic thrust of the heart against the chest wall coincides with a loud systolic sound [12].

    * e) The apex cardiogram shows a peak of rapid early outward movement at the time of the S_3. When marked, this peak is palpable and is then accompanied by a loud S_3.

    * Note: There is no feature of the LV pressure curve that corresponds to the rapid filling wave of an apex cardiogram [20].

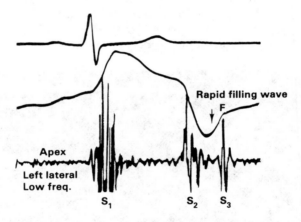

The S_3 occurs at the peak of the rapid filling wave of the apex cardiogram.

    f) The loudness of the S_3 is very dependent on how well the apex beat comes out between the ribs and how close the heart is to the chest wall.

    * g) In dogs with empty hearts, an S_3 can be recorded as long as the heart is beating vigorously [26].

2. What is the external production theory for the S_3?

    ANS.: During contraction the heart rotates counterclockwise, as viewed from the apex. The momentum of its rotation keeps it rotating in the same direction until the time of early diastole. Its rotation is also twisting the great vessels and stretching the restraining elastic structures that are working to limit its rotation. If the heart rotates with enough energy, its momentum may stretch the restraining structures to such an extent that there is a sudden recoil at the end of its rotation in early diastole. This recoil may throw the heart against the chest wall hard enough to produce a sound, or the recoil movement itself may cause the whole heart to shudder, producing the vibrations of an S_3.

THE PHYSIOLOGICAL S₃

1. How common is the physiological S_3 in normal subjects?

    ANS.: In one study it was recorded on a phonocardiogram near the apex in one-third of normal subjects under age 16 [24]. (This is not to say that it was audible in all cases in which it was recorded.) It is rarely audible or recordable in normal subjects over age 30. It may persist into the fifth decade in some women.

2. What cardiovascular conditions tend to produce an audible S_3 in the normal heart?

    ANS.: Anything that increases the velocity of ventricular expansion and recoil, such as an increase in flow or sympathetic stimulation, e.g., tachycardias.

    *Note: There is some physiological proof that the more energetic the expansion of the LV, the more likely is the presence of an S_3.

    a) The S_3 usually occurs only if atrial pressure is *more than slightly* higher than ventricular pressure near the end of rapid ventricular filling. The more vigorously the ventricle expands, the greater will be the pressure gradient between the left atrium and the left ventricle, and the more likely will there be an S_3.

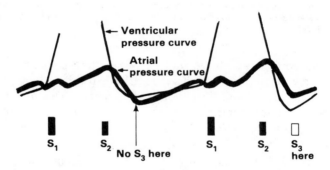

When the LV expands with enough energy to create a gradient between it and the left atrium, an S_3 occurs.

    b) The peak slope of the Y descent of the left atrial pressure pulse has been shown to be steeper than normal in subjects with heart failure and an S_3 [25].

3. What does the presence of a physiological S_3 tell you about the patient's circulation time?

    ANS.: It suggests at least a normal **circulation time**. The sympathetic tone and catecholamines that produce the rapid early expansion necessary for the S_3 will also increase the cardiac output and accelerate the circulation time.

    Note: A venous hum in the neck implies a normal or rapid circulation time, and its presence helps to confirm that the S_3 is physiological and is not associated with heart failure. (See page 352 for a method of eliciting a venous hum.)

4. When will a tachycardia produce a loud physiological S_3 in a normal patient over age 30?

    ANS.: There will be a loud S_3 if the rapid filling phase of ventricular expansion is augmented by atrial contraction. The gallop rhythm that results is then known as a summation gallop. This will occur when atrial contraction occurs in the early part of diastole, as with a marked tachycardia or with a moderate tachycardia together with a first-degree atrioventricular (AV) block (long P–R interval).

> * *Note:* It has been calculated that with a P–R of 0.14 sec, a tachycardia of 120 beats per minute may produce a summation gallop; with a P–R of 0.16 sec, the summation rate is 115; with a P–R of 0.18, it is 110; and with a P–R of 0.20, it is 105 [11].

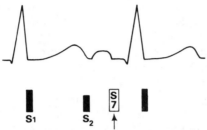

Simultaneous occurrence of atrial contraction and early rapid filling produces a summation sound facetiously called the "S₇" (S₃ + S₄). This usually requires a prolonged P–R interval.

5. How can you tell whether or not a triple rhythm is due to a summation gallop?

   ANS.: If you can slow the heart rate by carotid sinus pressure, diastole will be lengthened, and the gallop will disappear. This occurs because slowing the heart rate separates atrial contraction, which is late in diastole, from the early rapid filling phase.

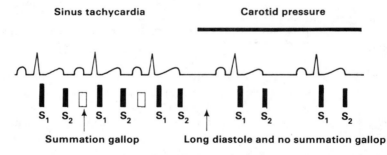

Carotid pressure slows the heart rate and separates the time of atrial contraction from the time of early rapid ventricular filling, thus eliminating a summation gallop. (See also Fig. 12-7.)

6. Is the summation sound soft or loud?

   ANS.: It is nearly always very loud.

   > *Note:* If an S₄ is made louder by occurring during the early rapid filling phase, the rhythm is called an augmented gallop [11]. (See figure on page 278.) If a pathological S₃ is made louder by an early atrial contraction, that triple rhythm may also be called an augmented gallop.

LOUDNESS OF THE S₃

1. Which chest piece and degree of stethoscope pressure best bring out the S₃?
   ANS.: The bell, applied with light to moderate pressure so that the low frequencies will not be damped out. (See note on page 270 for the rare exceptions to the last statement.)
2. Can an S₃ be made louder by tachycardia or bradycardias? Why?
   ANS.: Tachycardias can make the S₃ louder because more blood is received by the ventricle due to the increased cardiac output that occurs with tachycardias. (This statement assumes that the heart rate is not too rapid because a very fast rate can actually lower cardiac output.)
3. What increases the loudness of the S₃, inspiration or expiration?
   ANS.: Either. Expiration can make the S₃ sound louder by
      a) Squeezing blood out of the lungs into the left atrium and ventricle.
      b) Bringing the stethoscope closer to the heart.

   Inspiration can make it louder by increasing sympathetic tone to the heart **(sinus arrhythmia),** and speeding up the heart rate and blood flow through the mitral valve.

   Note: Either inspiration or expiration can make the S₃ louder by causing the apex beat to emerge between the ribs in any particular patient. In some patients the apex beat comes out between the ribs on inspiration, and in others it does so on expiration. If on inspiration it comes out one interspace lower than it does on expiration, the S₃ will sound louder one interspace lower on inspiration than it does on expiration.
4. Because the proximity of the apex beat to the stethoscope appears to be a factor in intensifying the loudness of the S₃, how can you bring the apex beat closer to the chest wall?

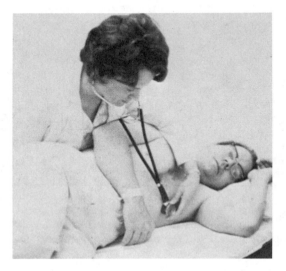

In the left lateral decubitus position shown, the apex of the heart is brought as close to the stethoscope as possible. This is an absolute necessity for hearing a soft S₃, because it is sensitive to proximity.

ANS.: By turning the patient into the **left lateral decubitus position.**
> *Note:* The occasional soft S₃ is heard better with moderate than with light pressure especially in chests in which it is difficult to place the stethoscope close to the apex beat owing to thick layers of muscle or fat.

5. What proof is there that ventricular volume and flow control the audibility of the S₃?
    ANS.: a) Conditions that increase the volume of flow make the S₃ louder; e.g., exercise or mitral regurgitation.
    b) Conditions that decrease flow to the heart and decrease ventricular volume cause decreased audibility of the S₃ (e.g., standing up, venous tourniquets, or the water-loss effect of diuretics [14]).
    > *Note:* One of the characteristics that is most confusing to the beginner when listening to a soft S₃ is its intermittent audibility—i.e., it waxes and wanes in and out of one's hearing threshold. This probably occurs because its loudness is very sensitive to slight changes in proximity and volume caused by respiration.

THE EXAGGERATED PHYSIOLOGICAL S₃

1. What can exaggerate the physiological S₃?
    ANS.: Any condition that causes excessive blood flow through the mitral valve.
    > *Note:* Increased flow into the LV through the aortic valve, as with aortic regurgitation (AR), does not exaggerate the physiological S₃ unless the AR is severe. Sudden severe AR usually does produce an S₃.

2. List the common shunts and the valvular lesion that may cause excessive flow through the mitral valve, therefore exaggerating or bringing back the physiological S₃.
    ANS.: a) The two left-to-right shunts, **ventricular septal defect** (VSD) and **persistent ductus arteriosus** (PDA). (**Atrial septal defects** [ASDs] do not increase flow through the mitral valve.)

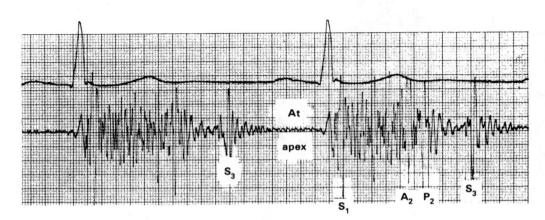

Low-frequency phonocardiogram from a 15-year-old girl with severe rheumatic MR. Besides the loud MR murmur and S₃, note the following: (1) The widely split S₂ (A₂P₂) expected in moderate to severe MR is present. (2) The P₂ is well heard at the apex, and should make you suspect some pulmonary hypertension. The patient's pulmonary artery systolic pressure was 35 mm Hg (upper normal is 25 mm Hg).

b) An incompetent mitral valve, that is, mitral regurgitation (MR).

Note: Excessive flow through a tricuspid valve does not usually cause a right-sided S_3, i.e., there is no physiological right-sided S_3. The right ventricular S_3 requires not only a large right ventricle (RV) but also a high right atrial pressure. For example, in an uncomplicated ASD with a very large flow through the tricuspid valve, there is usually no S_3. It seems that the right ventricular S_3 occurs only when there is an abnormal relation between the rate of rapid filling and the ventricle's ability to accommodate its increasing diastolic volume, i.e., only when there is reduced compliance [10]. The normal RV is more compliant than the LV and, unless it is also pressure-overloaded, it expands easily to accommodate increased flow.

* 3. How can the detection of a LV S_3 tell you whether the pulmonary hypertension in a patient with a VSD or PDA is due to an increased flow (hyperkinetic) or to a fixed irreversible resistance?

ANS.: The presence of a LV S_3 signifies that there is increased flow through the pulmonary circuit and that therefore the pulmonary hypertension is hyperkinetic and not fixed. This means that surgical closure of the VSD or PDA may lower the pulmonary artery pressure to normal [28].

THE PATHOLOGICAL S_3

1. What are the commonest associated cardiac findings in subjects with a pathological S_3?

ANS.: A high mean left atrial pressure due to a high V wave, a noncompliant LV, and a large ventricle resulting from a poor **ejection fraction**.

* Note: Noncompliance of the distended ventricle is part of the mechanism that produces an S_3. This fact is suggested by its occurrence in a considerable proportion of patients with **hypertrophic subaortic stenosis** (HSS), who have very thick, noncompliant (but not very dilated) ventricles. Low as well as high filling rates have been found in patients with a pathological S_3 [20].

2. What pathological cardiac condition is generally present when an S_3 occurs in the presence of a high left atrial pressure due to a low ejection fraction?

ANS.: A **cardiomyopathy,** most often idiopathic or due to extensive ischemic heart disease. Much more rarely, it is due to an infiltrate such as amyloid or sarcoid.

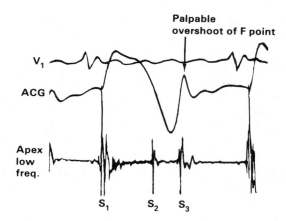

Palpable
overshoot of F point

V₁

ACG

Apex
low
freq.

S₁   S₂   S₃

This apex cardiogram and simultaneous apex phonocardiogram is from the same 20-year-old man as in the echocardiogram on p. 249. The pathological S₃ was extremely loud and could be heard anywhere on his chest. It is difficult to say whether it was the overshoot of the rapid filling wave (F point) or the vibrations of the S₃ that was palpable.

*3. What is the significance of an S₃ in a patient with mild or severe AR?

ANS.: It usually means LV dysfunction. An S₃ in a patient with AR correlates with an increased LV residual volume and not with the severity of AR [1].

THE PHYSIOLOGICAL VERSUS THE PATHOLOGICAL S₃

1. What is the difference in timing and quality between the physiological and the pathological S₃?

ANS.: None, except that the S₃ found in **constrictive pericarditis** may occur earlier than usual.

2. How can you usually tell a physiological S₃ from a pathological S₃?

ANS.: Only by knowing the circumstances under which it occurs, i.e., by finding the reason for the pathological S₃, such as symptoms and signs of heart failure or myocardial abnormalities.

*Note: Some patients with a pathological S₃ secondary to a past infarction are relatively asymptomatic, i.e., they do not seem to have the decreased exercise tolerance that is the usual consequence of a high left atrial V wave. The S₃ in these patients is often associated with a ventricular aneurysm or a large akinetic area. The mechanism for this S₃ is unknown.

3. Is the physiological S₃ ever as loud as the loudest pathological S₃?

ANS.: Almost. Conversely, a pathological S₃ may be very faint.

4. What is the difference between the physiological S₃ and the pathological S₃ in their response to pooling of blood in the legs by standing?

ANS.: Because pooling of blood in the legs is much more difficult in the patient who has congestive failure with edema and high venous pressure, standing will have less of an attenuating effect on the S₃ than usual in such patients.

5. What noise may follow the pathological S_3? When is this heard with the physiological S_3?

ANS.: A short diastolic rumble is often heard following the pathological S_3. It is also heard with the torrential flow through the mitral valve that occurs when the physiological S_3 is exaggerated either by MR or by a PDA. It is also sometimes heard in young children following their normal S_3. This low-frequency diastolic murmur following the S_3 occurs while the mitral valve leaflets are being rapidly swung into their semiclosed position by eddy currents under the mitral leaflets.

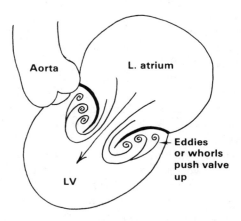

If the flow is fast, eddy currents may push the valve up enough to create a partial obstruction and so produce turbulent flow and a short diastolic murmur.

The flow under high pressure through the semiclosed AV valve presumably produces this rumble because rapid ventricular filling continues for a short time after the S_3.

Note: a) The short diastolic murmur following the pathological or physiological S_3 should not be mistaken for the much longer mumur of mitral stenosis. (See page 375 for method of distinguishing this murmur from the murmur of MS.)

*b) In the presence of sudden severe AR, LV pressure may rise so rapidly and steeply in diastole that it will produce a mid-diastolic closure of the mitral valve with a mid-diastolic S_1, which could be mistaken for an S_3. The first heart sound produced by ventricular contraction may be very soft and may be due entirely to tricuspid closure [22].

6. Does a high **filling pressure** always mean LV dysfunction and low ejection fraction?

ANS.: Not if it is caused primarily by a high A wave, because a strong left atrial contraction can produce a high A wave at the end of diastole and so cause a high filling pressure despite a normal ejection fraction. This is because it is the *mean* and not the *end-diastolic* filling pressure that best correlates with cardiac dysfunction. For example, in severe aortic stenosis there may be a 20-mm LV end-diastolic pressure but a mean left atrial pressure of 10 mm and therefore no decreased function.

THE RIGHT VERSUS THE LEFT VENTRICULAR S₃

1. How can you tell a RV from a LV S₃?

    ANS.: a) An S₃ generated by the RV is louder over the RV area, i.e., near the lower sternal area or epigastrium, unless the ventricle is markedly enlarged, in which case it may be loud anywhere on the part of the chest wall that overlies the RV. This includes those parts of the precordium usually occupied by the LV.

    b) A RV S₃ is usually louder on inspiration because there is more flow into the RV. The LV S₃ may be louder on either inspiration or expiration. (See page 253 for explanation.)

    c) An S₃ from the RV is usually associated with a RV heave or rock (see p. 131), a large jugular V wave, and a rapid Y descent.

2. List some of the common causes of an S₃ generated by the RV.

    ANS.: The common causes are right ventricular dilatation and high right atrial pressures secondary to

    a) severe tricuspid regurgitation due to pulmonary hypertension.

    b) sudden RV outflow obstruction, as in massive pulmonary embolism.

    *Note: Although pulmonary stenosis is also an outflow obstruction, it requires chronic stenosis that is severe enough to produce RV failure before the RV will dilate and cause an S₃. This occurs rarely because the compensatory mechanism for a chronic obstruction to outflow from birth is hyperplasia as well as hypertrophy, both of which are well able to overcome all but the most severe obstruction.

THE S₃ VERSUS THE OPENING SNAP

1. What is the difference between the A₂–OS interval and the A₂–S₃ interval?

    ANS.: The A₂–OS interval is rarely more than 100 msec (0.10 sec), whereas the shortest A₂–S₃ interval is usually 120 msec (0.12 sec). The difference between 100 and 120 msec is merely the difference between saying "pa-pa" as quickly as possible and saying it at a normal speaking rate.

    *Note: a) There are rare exceptions to both these figures; for example, by phonocardiogram the A₂–OS has been seen to be as long as 120 msec, and the S₃ in constrictive pericarditis or the tumor plop of left atrial myxoma may occur as early as 100 msec after the S₂.

    b) A "tumor plop" is the early diastolic sound produced when a left (or right) atrial myxoma attached to a stalk prolapses through the mitral (or tricuspid) valve in diastole. This early diastolic sound can occur at the time one would expect of either an OS or an S₃. It may be intermittent or may vary in loudness and may even vary its time relationship to the second sound [10]. It may differ from an S_3 even if it occurs at the same interval from the A_2 as the usual S_3 by being

a) Louder than expected.

b) More easily heard at the left lower sternal border than expected. (An S_3 is not usually heard at the left lower sternal border unless it is extremely loud.)

2. How does the quality or pitch of the S_3 help to distinguish it from the OS?

ANS.: The S_3 is low in pitch, sounds like a thud or boom, and is best heard with the bell. The OS, on the other hand, is usually a high-frequency, short clicking sound, best recognized with the diaphragm.

*Note: Occasionally the OS is atypical and deceptively low in pitch. This occurs when the mitral valve is very calcified or if early ventricular expansion is very poor due to severe myocardial damage.

3. How does the site of best auscultation help to distinguish an S_3 from an OS?

ANS.: An OS is commonly loudest at some point between the apex and the left sternal border, whereas the S_3 is almost always loudest at the apex unless it is a right-sided S_3.

*Note: a) The right-sided S_3 will be loudest along the left sternal border.

b) If there is a large LV, the OS may be as loud at the apical area as at the left sternal border.

c) If there is constrictive pericarditis, the early S_3 or pericardial knock may be loudest at the left sternal border, possibly because the RV also produces an S_3 in this condition [15].

*4. Why will pericardial constriction produce an early and loud S_3?

ANS.: Pericardial constriction is the only condition besides tamponade in which, despite normal AV valves, there is a high pressure V wave in the atrium proximal to a ventricle that may be normal in size and function. Because the ventricle is restricted in the extent to which it can expand, it reaches its maximum state of expansion early and rapidly, and the high filling pressure causes it to expand with more energy, generating a loud sound. There is also some suggestion from systolic time interval studies that in constrictive pericarditis there is an excessive effect of catecholamines on the LV. (See page 260 for an explanation of why tamponade does not favor the production of an S_3.)

Note: a) Cineangiograms of patients with constrictive pericarditis show that this early filling of the LV is accomplished with exceptional rapidity.

b) The early S_3 of constriction may be very faint or absent. It may be brought out by squatting, increasing the blood volume, or increasing the afterload, as with phenylephrine. It may be obliterated by decreasing venous return, as with nitroglycerin [17].

c) A relatively early S_3 may occur with ruptured chordae, i.e., it is usually less than 150 msec from the A_2. With rheumatic MR, the A_2–S_3 interval is almost always more than 150 msec [13].

d) In restrictive cardiomyopathies the hemodynamic picture is quite similar to that seen in constriction, and the S_3 can also occur as early as in constrictive pericarditis. This S_3 is usually loud and is best heard at the apex [4].

5. What has the loud S_3 of pericardial constriction been called?

ANS.: A pericardial knock, because it is very loud.

Note: a) The pericardial knock is not present in **tamponade** because early rapid expansion of the ventricles is markedly blunted by the fluid [8]. However, in patients with the effusive-constrictive type of pericarditis, the pericardial knock is usually present.

* b) If a pericardial knock occurs early enough, as with severe constriction, it can come at the end of maximum opening of the mitral valve, i.e., at the time of the E point of the mitral echo, which is analogous to the timing of the OS.

* c) Although the usual pericardial knock occurs early, i.e., 100–110 msec after the A_2, it may occur at the usual S_3 time, i.e., 120 msec after the A_2, presumably due to a concomitant cardiomyopathy that slows early ventricular expansion.

6. How may the quality of the S_1 help to verify whether the sound you hear after the S_2 is an S_3 or an OS?

ANS.: An OS is almost always associated with a loud, snapping first sound, i.e., the S_1 is short and high-pitched (the "closing snap"). Therefore, a soft or muffled first sound tends to deny the presence of an OS.

Note: Unfortunately, constrictive pericarditis is frequently associated with a loud S_1, thus causing the early pericardial knock to seem even more like an OS [16].

*7. When can both an OS and an S_3 be present in the same person?

ANS.: If a mobile anterior leaflet is associated with severe MR, and the posterior leaflet is even slightly fibrosed and fixes the edges of the anterior leaflet, the normal anterior leaflet belly will produce a snap as it opens, and the severe MR will produce the exaggerated physiological S_3.

8. What is the rhythm of an S_1 followed by an S_2, OS, and S_3? Can you make a rhythmic phrase that fits?

ANS.:   Tum   Tu Du Boom   Tum   Tu Du Boom
          1   2   OS   3   1   2   OS   3

*9. How can an apex cardiogram help to distinguish an S_3 from an OS?

ANS.: The OS will fall near the O point, and the S_3 will fall near the peak of the early rapid filling wave of the apex cardiogram. (See figure on pp. 256 and 367.)

Summary of How to Tell an S_3 from an Opening Snap

1. The OS is not usually more than 100 msec (a rapid "pa-pa") from the S_2. The S_3 is rarely less than 120 msec (0.12 sec) from the A_2 (usually 140 msec).
2. The OS is usually a short, sharp click, best heard with the diaphragm near the left sternal border; the S_3 is a thud or boom, best heard by applying light or moderate pressure with the bell near the apex.
3. The OS is associated with a sharp, loud S_1. The S_3 may or may not have a loud S_1.
*4. An OS will separate further from the A_2 when the patient stands. An S_3 will not change its distance from the A_2 on standing.
5. An apex cardiogram will show the OS occurring at or near the O point, whereas the S_3 occurs at or near the peak of the rapid filling wave, or F point.

THE S₃ AND MITRAL STENOSIS

1. Why is a left ventricular S_3 not to be expected in significant MS?

    ANS.: Mitral valve obstruction tends to prevent rapid filling of the LV in early diastole, despite a high left atrial pressure. Without rapid early filling, an S_3 is an unexpected finding.

2. When does an S_3 begin the MS diastolic murmur?

    ANS.: If the mitral diastolic murmur begins with a loud sound, that sound is probably an S_3. One recent study showed that when the S_3 was recorded in MS, its presence and intensity were independent of the severity of the MS. The S_3 varied only with the intensity of LV expansion and recoil in early diastole and could be present even in severe MS with reduced flow. The S_3 probably reflects good LV function, i.e., the LV can expand rapidly and produce a good recoil effect.

    *Note: In the French literature, the loud S_3-like beginning of the diastolic murmur has been called the "initial jerk" of the MS murmur.

3. When may a right ventricular S_3 be heard in MS?

    ANS.: If the right atrial pressure is high and the RV is dilated owing to pulmonary hypertension and congestive failure. If the enlarged RV usurps the apex area, the S_3 may be heard well into the middle of the left thorax and may be mistaken for a LV S_3.

REFERENCES

1. Abdulla, A. M., et al. Clinical significance and hemodynamic correlates of the third heart sound gallop in aortic regurgitation. *Circulation* 64:464, 1981.
2. Arevalo, F., et al. Hemodynamic correlates of the third heart sound. *Am. J. Physiol.* 207:319, 1964.
3. Arevalo, F., and Sakamoto, T. On the duration of the isovolumetric relaxation period (IVRP) in dog and man. *Am. Heart J.* 67:651, 1964.
4. Chew, C. Y. C., et al. Primary restrictive cardiomyopathy. Non-tropical endomyocardial fibrosis and hypereosinophilic heart disease. *Br. Heart J.* 39:399, 1977.
5. Coulshed, N., and Epstein, E. J. Third heart sound after mitral valve replacement. *Br. Heart J.* 34:301, 1972.
6. Dock, W. The forces needed to evoke sounds from cardiac tissues, and the attenuation of heart sounds. *Circulation* 19:376, 1959.
7. El Gamal, M., and Smith, D. R. Occurrence of a left ventricular third heart sound in incompetent mitral heterografts. *Br. Heart J.* 32:497, 1970.
8. Firestein, G., Hensley, C., and Varghese, P. J. Left ventricular function in presence of small pericardial effusion. *Br. Heart J.* 43:382, 1980.
9. Gianelly, R. E., Popp, R. L., and Hultgren, H. N. Heart sounds in patients with homograft replacement of mitral valve. *Circulation* 42:309, 1970.
10. Goldschlager, A., et al. Right atrial myxoma with right to left shunt and polycythemia presenting as congenital heart disease. *Am. J. Cardiol.* 30:82, 1972.
11. Grayzel, J. Gallop rhythm of the heart. *Circulation* 20:1053, 1959.
12. Kay, C. F., et al. The "late systolic heartbeat" of pericardial effusion. *Am. Heart J.* 72:7, 1966.
13. Kinoshita, M., et al. Phonocardiographic findings of mitral insufficiency due to ruptured chordae tendineae. *Cardiovasc. Sound Bull.* 5:263, 1975.
14. Leonard, J. J., Weissler, A. M., and Warren, J. V. Modification of ventricular gallop rhythm induced by pooling of blood in the extremities. *Br. Heart J.* 20:502, 1958.

15. Matsuzaki, M., et al. A study of abnormal interventricular septal motion: Influence of position of interventricular septum in end-diastole. *J. Cardiography* 7:153, 1977.
16. Moreyra, E., Knibbe, P., and Segal, B. L. Constrictive pericarditis masquerading as mitral stenosis. *Chest* 57:245, 1970.
17. Nicholson, W. J., et al. Early diastolic sound of constrictive pericarditis. *Am. J. Cardiol.* 45:378, 1980.
18. Nixon, P. G. F., Wooler, G. H., and Radigan, L. R. Mitral incompetence caused by disease of the mural cusp. *Circulation* 19:839, 1959.
19. Ozawa, Y., Smith, D., and Craige, E. Origin of the third heart sound. *Circulation* 67:399, 1983.
20. Prewitt, T., et al. The "rapid filling wave" of the apex cardiogram. Its relation to echocardiographic and cineangiographic measurements of ventricular filling. *Br. Heart J.* 37:1256, 1975.
21. Reddy, P. S., et al. The genesis of gallop sounds: Investigation by quantitative phono- and apexcardiography. *Circulation* 63:922, 1981.
22. Rothbaum, D. A., DeJoseph, R. L., and Tavel, M. Diastolic heart sound produced by mid-diastolic closure of the mitral valve. *Am. J. Cardiol.* 34:367, 1974.
23. Sakamoto, T., et al. Genesis of the third heart sound. Phonoechocardiographic studies. *Jap. Heart J.* 17:150, 1976.
24. Schwartze, D. Frequency of the normal third heart sound in childhood. *Zeit. Kreislaufforschung* 55:306, 1966.
25. Shah, P. M., and Yu, P. N. Gallop rhythm: Hemodynamic and clinical correlation. *Am. Heart J.* 78:823, 1969.
26. Smith, J. R. Observations on the mechanism of the physiologic third heart sound. *Am. Heart J.* 28:661, 1944.
27. Wiggers, C. J. Studies on the consecutive phases of the cardiac cycle. *Am. J. Physiol.* 56:415, 1921.
28. Wood, P. The Eisenmenger syndrome or pulmonary hypertension with reversed central shunt. *Br. Med. J.* 2:701, 1958. Classic article.

12. *The Fourth Heart Sound (S₄)*

NOMENCLATURE

1. What has the triple rhythm produced by the sequence of a fourth heart sound, the S_1, and the S_2 been called?

    ANS.: An atrial gallop, a presystolic gallop, or an S_4 gallop.

    Note: a) The term *atrial gallop* implies that the atrium itself is the source of the extra sound. Atrial contraction itself is not audible with the stethoscope.

    b) The term *presystolic gallop* is misleading because the gallop sound produced by an S_3 may also be "presystolic," during a tachycardia, when the first sound follows very shortly after the S_3.

2. What is the advantage of the term S_4?

    ANS.: It specifies exactly which extra sound is thought to be producing the triple rhythm, regardless of diastolic length and without reference to exact mechanisms. It enables you to refer to the single sound S_4 without the necessity of always using the term *gallop,* which by definition implies at least three sounds.

*THE INAUDIBLE S₄ COMPONENT

*1. Does the atrial muscle itself produce vibrations as it contracts?

    ANS.: Yes, but such vibrations are usually inaudible because they are too low in frequency and amplitude. They can be picked up by placing a phonocatheter inside the atrium or in the esophagus.

    Note: a) The interval from the onset of the P of the ECG to the onset of the audible S_4 (henceforth simply called the S_4) averages 160 msec (120–200 msec). It occurs about 40 msec after the inaudible component.

    b) Contractions of an atrium may cause an audible sound in complete atrioventricular (AV) block or junctional rhythm. These vibrations can sometimes be recorded at the apex during systole as the atrium contracts against the closed AV valves.

    c) In some cases of atrial flutter in patients in heart failure, clicking sounds, which are loudest at the base of the heart, occur just after each F wave [12]. They can be heard during both systole and diastole and may become louder during diastole.

    Since the only chamber in which such sounds can be recorded by intracardiac phonocatheter is the atrium, they would appear to

---

*Material marked with an asterisk is for reference and for advanced students in cardiology.

represent the effect of atrial contraction itself [30]. They have also been heard during atrial fibrillation [32]. Echocardiograms have shown simultaneous fluttering motions of the aortic wall, aortic leaflets, mitral annulus, ventricular septum, and both mitral and tricuspid leaflets in patients with atrial fibrillation [3].

THE AUDIBLE PHYSIOLOGICAL AND PATHOLOGICAL S_4

Mode of Production

1. Where is the S_4 best recorded by an intracardiac phonocatheter, in the atrium or in the ventricle?
   ANS.: In the ventricle.
*2. What does the apex cardiogram show at the time of the S_4?
   ANS.: It shows a hump just before the systolic outward impulse. This presystolic hump or A wave is often large enough to be palpable.
      Note: The peak of the atrial hump coincides with the largest vibration of the S_4.

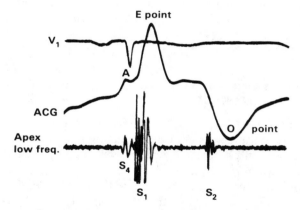

Apex cardiogram and phonocardiogram from a 50-year-old man with a previous infarction. The S_4 is simultaneous with a large palpable atrial hump (A wave) on the apex cardiogram. The A wave is 15% of the total apex pulse amplitude, or vertical E to O distance. Atrial humps of 15% or more of the E–O amplitude are usually palpable.

3. What causes this A wave or end-diastolic outward movement on the apex cardiogram?
   ANS.: It is the effect of left atrial contraction, causing a slight increase in the volume of the left ventricle (LV) at the end of diastole. This slight increase in volume before the ventricle contracts can be seen even in normal subjects on a cineangiogram with contrast material in the LV.
      Note: a) An apical A wave may be palpable even when the S_4 may be too low in frequency to be audible. On the other hand, a pathological S_4 may be heard in the absence of a palpable A wave. This is obvious when you realize that only a chest that allows an apex beat

to be easily palpated will allow you to palpate the A wave, yet the S_4 sound may still be heard. There are many cardiologists who believe that you should never call an S_4 pathological unless you can find a palpable A wave with it [39]. If you follow this teaching, you will misinterpret every pathological S_4 in which the apex beat is difficult to palpate.

b) An A wave of more than 12 percent of the total apex cardiogram movement is probably abnormal, and if it is 14 percent or more, it will probably be palpable [14]. (See figure on pages 264 and 273.)

c) The greater the loss of compliance of the LV, the earlier the S_4 occurs on the A wave of the LV pressure curve [33].

4. Can an S_4 be produced by an atrium that is contracting against a stenotic atrioventricular (AV) valve as in mitral stenosis (MS)?

ANS.: No.

Note: The atrium must be able to transmit its pressure freely to the LV, or else only a presystolic murmur will be heard.

5. What theory could account for the production of an audible S_4 if it (a) occurs at the peak of atrial contraction, (b) causes such an increase in LV end-diastolic volume that it produces a recordable and often palpable systolic outward movement, (c) occurs when atrial pressure is higher than ventricular pressure, (d) sounds the same as an S_3, and (e) cannot occur if the AV valves are closed or stenotic?

ANS.: Atrial contraction, by causing eddy currents on the undersurface of the AV valves, tends to hold them upward. However, since atrial contraction also raises the volume in the ventricle, the chordae tendineae and papillary muscles are stretched at exactly the same time as the AV valves are being pulled up or held in the opposite direction. If it has enough energy, this tug on the chordae and papillary muscles could account for the sound.

RECOGNIZING THE RHYTHM OF THE S_4 GALLOP

If you remember that the P wave indirectly produces the S_4 and the QRS is responsible for the S_1, then, if you know that the S_2 occurs at the end of the T, the rhythm of S_4, S_1, and S_2 is the same as that of P, QRS, and end of T.

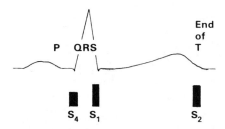

If you realize that the T wave is a *systolic* event, it will be easy to remember that the S_2 comes at the end of the T wave. Thus, the rhythm of an S_4 gallop is the rhythm symbolized by P,R---T, where R represents the QRS complex and T represents the end of the T.

Because the P is closer to the QRS than the QRS is to the end of the T, the rhythm or cadence is a pair of sounds close together followed by a pause, then the second sound. Therefore, the rhythm of the two cycles would be as follows: 4–1– – – –2   4–1– – – –2.

Vocal imitations of the heart sounds can help in perceiving the actual phenomena. Because the S_4 is low-pitched, you should practice imitating the S_4–S_1– – – –S_2 by saying "huh-one– – – –two." Place the "huh" as closely as possible to the "one," so that they are practically one word, "huh-one." Also, say the "huh" as softly as possible, because the S_4 is often just within the realm of audibility and, in fact, like the S_3, tends to range in and out of audibility from beat to beat when it is soft.

THE PHYSIOLOGICAL S₄

1. Can an S_4 be heard in normal subjects?

   ANS.: It can occasionally be heard in some normal subjects in all age groups. However, it is so rarely normal that unless it is heard in a young person with a concomitant physiological S_3 or in an athlete with physiological hypertrophy, you should suspect that it is an abnormal finding.

   *Note: About 50 percent of tall athletes (e.g., basketball professionals) have a physiological S_4. Almost all of those with an S_4 show some ECG or vectorcardiographic evidence of left ventricular hypertrophy (LVH) [35]. It can be recorded in almost two-thirds of young boys with a high-gain, low-frequency phonocardiogram [6] and in 35–70 percent of apparently normal subjects over age 40 [2, 34]. This may mean only that different equipment has different recording capabilities for low frequencies and does not necessarily mean that these vibrations are audible. In one study, asymptomatic patients over age 40 with a recorded S_4 had positive treadmill tests; therefore it is questionable how often a physiological S_4 is heard in perfectly normal hearts in persons over age 40 [2].

2. Why is the physiological S_4 so rarely heard?

   ANS.: a) It is usually too soft and too low-pitched.

   b) It is often too close to the S_1 to be separated from it by ear. It is then called the atrial component of the S_1, and it will be seen to begin just before the QRS on a simultaneous phonocardiogram and ECG.

*3. What is the mechanism of the physiological S_4?

   ANS.: The normal atrium may contract in a peristaltic fashion toward the ventricle. Therefore, by the time atrial contraction has caused the ventricle to reach its peak presystolic pressure, most of the atrium is relaxed and has a lower pressure (X descent). At this time, however, the ventricle is not relaxing, and there is a momentary reversal of the pressure gradient. This reversal of pressure will tend to close the mitral leaflets, pull up on the chordae tendineae, and produce a sound [20]. This peristaltic atrial movement is probably not present in a hypertrophied, strongly contracting atrium and is probably not the mechanism for the pathological S_4.

Note: a) The physiological S_4 has been correlated with echocardiographic closure of the mitral valve at the completion of atrial relaxation in patients with AV block [7].

b) This method of AV valve closure for the physiological S_4 is probably a different mechanism than that for the pathological S_4, as suggested by the following factors:

1) In complete AV block with myocardial damage, split S_4 sounds are frequently audible; the first component of the split occurs at the usual distance of an S_4 after the P wave, and the second one occurs 200 msec or more from the P wave. (The pathological S_4 is rarely more than 140 msec from the beginning of the P wave.)

2) The atrial pressure is higher than the ventricular pressure at the time of the usual pathological S_4, but is lower than ventricular pressure at the time of the second S_4 component in complete AV block in both animals and humans. (See figure on page 268.)

*4. When an S_4 is very close to the S_1, how can you distinguish clinically and by phonocardiogram between the physiological and the pathological S_4?

ANS.: a) Pressure on the carotid sinus does not change the intensity or position of the physiological S_4 but will cause the pathological S_4 to fade or disappear into the S_1.

b) If the S_4 is more than 70 msec from the S_1, it is likely to be a pathological S_4 [6].

THE PATHOLOGICAL S_4

Causes and Associated Conditions

1. After what age is an S_4 most likely to be pathological?

ANS.: After age 20. You should, however, consider any S_4 possibly pathological, even in a young subject, until proved otherwise. This means that before you call it physiological in the younger age group, you should probably hear a physiological S_3 and a physiologically split S_2, feel a normal apex beat, hear a venous hum in the neck (see p. 353), and obtain a normal ECG and chest x-ray. An echocardiogram should also probably be done to rule out a hypertrophic cardiomyopathy.

2. What kind of atrial contraction is necessary for the production of an audible S_4?

ANS.: A strong atrial contraction is the most important requirement for an audible S_4.

3. What condition generates a strong atrial contraction?

ANS.: Any condition in which the ventricle is "stiffer" than normal, i.e., in which the ventricle has decreased distensibility or **compliance.**

4. How does loss of distensibility of a ventricle cause a strong atrial contraction, i.e., how does the atrium "know" it must contract more strongly when the ventricle has lost compliance?

Boldface type indicates that the term is explained in the Glossary.

ANS.: The left atrium and left ventricle are one chamber in diastole, i.e., while the mitral valve is open, pressures are almost equal in both atrium and ventricle. This common chamber may be called an atrioventricle during diastole. If the LV is poorly distensible, as with LVH, the pressure rise due to filling of the atrioventricle from the pulmonary veins is steep. By the time the P wave and its subsequent atrial contraction occur, the atrial pressure is so high that it has a strong **Starling effect,** and the atrium will contract with greater energy than normal.

5. What conditions cause a decreased compliance of the ventricle?

ANS.: Those in which the ventricle is

   a) Thickened by LVH, as when it is laboring under a chronic **pressure load,** e.g., hypertension (the commonest cause of LVH in which an S₄ is heard).

   b) Stiffened by replacement of myocardium by fibrous tissue or infiltrate, e.g., amyloid heart disease or an old myocardial infarction.

   c) Stiffened by **ischemia** due to angina or acute infarction. (Subtotal or total acute coronary occlusions in dogs can be shown to increase the stiffness of the LV [39].)

6. How can a strong atrial contraction at the end of diastole cause a stronger contraction in a poorly compliant ventricle?

ANS.: Forcing blood into the ventricle just before the ventricle contracts produces an extra stretch of the ventricular myocardium. Starling's law tells us that such an extra stretch will give a stronger contraction.

   Note: A patient whose filling pressure is elevated by a strong atrial contraction will be less dyspneic than one who has the same high filling pressure due to a high V wave because a high A wave starting from a low left atrial pressure will result in a lower mean left atrial pressure than will a high V wave falling to a high left atrial pressure.

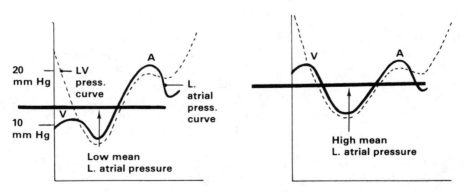

A low V wave and a disproportionately high A wave are seen on the left. These give a lower mean left atrial pressure and therefore less dyspnea than do both a high V wave and a relatively poor atrial contraction, as seen on the right.

7. What can prevent the effect of even a strong left or right atrial contraction from being transmitted to its respective ventricle?

ANS.: Mitral or tricuspid stenosis.

   Note: If the mitral obstruction is due to a left atrial myxoma, an S₄ can occur, presumably because either the atrial contraction has some effect on the tumor, or the atrial contraction can transmit its pressure to the LV by way of the atrial tumor.

8. What causes an atrium in sinus rhythm to be too weak to help out a ventricle?

ANS.: a) If the atrium is too large, as in chronic severe rheumatic mitral regurgitation (MR), the atrium may be overstretched and may therefore contract less efficiently. This can also occur when the left atrium is severely damaged by myocarditis, infarction, or infiltrate. It may be the damage rather than the enlargement that prevents an efficient contraction under these circumstances.

b) The atrium may also be weak if there is excess vagal stimulation [19].

c) Too little blood in the atrium also weakens it, i.e., decreased venous return due to either diuresis or having the patient stand.

9. How can the S_4 assist in the diagnosis of **constrictive pericarditis** or **tamponade?** Explain.

ANS.: An S_4 is not heard in constriction or tamponade. This seems surprising at first, because in tamponade the pressure rises quickly to a high point in the "atrioventricle" during diastole, and you would think that the stretch of the atrium would stimulate it to contract strongly. On the other hand

a) The inability of the ventricle to expand at the end of diastole due to the constriction could account for the loss of the forces necessary to produce an S_4.

b) The LV pressure rises so high at the end of diastole that the left atrium may not be able to open the mitral valve well.

c) The atrium may be so tethered by the constrictive process that it cannot contract well.

The S_4 in Myocardial Infarction and Angina

1. What proportion of patients with acute myocardial infarction have an S_4?

ANS.: Almost all will have a phonocardiographic S_4 unless they have MS or atrial infarction. It is heard by auscultation in about a half of the patients during the first few days following infarction [39]. Although this hyperacute S_4 may disappear, it will rarely ever do so if it remains beyond the first few days.

Note: The frequent S_4 heard in the first few days following infarction is partly explained by one study in which it is claimed that the infarcted area, whether dyskinetic (bulges out like an **aneurysm** in systole) or akinetic (no movement during systole), causes loss of compliance of the LV [21]. Also, it has been shown that ischemia or the presence of excess catecholamines in the first few days of infarction can also cause a loss of compliance of the LV [10].

2. Why may patients with angina have an S_4 only during an attack of chest pain?

ANS.: There is a marked increase in stiffness of the LV during angina, both at the beginning and at the end of diastole [4, 39].

The S_4 In Volume Overload

1. When is ventricular enlargement usually associated with a normally compliant ventricle and therefore with an absent S_4?

ANS.: When the volume overload is chronic due to regurgitant or shunt flows, e.g., in **ventricular septal defect** (VSD), **persistent ductus arteriosus,** chronic aortic regurgitation (AR), or chronic MR.

Note: An S_4 can, however, occur with the volume overloads that occur in hyperthyroidism or severe anemia [1]. In these conditions there is a relative loss of compliance of the LV due either to the effect of catecholamines on a recently volume-overloaded LV or perhaps to lack of adequate dilatation to accommodate the increased volume.

2. When will there be an S_4 in a subject with MR?

ANS.: When the MR is

a) Secondary to papillary muscle dysfunction or LV dilatation due to fibrosis or ischemia.

b) Sudden and severe due to ruptured chordae. In this case, the left atrium and ventricle are enlarged only moderately despite the massive volume overload, probably because the pericardium resists acute stretching.

Note: In rheumatic, chronic MR, there is almost never a left-sided S_4 because the left atrium is dilated, damaged, and hypocontractile.

LOUDNESS AND AUDIBILITY OF THE S_4

1. Where is the LV S_4 usually best heard?

ANS.: At the apex, when the patient is in the **left lateral decubitus position.**

* *Note:* The LV S_4 is occasionally better heard at the left lower sternal border than at the apex. The reason for this is unknown, but it occurs mostly in patients with angina or a past history of infarction [41].

2. Why should you usually use the stethoscope bell to bring out the S_4?

ANS.: Most of the energy of the S_4 (as of the S_3) is in the low-frequency range. The diaphragm is designed to dampen low frequencies.

* *Note:* An S_3 or an S_4 may occasionally be heard better with firm bell pressure because

a) When the S_3 or S_4 is loud, high frequencies develop, and attenuating the low frequencies by firm bell pressure can then sharpen the perception of the extra sounds by helping to separate them from the S_1 or S_2, especially during tachycardia [28].

b) With heavy bell pressure, the volume inside the bell is reduced. It may be that volume displacement by the A wave into a smaller total volume produces a greater effect on the eardrum.

3. What are the pitfalls of using held expiration as a means of bringing the stethoscope closer to the heart to help hear the S_4?

ANS.: Held respiration (apnea) will decrease venous return because the lungs act like a pump and help speed up the circulation time. The soft S_4 is very sensitive to blood volume.

4. How can the S_4 be made louder?

ANS.: a) By increasing blood flow to the atrium.

b) By increasing the pressure in the left atrium so that there is a greater stretch force on the atrial walls.

c) By bringing ventricular movements closer to the stethoscope.

5. Besides having the patient exercise, how can you increase the flow to the atrium?

ANS.: a) By asking the patient to release a Valsalva strain that has been maintained for at least 10 sec. This will cause a sudden rush of blood to the RV and a few seconds later to the LV, which then also must pump against an increased resistance for several seconds after the Valsalva.

b) By asking the patient to cough several times. This is really another form of exercise as well as a mini-Valsalva maneuver.

c) By asking the patient to take four or five deep, rapid breaths. This activates the lung pump and thus increases flow to the heart.

d) By asking the patient to squat. This can increase cardiac output for a few beats.

e) By isometric contraction through a handgrip (see below for hemodynamics). This increases cardiac output as well as blood pressure.

6. How can you bring ventricular movements closer to the stethoscope?

ANS.: Turn the patient into the left lateral decubitus position. If you listen immediately afterward, the effect of the exertion will be operative for a few beats.

Note: When all these maneuvers fail to produce an S_4 that is suspected, have the patient change from a standing to a left lateral decubitus position. This often produces an S_4 for a few beats.

HANDGRIP AND THE S_4

1. When does isometric handgrip contraction, such as when one squeezes a folded towel with one hand, bring out an S_4?

ANS.: A handgrip has this effect only if it raises pressure at the end of diastole in the LV. This occurs under two circumstances:

a) If there is abnormal LV function. In one study, when an S_4 occurred after 3 to 4 minutes of 25 percent maximum voluntary contraction or after about 30 sec of 50 percent maximal voluntary contraction, abnormal LV function was more likely than when an S_4 occurred at rest [31].

*b) If LV function is normal but severe MR or AR is present, probably because isometric contraction increases the regurgitation by increasing blood pressure.

2. When and how does handgrip contraction increase blood pressure?

ANS.: A handgrip produces local ischemia, which generates reflexes whose apparent purpose is to supply more blood flow to the ischemic area. In most subjects, handgrip transiently increases cardiac output through an augmentation of heart rate and contractility [18, 26]. It also increases peripheral resistance [23] in hypertensive patients, in patients with a reduction in cardiac reserve, and in patients with significant obstructive lesions, as in MS.

Note: a) Handgrip has been widely recommended to bring out an S_3 and an S_4. It does not always help for this purpose, probably because the increased contractility of the LV reduces the need for both an S_4 and the high left atrial pressure that is necessary for the S_3. If, however, the patient has angina or a pressure-loaded LV, as in aortic stenosis or elevated blood pressure, the end-diastolic pressure will usually be elevated by handgrip, and an S_4 will be brought out, especially if the heart is small [9, 26].

    b) The strength of the handgrip does not control the peak heart rate and blood pressure rise as long as equal degrees of fatigue are produced. The strength of the handgrip controls only the rate of development of the peak heart rate and blood pressure. For example, a 75 percent maximum voluntary contraction for 1 minute achieves about the same effect as a 25 percent effort for 5 minutes.

DIFFERENTIATION FROM THE S₃

1. How does the quality or the pitch of the S_4 differ from that of the S_3?

    ANS.: They do not differ. They may both be described as a low-pitched thud or boom. Because of their very low frequency of vibrations, they often feel more like a physical movement felt by the eardrum than like a sound heard by the auditory system.

2. When is it difficult to tell an S_3 from an S_4?

    ANS.: During tachycardia.

3. How can you tell without a phonocardiogram or pulse tracing whether an S_3 or an S_4 is present with a tachycardia?

    ANS.: a) If you can slow the rate with carotid sinus pressure, you may be able to discern that the extra sound keeps a constant relationship with the S_1, in which case it is an S_4. If it maintains a constant relationship with the S_2 and moves away from the S_1, it is an S_3.

        b) Wait for a pause following a premature beat. An S_4 will obviously precede the S_1 that ends the pause.

        Note: The long diastole after a premature ventricular contraction does not always allow you to hear an S_4. This is unfortunate because if it did, it would always separate an S_3 from an S_4 or from a summation gallop. Often the S_4 disappears at the end of a long diastole, possibly because of the reduced afterload.

*4. How can you tell by a phonocardiogram whether an extra sound is an S_3 or an S_4?

    ANS.: a) Because the longest distance between an S_2 and an S_3 is 200 msec, any interval longer than this suggests that the extra sound is an S_4.

        b) Because the shortest distance between a P wave and an S_4 is 60 msec, any interval less than this suggests that the extra sound is an S_3.

        c) A simultaneous phonocardiogram plus apex cardiogram will show the S_3 at the peak of the early rapid filling wave, whereas an S_4 occurs at the peak of the atrial hump or A wave. (See figure on page 273.)

5. If both an S_3 and an S_4 are present, what is the rhythm called?

    ANS.: Quadruple rhythm, train-wheel rhythm, or double gallop.

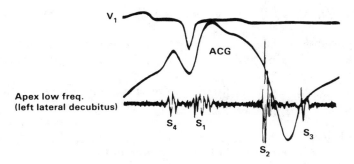

Apex cardiogram and phonocardiogram from a 55-year-old male with two previous infarctions. Surprisingly, despite his S_3 and S_4, or double gallop, he was almost asymptomatic without treatment. His atrial hump was easily palpable.

DIFFERENTIATION OF AN S_4–S_1 FROM A SPLIT S_1 (M_1–A_1 OR M_1–T_1)

1. When is an S_4–S_1 difficult to distinguish from a split S_1 due to an M_1–A_1 or M_1–T_1?
   ANS.: When the S_4 is very close to the S_1.
   * *Note:* Even experienced auscultators can mistake a split S_1 for an S_4–S_1 as shown by the study in which they were asked to record whether or not an S_4 was heard in 200 consecutive patients over age 50. Among 34 patients without an S_4 on phonocardiogram, there were 56 percent false-positive answers [34].

   How can you cause an S_4 to occur farther from the S_1 and so make the gallop rhythm more apparent?
   ANS.: a) By increasing venous return, e.g., by having the patient exercise or squat, or by the post-Valsalva strain effect.
   b) By increasing the work of the LV, e.g., by raising peripheral resistance with drugs, squatting, or handgrip. (See page 271 for a description of the type of patient in which handgrip will raise resistance.)

3. What is the difference in quality between an S_4 and the first major component of a split S_1, i.e., the M_1?
   ANS.: When the S_4 is loud, it is difficult to tell the difference in quality between an S_4 and an M_1, but when soft, the S_4 has fewer high frequencies, so that it is often inaudible when the diaphragm is pressed hard against the chest. The M_1 is usually heard almost as well with the diaphragm and firm pressure as with the bell, regardless of whether it is loud or soft.

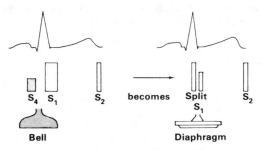

Pressure with the bell or the use of a diaphragm will eliminate most soft S_4s and may bring out the narrow, sharp, clicking physiological split of S_1.

4. How can the site of auscultation tell you whether you are listening to an S_4–S_1 rather than to a split M_1–A_1 or M_1–T_1?

   ANS.: The S_4 tends to disappear anywhere away from the apex beat. Therefore, a split S_1 that sounds the same at the left sternal border as at the apex has an M_1 as the first component.

5. How do changes from cycle to cycle tell you that the patient probably has an S_4 instead of an M_1–A_1?

   ANS.: A soft S_4 tends to disappear from perception from beat to beat; an M_1 does not characteristically do this. The change from beat to beat is due to the fact that the S_4 is very sensitive to changes in volume in the LV, as well as to proximity of the LV to the stethoscope. Both of these parameters are affected by respiration.

6. How can postural volume changes differentiate an S_4–S_1 from an M_1–A_1?

   ANS.: Because the S_4 is very sensitive to blood volume changes, standing will generally make it disappear. The M_1–A_1 may even become more apparent on standing because the M_1–A_1 interval represents **isovolumic contraction** time, which can be prolonged by standing, and wide splits are more obvious to the ear.

   Note: A general principle that helps you to distinguish an S_4 from an M_1 is that it is easy to get rid of an S_4 and difficult to get rid of an M_1. If the first component of what sounds like a split S_1 disappears on decreasing blood volumes, on increasing stethoscope pressure, or by moving away from the apex, you are dealing with an S_4. If the S_4 is so loud that none of the above maneuvers diminish it, it will usually be palpable as an atrial hump or A wave on the apex beat's pulse contour when it is palpated with the patient in the left lateral decubitus position.

*7. How can you distinguish between an S_4–S_1 and an M_1–ejection sound by phonocardiogram and pulse tracings?

   ANS.: a) If a phonocardiogram is taken simultaneously with an ECG, a sound that starts before the QRS is an S_4. (An S_4, however, need not necessarily begin before the QRS.)

   b) By taking a phonocardiogram simultaneously with an apex cardiogram, the S_4 is always recorded as a vibration that is simultaneous with the peak of the atrial hump or A wave of the apex cardiogram; the S_1 always appears after this atrial hump. The A_1, or aortic ejection sound, tends to occur at or near the peak of the upstroke of the apex cardiogram.

SEVERITY OF CARDIAC DYSFUNCTION AND PRESENCE OF AN S_4

1. When does an S_4 occur with the pressure overloads caused by *mild* aortic stenosis (AS) or *mild* systemic hypertension?

   ANS.: Only when enough myocardial damage has resulted from some other disease such as ischemic heart disease so that LV compliance is sufficiently diminished to cause an S_4.

*2. When is a right-sided S_4 not expected despite severe pulmonary hypertension?

   ANS.: When the contraction of the right atrium can decompress itself through a large atrial septal defect (ASD) or VSD.

Note: In the occasional ASD a presystolic murmur instead of an S_4 may be produced by atrial contraction.

3. What does the presence of an S_4 indicate about the gradient in (a) AS and (b) pulmonary stenosis (PS)?

ANS.: a) In valvular AS it suggests a severe gradient of at least 70 mm Hg across the aortic valve. (This should refer to an audible and not just a phonocardiographic S_4.) This is not valid either in subjects with angina in whom ischemic heart disease may be an additional cause of an S_4 or in subjects with **hypertrophic subaortic stenosis** (HSS) who may have an S_4 with any gradient [16].

b) In PS it suggests a gradient across the pulmonary valve or **infundibulum** of at least 70 mm Hg [42].

Note: In severe PS a strong right atrial contraction may actually open the pulmonary valve and produce a presystolic murmur or even a presystolic pulmonary valve opening click. The presystolic click often occurs between the S_4 and the S_1 and signifies severe PS, just as the S_4 does.

4. What proportion of hypertensive patients with a diastolic pressure of more than 100 mm Hg will have an audible S_4?

ANS.: About half.

5. Which is a more serious sign of heart disease, the pathological left-sided S_3 or the S_4?

ANS.: A pathological S_3 is more serious because it is associated with an increase in left atrial V wave pressure, which is a sign of decompensation at rest. An S_4, on the other hand, merely means that a poorly compliant ventricle is "calling on the atrium for help" and has only a high A wave pressure. The help it receives may be enough to keep the output adequate, even with moderate exercise.

6. What happens to the S_4 when failure becomes severe and an S_3 develops?

ANS.: After a stage in which both an S_3 and an S_4 may be present, the S_4 tends to soften and then disappear, and the patient with severe failure may be left with only an S_3 [5].

*7. When is an S_4 heard in the neck? Why?

ANS.: When a right atrial contraction is so strong (as in PS or pulmonary hypertension) that it produces a forceful jugular A wave that strikes the stethoscope chest piece, producing a sound with the timing of an S_4. It is not surprising that the effect of a strong right atrial contraction can be heard in the neck because sudden tensing of strips of various tissues has shown that the superior vena cava produces the loudest sounds among all cardiac tissues that have been tested, e.g., pulmonary artery, aorta, valves, and the walls of the ventricles [11].

Note: a) Right-sided S_4s are heard under the same circumstances at the right side of the heart as are left-sided S_4s at the left side. Therefore, they are heard in the presence of RV overloads that cause loss of compliance of the RV such as severe PS and pulmonary hypertension. They are also heard in sudden, severe tricuspid regurgitation due to ruptured chordae or endocarditis. (Right-sided endocarditis is usually seen only in heroin addicts.)

b) A P–S_4 of more than 160 msec is usually associated with a left-sided S_4. Right-sided P–S_4 intervals are rarely if ever that long. This implies that S_4–S_1 intervals on the right side are usually relatively long.

SEVERITY OF THE CARDIAC DYSFUNCTION AND TIMING AND AMPLITUDE OF THE S_4

1. What is the relation between the P–S_4 interval and the severity of the loss of compliance present?

   ANS.: The shorter the P–S_4 interval, the more severe the loss of compliance [13]. (If the P–S_4 interval is short, the S_4–S_1 interval will be long.)

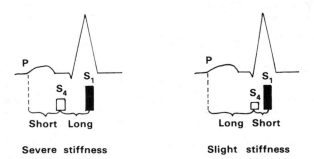

The longer the S_4–S_1 interval, the greater is the loss of compliance of the LV (provided the P–R interval is not prolonged) and usually the louder is the S_4.

*2. How can a P–S_4 interval be used to tell a pathological S_4 from a physiological S_4?

   ANS.: In one study, a P–S_4 of less than 130 msec was associated with abnormal LV compliance. Between 130 and 140 msec was equivocal, and more than 140 msec implied normal LV compliance as reflected by LV end-diastolic pressures [37].

3. What will happen to the S_4–S_1 interval in a patient who is hypertensive and is either made normotensive with an antihypertensive agent or has the flow to the heart decreased by asking him to stand up?

   ANS.: Both of these maneuvers will cause a narrow S_4–S_1 interval—i.e., the S_4 moves toward the S_1 and may join with it, becoming indistinguishable [22]. This could explain why an S_4–S_1 interval may be narrow despite hypertension or AS if the flow is decreased due to diuretics or heart failure.

   Note: a) The earlier the S_4, the louder it becomes. By electrical pacing of dogs' atria it has been shown that the earlier in diastole the atrium contracts, the more powerfully it contracts. It has also been shown that long S_4–S_1 intervals result in a more energetic ventricular contraction than do short S_4–S_1 intervals.

   b) As the S_4 moves farther from the S_1, the S_1 becomes softer [22, 27]. If the atrium reaches its peak pressure early, it may allow left atrial relaxation (X descent) to reach low levels early, and left atrial pressure will be relatively low when the ventricle starts to contract. Therefore, the LV will close the mitral valve at the slowest part of its acceleration curve. (See figure on page 181.)

   *c) The S_4–S_1 interval in hypertensive patients with LVH should be well separated even if the P–S_4 interval is not shortened, because in LVH the Q–M_1 interval is prolonged due to prolongation of the electromechanical interval [5].

*5. Why will acute myocardial infarction tend to narrow the S_4–S_1 interval, even if the P–S_4 is shortened?

ANS.: Catecholamines, which reach a high level in acute infarction, tend to shorten the Q–M_1 interval.

SUMMATION AND AUGMENTED GALLOPS

1. Why can a first-degree AV block augment the S_4?

ANS.: A first-degree AV block, i.e., in which the P wave comes very early in diastole and the QRS comes very late, may cause the atrium to contract early enough to coincide with rapid ventricular filling. Atrial contraction occurring at this time squeezes blood into the ventricle at the same time that rapid ventricular expansion is also drawing blood into the ventricle. Thus, a soft S_4 can become very loud. Unless the P–R interval is extremely prolonged, this contraction of the atrium at the time of rapid ventricular filling will occur only with a tachycardia.

2. What is the gallop rhythm called when the high flow of the early rapid filling phase of the LV is augmented by atrial contraction, as with first-degree AV block and tachycardia?

ANS.: A summation gallop, i.e., it is the summation of the mechanism for the production of an S_3 with the mechanism for the production of an S_4, to make an audible sound (this has facetiously been called the S_7). (See figure on page 252.)

Note: A summation gallop is physiological if neither an S_3 nor an S_4 would be present without the first-degree AV block and tachycardia.

*3. When are summation gallops pathological?

ANS.: When a pathological S_3 is augmented by atrial contraction occurring very early in diastole or when a pathological S_4 is augmented by occurring during the early rapid filling phase. These are then called "augmented gallops" [17]. This implies that an S_3 or an S_4 was augmented by the fortuitous assistance of a marked tachycardia or a prolonged P–R interval. Thus, an augmented gallop is a pathological type of summation gallop.

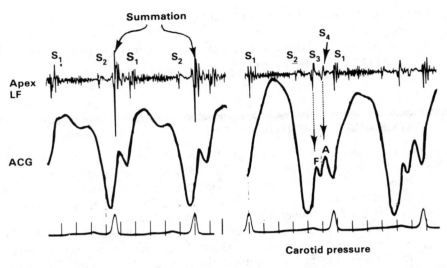

In this patient with heart failure and AS, a tachycardia of 115 with a P–R of 150 msec (0.15 sec) causes a summation gallop. When the rate is slowed by carotid pressure, both an S₃ and an S₄ appear. Therefore, this is an *augmented* type of summation gallop.

4. What may you hear if the heart rate of a patient with a summation gallop is slowed by carotid sinus pressure?

ANS.: You may hear either nothing or a pathological S₃, a pathological S₄, a physiological S₃, or both a pathological S₃ and S₄, i.e., a double gallop.

   *Note: How long a P–R interval is necessary for a summation gallop to occur depends on the length of diastole. (See page 252 for actual P–R intervals that will produce summation for various heart rates.)

THE PACEMAKER S₄-LIKE CLICK

*1. When can an electronic pacemaker produce an extra sound? When does the extra sound occur?

ANS.: When it causes intercostal skeletal muscle contraction, it can produce a high-pitched, clicking sound just preceding the M₁, so that it sounds like a widely split S₁ [24, 25]. It is accentuated by inspiration and occurs about 6 msec after the pacing stimulus [8].

Perforation of the myocardium of the RV by a transvenous pacing electrode should be suspected when the pacemaker-induced sound occurs. This, however, is not a necessary concomitant.

*2. Where on the chest are pacemaker sounds best heard?

ANS.: Sometimes at the apex and sometimes at the left lower sternal border. They are occasionally audible only in the left lateral decubitus position.

*3. Where has the pacemaker been situated when it produced a click plus diaphragmatic contraction with each click, without perforation of the heart?

ANS.: a) In the coronary sinus, where it stimulated the left hemidiaphragm, according to one report [38].

b) In the RV posteroinferior apical region in close proximity to the left hemidiaphragm, according to another report.

c) At the apex of the RV anteriorly, where it caused diaphragmatic stimulation that was distressing to the patient [15].

*Note: An atrial click also occurs 100 to 200 msec after a P wave, most often in patients with many different cardiac conditions such as ASD, thoracic deformities, hyperthyroidism, idiopathic cardiomyopathies, pericardiectomy, and pericarditis [36].

REFERENCES

1. Argano, B. J. Phonocardiographic findings in anemia. *Chest* 60:599, 1971.
2. Aronow, W. S., Cassidy, J., and Uyeyama, R. R. Effects of position on the resting and postexercise phonocardiogram. *Chest* 61:439, 1972.
3. Bamrah, V. S., Hughes, C. V., and Tristani, F. E. Mechanism of atrial sounds in atrial fibrillation. Phonoechocardiographic correlation. Report of a case. *Circulation* 53:569, 1976.
4. Barry, W. H., et al. Changes in diastolic stiffness and tone of the left ventricle during angina pectoris. *Circulation* 49:255, 1974.
5. Bethell, H. J. N., and Nixon, P. G. F. Understanding the atrial sound. *Br. Heart J.* 35:229, 1973.
6. Bridgman, E. W. Notes on a presystolic sound. *Arch. Intern. Med.* 14:474, 1914.
7. Brockman, S. K. Dynamic function of atrial contraction in regulation of cardiac performance. *Am. J. Physiol.* 204:597, 1961.
8. Cheng, T. O., Ertenm, G., and Vera, Z. Heart sounds in patients with cardiac pacemakers. *Chest* 62:64, 1972.
9. Cohn, P. F., et al. Diastolic heart sounds during static (handgrip) exercise in patients with chest pain. *Circulation* 47:1217, 1973.
10. Diamond, G., and Forrester, J. S. Effect of coronary artery disease and acute myocardial infarction on left ventricular compliance in man. *Circulation* 45:11, 1972.
11. Dock, W. The genesis of diastolic heart sounds. *Am. J. Med.* 50:178, 1971.
12. Dolara, A., and Tardini, B. Atrial flutter sounds: Report of a case. *Am. Heart J.* 78:369, 1969.
13. Duchosal, P. A study of gallop rhythm by a combination of phonocardiographic and electrocardiographic methods. *Am. Heart J.* 7:613, 1932.
14. Epstein, E. J., et al. The "A" waves of the apex cardiogram in aortic valve disease and cardiomyopathy. *Br. Heart J.* 30:591, 1968.
15. Gaidula, J. J., and Barold, S. S. Diaphragmatic origin of the pacemaker sound. *Chest* 61:195, 1972.
16. Goldblatt, A., Aygen, M. D., and Braunwald, E. Hemodynamic phonocardiographic correlations of the fourth heart sound in aortic stenosis. *Circulation* 26:92, 1962.
17. Grayzel, J. Gallop rhythm of the heart. *Circulation* 20:1053, 1959.
18. Grossman, W., et al. Changes in the inotropic state of the left ventricle during isometric exercise. *Br. Heart J.* 35:697, 1973.
19. Harris, W. S., Robin, P., and Tabatznik, B. Modification of the atrial sound by the cold pressor test, carotid sinus massage, and the Valsalva maneuver. *Circulation* 28:1128, 1963.
20. Herbert, W. H. Basis for effects of atrial dynamics on ventricular function. *N.Y. State J. Med.* 67:675, 1967.
21. Hood, W. B., Jr., et al. Experimental myocardial infarction, reduction of left ventricular compliance in healing phase. *J. Clin. Invest.* 49:1316, 1970.
22. Kincaid-Smith, P., and Barlow, J. The atrial sound in hypertension and ischaemic heart disease. *Br. Heart J.* 21:479, 1959.
23. Kivowitz, C., et al. Effects of isometric exercise on cardiac performance. *Circulation* 44:994, 1971.

24. Kluge, W. F. Pacemaker sound and its origin. *Am. J. Cardiol.* 25:362, 1970.
25. Kramer, D. H., Moss, A. J., and Shah, P. M. Mechanisms and significance of pacemaker-induced extracardiac sound. *Am. J. Cardiol.* 25:367, 1970.
26. Krayenbuehl, H. P., et al. Evaluation of left ventricular function from isovolumic pressure measurements during isometric exercise. *Am. J. Cardiol.* 29:323, 1972.
27. Leonard, J. J., Weissler, A. M., and Warren, J. V. Observations on the mechanism of atrial gallop rhythm. *Circulation* 42:1007, 1958.
28. Luisada, A. A., and Bartolo, G. High frequency phonocardiography. *Am. J. Cardiol.* 8:51, 1961.
29. Marsicano, T. H., et al. Myocardial mechanics and subtotal coronary occlusion. Circulation (Abstracts) (Suppl. III) 55 & 56:126, 1977.
30. Massumi, R. A., et al. The audible sound of atrial tachyarrhythmia (flutter?). *Circulation* 33:607, 1966.
31. Matthews, O. A., et al. Left ventricular function during isometric exercise (handgrip): Significance of an atrial gallop (S₄). *Am. Heart J.* 88:686, 1974.
32. Neporent, L. M., and DaSilva, J. A. Heart sounds in atrial flutter-fibrillation. *Am. J. Cardiol.* 19:301, 1967.
33. O'Rourke, R. A. The atrial sound. Factors regulating its occurrence and timing. *Am. Heart J.* 80:715, 1970.
34. Rectra, E. H., et al. Audibility of the fourth heart sound, a prospective, "blind" auscultatory and polygraphic investigation. *J.A.M.A.* 221:36, 1972.
35. Roeske, W. R., et al. Noninvasive study of athletes' hearts. *Circulation* 53:287, 1976.
36. Sakamoto, T., et al. Clinical observations of atrial click. *CV Sound Bull.* 5:275, 1975.
37. Schapira, J. N., et al. The atrial gallop: determination of its clinical significance. Circulation (Abstracts) 57 & 58:75, 1978.
38. Schluger, J., and Wolf, R. E. Sound caused by diaphragmatic contraction resulting from transvenous cardiac pacemaker. *Chest* 61:693, 1972.
39. Stock, E. Auscultation and phonocardiography in acute myocardial infarction. *Med. J. Aust.* 1:1060, 1966.
40. Tavel, M. E. The fourth heart sound—A premature requiem? *Circulation* 49:4, 1974.
41. Turner, P. P., and Hunter, J. The atrial sound in ischaemic heart disease. *Br. Heart J.* 35:657, 1973.
42. Vogelpoel, L., and Schrire, V. Auscultatory and phonocardiographic assessment of pulmonary stenosis with intact ventricular septum. *Circulation* 22:55, 1960.

13. *Ejection Murmurs*

PHYSICAL CAUSES

1. What is the cause of murmurs?
   ANS.: Sufficient flow in the cardiovascular system to generate enough turbulent energy in the walls of the heart or blood vessels to produce sounds.
2. What anatomical situations tend to produce high energy turbulence?
   ANS.: a) Obstruction to blood flow, caused either by circumferential narrowing or by a local protrusion into the bloodstream.
   b) Flow into a distal chamber of larger diameter than the proximal one.

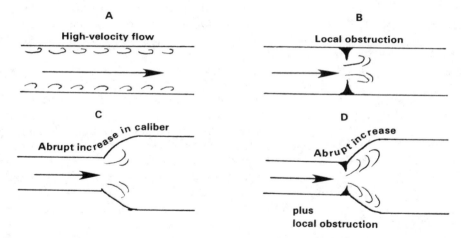

Causes of turbulence. In A, turbulence occurs in fluids flowing at high velocity through tubes of uniform caliber, according to the formula for Reynolds numbers. In B and C, either a local obstruction or fluid flowing into a channel of larger diameter can produce turbulence at much less flow velocity. In D, a combined effect of obstruction and abrupt increase in caliber, as in post-stenotic dilatation, produces turbulence at relatively low flow velocity.

3. What happens to the velocity of flow at an orifice?
   ANS.: It increases, just as it does when you narrow the nozzle of a hose.
4. How does the area of an orifice affect the volume of flow across it, the rate of flow across it, and the loudness of the murmur?
   ANS.: With a decrease in orifice area and given enough time, the volume of flow will tend to be maintained by a compensatory increase in pressure upstream from the stenotic area. The smaller the orifice, the greater the velocity of flow at the orifice and the greater the turbulence and the loudness of the murmur.
   Note: Turbulence is also affected by the following factors:

*Material marked with an asterisk is for reference and for advanced students in cardiology.

   a) Viscosity. The greater the viscosity, the less the turbulence. It is to be expected, then, that the high hematocrit present in patients with cyanotic congenital heart disease can increase blood viscosity enough to attenuate murmurs.
   b) The irregularity and sharpness of the edge of the orifice. The greater the irregularity sharpness at the orifice edges, the louder the murmur.

*5. What is a Reynolds number, and how does it apply to murmurs in humans?

   ANS.: Turbulence in a tube is calculated by the Reynolds number formula, which includes diameter, viscosity, and velocity. The greater the Reynolds number, the greater the turbulence. Because the Reynolds number theory pertains only to smooth tubular vessels, it is not surprising that the production of acoustic phenomena through orifices has been found to be independent of the Reynolds number in both *in vivo* and *in vitro* studies [41] and that the Reynolds number in the cardiovascular system is rarely great enough to produce a murmur [8, 41].

*6. What is the vortex or eddy theory of the cause of murmurs?

   ANS.: Turbulence sets up vortices or eddies, and these can strike the walls of the vascular system to produce vibrations that have frequencies and amplitudes that are compatible with actual murmurs.

   Note: A good analogy for eddies is that they are like smoke rings. (See figure on page 257.)

7. How does the frequency or pitch of a murmur relate to the (a) **gradient** and (b) flow?

   ANS.: a) The greater the gradient, the higher the frequency and pitch produced. High gradients with little flow volume produce "blowing" murmurs.
   b) The greater the flow, the more are low and medium frequencies produced, i.e., "the greater the flow, the more the low." When low gradients produce murmurs that are highly dependent on flow, the result is a "rumbling" murmur.
   c) A combination of high gradient and high flow produces mixed frequencies that, if loud, can result in harsh murmurs.

CHARACTERISTICS OF THE EJECTION MURMUR

1. What valvular flow event is implied by the term *ejection* murmur?

   ANS.: The term implies a murmur that is produced by blood flowing forward through a *semilunar valve* during systole.

2. What is characteristic of ejection murmurs on a phonocardiogram?

   ANS.: They start with the final component of the first heart sound (S_1), are diamond- or kite-shaped, and finish before the second sound of the side of the heart from which the murmur originates. This means that a left-sided ejection murmur will finish before the A_2, and a right-sided ejection murmur will finish before the P_2.

Boldface type indicates that the term is explained in the Glossary.

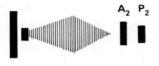

This murmur could be either pulmonary or aortic, since it ends before both components of the second sound.

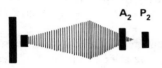

This murmur can be a pulmonary ejection murmur, since although it extends beyond the A_2, it finishes before the P_2.

3. Why must an ejection murmur be crescendo-decrescendo in loudness?

ANS.: The configuration of the loudness of a murmur across a valve is controlled mainly by the shape of the gradient. This gradient is controlled by the velocity and acceleration of flow, i.e., the greater the velocity and acceleration of flow, the greater the gradient and the louder the murmur.

In aortic stenosis (AS), as the pressure in the left ventricle (LV) rises to just above diastolic pressure in the aorta, it takes a short time to overcome the inertia of the aortic blood and walls. Therefore, the initial gradient across the aortic orifice is slight, and the murmur starts softly. The pressure gradient and velocity of flow then increases toward midsystole, as does the murmur. As soon as the ventricle begins to reach the state of reduced ejection, just past the middle of systole, the flow decreases, the gradient decreases, and the murmur decreases.

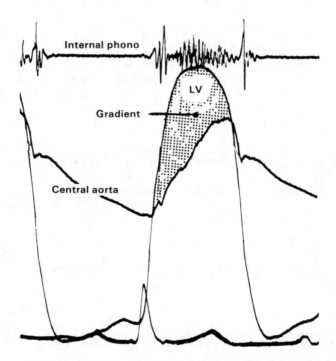

A simultaneous aortic and LV pressure tracing (taken with a catheter tip micromanometer to eliminate time delays through tubes) in a subject with valvular AS. The shape of the murmur follows the shape of the gradient (shaded area).

4. Why does an aortic or pulmonary ejection murmur sound to the ear as if it ends before the semilunar valve closure sound of its side even though on phonocardiograms the murmur often reaches the S_2?

ANS.: Just before the valve closes, the velocity of forward flow has decreased so much that even if the murmur does extend to the second sound by phonocardiogram, the ear cannot hear the very end of this faint decrescendo part of the murmur.

5. What happens to the loudness of an ejection murmur after a long diastole, as in the long pause after a premature ventricular contraction or after the long diastoles of atrial fibrillation? Why?

ANS.: It becomes louder. The main reason may be because the long period of diastole allows a larger volume to collect in the LV and stretch its walls. This increased volume is ejected during the next systole with increased energy by means of the Starling effect.

Note: One study could not show by ventriculography that the long diastole after a premature beat actually causes an increased volume in the ventricle [60]. This study implies that the reasons for an accentuated ejection murmur after a sudden long diastole are:

a) The **postextrasystole potentiation** following an early ventricular depolarization (as with a premature ectopic beat) produces a positive inotropic effect on the ventricle (believed to be due to a calcium flux effect) and contributes to the loudness of the ejection murmur after a long diastole. It has been shown in one study that the worse the myocardial function, the greater the postextrasystolic potentiation effect. This suggests that the greater the increase in loudness after a sudden long pause, the worse may be the myocardial function [49].

b) A long diastole allows more peripheral runoff and therefore a reduction in afterload. This causes an increase in the velocity of myocardial shortening and an increase in the volume of forward flow.

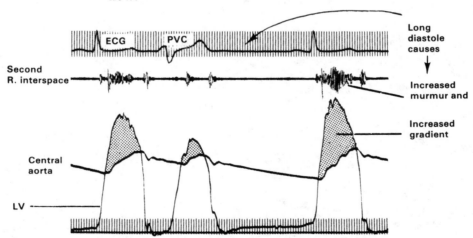

A phonocardiogram and simultaneous aortic and LV pressure tracing from a 16-year-old boy with valvular AS. Not only did the murmur and gradient increase after the long diastole, but the ejection sound also increased. Note that the small gradient of the premature ventricular contraction (PVC) itself produced only a short early systolic murmur.

6. Do the pitch or frequency characteristics of an ejection murmur change when the murmur is soft? Why?

ANS.: No, it retains the low (and medium) frequencies. (This is important because regurgitant murmurs do not do this.) Because ejection murmurs are produced by the entire stroke volume passing through the aortic or pulmonary valve with each systole, there will always be enough flow to produce low and medium frequencies, even when the obstruction or gradient across the valve is trivial.

7. How can you best define an ejection murmur?

ANS.: It is best defined as an "ejection murmur complex"—i.e., it is a murmur that begins at the end of the S_1, is crescendo-decrescendo, ends before the second sound of its side, becomes louder after long diastoles, and retains low and medium frequencies even when soft.

Note: The original meaning of the term *ejection murmur* was a midsystolic crescendo-decrescendo murmur that ended before the second sound of its side [37]. This definition ignores the following facts:

a) On phonocardiograms, most ejection murmurs can usually be seen to start without any pause after the S_1.

b) A regurgitant murmur may also be crescendo-decrescendo and may occasionally end before the S_2 of its side.

8. How can you tell by auscultation alone that a murmur is crescendo-decrescendo (diamond- or kite-shaped on a phonocardiogram)?

ANS.: A rhythmic cadence is created by the sequence of S_1 followed by the peak of the crescendo followed by S_2.

huh–huh–duh

peak
S_1 of S_2
diamond

Note: a) This rhythm should be thought of only as the background effect to the systolic noise that includes the S_1 and S_2. If an S_2 is missing, "huh–huh" tells you that the murmur is crescendo-decrescendo. If the S_1 is missing, the rhythm of "huh–duh" also tells you that the murmur is crescendo-decrescendo.

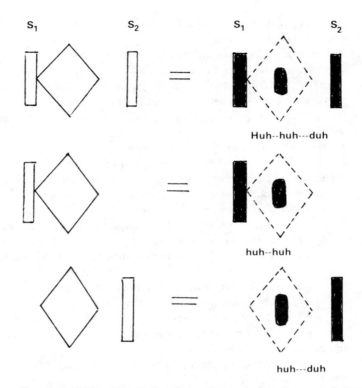

S_1 S_2 S_1 S_2

Huh--huh---duh

huh--huh

huh---duh

If you imagine the string section of an orchestra playing a long note during systole and the drums playing a rhythm of two or three notes, you will have the impression given by the peak of an ejection murmur plus either an S_1, an S_2, or both.

      *b) Because the pitch of an ejection murmur is also often crescendo-decrescendo, the shape of some ejection murmurs is sometimes best seen with the high-frequency band of a phonocardiogram [42].

9. How can the loudness of an ejection murmur tell you whether or not there is a significant gradient across a valve?

    ANS.: A soft murmur, i.e., grade 2 or less, is likely to occur with an unimportant gradient, provided that artifactual reasons for the softness, such as obesity or heart failure, are absent. If the murmur is very loud, i.e., grade 4/6 or more, the gradient is likely to be at least 20 mm Hg. Unfortunately, a loud murmur does not tell you how much over 20 mm Hg the gradient may be.

10. List some factors, besides a thin chest wall, that spuriously increase the loudness of systolic ejection murmurs, i.e., without reflecting the degree of the gradient.

    ANS.: a) The systolic expansion of a markedly dilated pulmonary artery or aorta, creating artifactual crackles or crunches by pressure against the surrounding lung tissue.

        b) Any cause of increased flow, such as exercise, thyrotoxicosis, arteriovenous fistula, anemia, shunt, excessive diastolic filling, as in bradycardia or aortic regurgitation.

TYPES OF EJECTION MURMURS

1. List the two common types of ejection murmurs.
   ANS.: 1) The systolic flow murmur, i.e., a murmur due to causes other than obstruction to flow.
   2) The aortic or pulmonary stenosis ejection murmur.
2. List the five types of systolic flow murmurs.
   ANS.: 1) The murmur due to the normal "impulse gradient," which is perceivable only because of a thin chest or a quiet room. A normal impulse gradient is the gradient produced by the normal acceleration of ventricular blood across a nonobstructed semilunar valve.
   2) The flow murmur due to increased stroke volume or rate of ejection.
   3) The murmur due to unknown anatomical causes of turbulence, namely, the innocent humming ejection murmur of childhood.
   4) The murmur due to **aortic sclerosis**.
   5) The murmur due to ejection into a dilated artery.
   Note: a) When flow suddenly enters a dilated chamber—i.e., a dilated pulmonary artery or aorta—it can produce turbulence that results in a murmur. The three major examples of this type of murmur are idiopathic dilatation of the pulmonary artery or of the ascending aorta, as with an **aneurysm,** and the pulmonary ejection murmur occurring in patients with severe pulmonary hypertension. These murmurs are very short, finishing at about midsystole [53].
   * b) It is possible that when these murmurs go beyond midsystole they are artifactually produced by adhesions between a dilated ascending aorta or main pulmonary artery and the surrounding pleura. (See page 290, Question 4.)

SYSTOLIC FLOW MURMURS

The Normal Impulse Gradient Murmur and the Increased Flow Murmur

1. How can a systolic murmur be produced across a normal semilunar valve?
   ANS.: There is always a forward pressure gradient across a semilunar valve, as there must be in any pipe with a forward flow.

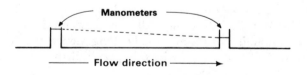

The gradient between the upstream and downstream manometers may not be measurable by the usual cardiac catheter techniques. If, however, the gradient is increased enough by obstruction to flow, a semilunar valve, or even a local protuberance from one wall, enough turbulence may occur to produce a murmur.

2. What is the relationship between the gradient across a semilunar valve and the shape of the murmur?

ANS.: The greater the gradient across a semilunar valve, the louder and longer the murmur and the later the peak of the crescendo–decrescendo.

* *Note:* Across a normal valve, however, the shape of the murmur is controlled entirely by the velocity of flow, and not by the shape of the gradient. The velocity of flow is crescendo–decrescendo with an early peak, i.e., it is mainly an *early* ejection murmur.

The normal peak gradient across a normal aortic valve (the impulse gradient) is earlier than the peak of velocity of flow because gradient is related to acceleration of flow, and acceleration peaks earlier than does velocity of flow in the absence of stenosis.

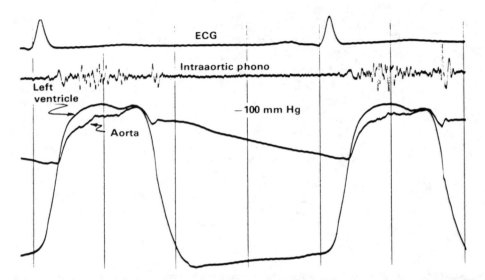

Aortic and LV pressure tracings together with a phonocardiogram from a 40-year-old man with an innocent aortic ejection murmur. Note the early systolic gradient between the LV and aorta, which is the normal impulse gradient found not only in normal left-sided chambers but also normally seen between the right ventricle and pulmonary artery. This tracing is taken by a single catheter with two end holes, in order to obtain absolutely accurate timing and pressure differences across the aortic valve.

3. In what percentage of normal subjects is the normal impulse gradient ejection murmur heard?

ANS.: In 100 percent, depending on

a) The soundproofing of the room. All normal subjects have an ejection murmur in a soundproof room, usually along the left sternal border but often only after elevation of the legs, hyperventilation, or mild exercise [26].

b) The physical or emotional state of the subject.

c) The degree to which the shape and thickness of the chest separate the stethoscope from the heart.

d) The age of the subject. About 96 percent of healthy children up to age 14 have ejection murmurs on ordinary clinical examination in a quiet but not soundproof room [38]. These murmurs are usually maximal at the left sternal border. About 15 percent of adults under age 40 have an innocent ejection murmur [12].

4. Why are young patients most likely to have an easily audible flow murmur, besides their thinner chests?

ANS.: Because of their more rapid **circulation time**.

*Note: Young patients with innocent murmurs have been shown in one study to have lower blood viscosity and lower hematocrits than patients without murmurs [52].

Ejection Murmurs Due to Increased Flow

1. What are the preferred terms for an easily audible ejection murmur that is produced by an increase in flow across a valve rather than by valve narrowing?

ANS.: a) *Systolic flow murmur* is the preferred term in speaking to physicians.

b) *Innocent murmur* is the preferred term when you are speaking to patients. This term implies that the prognosis is such that it will give the patient no trouble. This is a very reassuring term to use in speaking to a patient.

*Note: The term *relative stenosis* does not aptly explain the flow murmur shape across a normal valve because such a shape is more related to changes in velocity (acceleration) than to gradient. Therefore, the flow murmur is different from a stenosis murmur, in which the gradient, flow velocity, and murmur have the same shape.

2. Why is the term *benign* or *functional* not desirable when you are describing to the family a murmur that is not associated with any known cardiological abnormality?

ANS.: *Benign* implies that an abnormality is present but is not malignant. *Functional* may have no meaning to a layman, although to a physician it may mean "due to increased flow."

3. List the commonest causes of ejection flow murmurs due to increased stroke volume.

ANS.: 1) Shunt flow, e.g., an atrial or ventricular septal defect will produce pulmonary systolic flow murmurs.

2) Increased ventricular volumes due to regurgitant leaks such as aortic or pulmonary regurgitation will produce systolic flow murmurs.

3) Marked bradycardia, as in complete atrioventricular (AV) block.

4) Increased cardiac output, as in thyrotoxicosis, anemia, exercise, pregnancy, and systemic arteriovenous fistulas.

Note: a) Cardiac output is not significantly increased in anemia until the hemoglobin and hematocrit drop to about 50 percent of normal. Patients with anemia may have a lower viscosity than normal, and this may also increase turbulence.

b) About 90 percent of pregnant women have ejection murmurs due to increased blood volume [25].

c) Flow murmurs are more likely to occur across an aortic than across a pulmonic valve because peak velocity and turbulence intensity are higher across the normal aortic orifice than across the pulmonic valve, presumably because of the larger cross-sectional area of the pulmonic valve and the slightly longer duration of ejection through the pulmonic valve [58].

4. What is meant by a "hemic" murmur?

ANS.: A hemic murmur is any murmur that is present in the anemic state and disappears when the anemia is corrected. For example, mitral regurgitation (MR) may be heard only with the increased heart size, blood volume, and need for coronary flow caused by severe anemia [15].

Atrial Septal Defect Systolic Flow Murmurs

1. What causes a systolic murmur in patients with an uncomplicated ASD?

ANS.: Increased flow through the dilated main pulmonary artery.

2. Why is there no murmur through the defect in the atrial septum?

ANS.: Because there is almost no gradient across the defect. If the defect is large, the two atria act as a single chamber, so that the pressures on each side of the defect are almost equal. Even if the defect is small, the gradient between the left and right atria is never more than a few millimeters of mercury.

* Note: a) A soft murmur through an ASD might be inaudible even if one occurred at that site, because it has been shown that an acoustic signal produced artificially by a mechanical sound generator in the right atrium is almost completely dissipated before it reaches the chest wall [20].

b) A continuous murmur may be produced across an ASD in the presence of a small defect plus MR or rheumatic mitral stenosis (MS), which raises the pressure in the left atrium considerably higher than that in the right atrium. An ASD plus MS is called Lutembacher's syndrome.

3. Where is the ASD systolic ejection murmur best heard? What is notable about its radiation?

ANS.: The ejection murmur is best heard at the second or third left interspace. There is frequent transmission to the apex, even when the murmur is soft [37]. This is probably due to the dilated right ventricle (RV), which transmits all RV and pulmonary artery events to the apex.

* 4. What suggests that part of the pulmonary flow murmur of ASD is extracardiac, i.e., probably due to adhesions between the dilated pulmonary artery and the pleura?

ANS.: a) It is often crackly, crunchy, or scratchy [37].

b) Other causes of marked pulmonary artery dilatation sometimes produce this crackling or crunchy type of murmur (e.g., idiopathic dilatation of the pulmonary artery).

c) It is often louder and longer than a mere flow murmur should be despite the absence of pulmonary stenosis (PS).

d) In some ASDs there is no ejection murmur, despite at least a moderate shunt and a normal pulmonary artery pressure.

The Straight Back Syndrome Ejection Murmur

1. What is meant by the straight back syndrome?

ANS.: Compression of the heart due to loss of the normal dorsal curvature of the spine, resulting in a pulmonary ejection murmur that is usually mistaken for that of either PS or ASD [50].

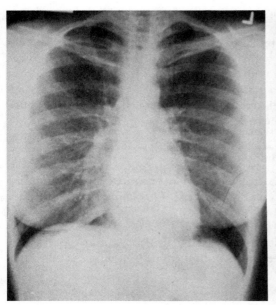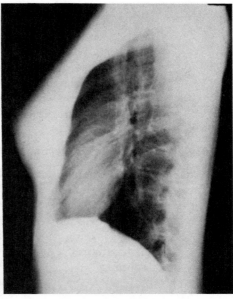

In this patient with the loss of dorsal curvature the anteroposterior diameter is one-third of the transverse diameter. The "straight front," plus the slight anterior bowing of the lower thoracic spine, probably contributed to the compression effect on the heart. (Courtesy of Dr. Antonio C. deLeon, Jr.)

2. What other palpatory and auscultatory findings in the straight back syndrome mimic ASDs?

ANS.: 1) An exaggerated left parasternal movement may be present.

2) The split of the S_2 may be wide and the second component of the split S_1 may be accentuated [17].

3) The systolic murmur is often scratchy or crunchy.

3. How loud is the ejection murmur of the straight back syndrome?

ANS.: It may range from grade 1/6 to grade 4/6. Even without a **pectus excavatum,** a markedly narrowed anteroposterior diameter can occasionally cause a murmur loud enough to have a thrill [13].

Note: a) The murmur has occasionally been noted to change markedly in intensity from grade 2 to grade 4 with stethoscope pressure.

* b) A short, early, grade 1/6, scratchy diastolic murmur that increases with inspiration is present in many patients with the straight back syndrome.

4. Why will loss of the normally gentle dorsal kyphosis cause a pulmonary ejection murmur?

ANS.: The upper mediastinal structures, including the pulmonary artery, may be compressed against the sternum, thus creating murmurs. In a small percentage of such patients there is actually a gradient of 5–15 mm Hg in the pulmonary outflow tract, apparently created by this compression.

Note: a) An anteroposterior chest diameter (back of sternum to front of vertebrae) that is one-third or less of the transverse diameter (from inside of the ribs), measured at just above the right dome of the diaphragm, is almost diagnostic of the straight back syndrome [13].

b) The objections to the term *straight back syndrome* are:

1) Many subjects with straight backs have an anteriorly bowed sternum that provides ample space for the heart and thus have no pseudocardiac disease [14].

2) Scoliosis as well as pectus excavatum are commonly found with the straight back syndrome.

The Humming Systolic Ejection Murmur

1. What adjectives have been used to describe the quality, or timbre, of the humming (innocent) ejection murmur that is found in children? What eponym has been used for it?

   ANS.: It has been described as a humming, buzzing, vibratory, twanging, moaning, or groaning murmur. It has also been called Still's murmur after the British author of a pediatric textbook published in 1918, who described it as "twanging."

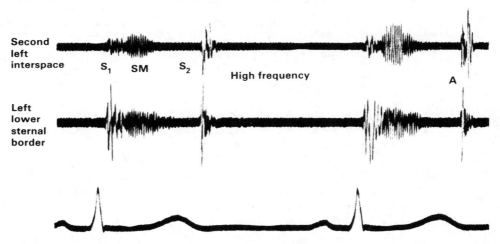

The regular vibrations on this phonocardiogram of a humming systolic murmur (SM) tell you that the murmur has a musical quality. The peak of the crescendo occurring in the first third of systole tells you that the gradient across the semilunar valve is probably trivial.

2. What does the humming or twanging character of an ejection murmur in childhood tell you about the gradient across the semilunar valve?

   ANS.: It means that there is only a slight gradient across the valve producing the murmur. It also suggests strongly that the murmur is innocent and will either disappear when puberty is complete or sound the same 15 years later [18].

3. Which valve appears to be the source of the humming murmur?

   ANS.: The aortic valve. A fine *thrill* can be recorded on the carotid tracings of some children with the murmur.

   * *Note:* It was once proposed that a taut pulmonary valve fibrous ring could

cause vibrations as blood passes through it. However, pulmonary hypertension or pulmonary artery dilatation from any cause that tenses the valve ring does not cause a humming murmur.

*4. What evidence suggests that this murmur does not come from the pulmonary area?

ANS.: a) Intracardiac phonocardiograms from the pulmonary artery in patients who have this murmur show only the same ejection murmur as that picked up in most normal persons, i.e., it is not vibratory either by paper recordings or when heard through a loudspeaker [65].

b) After a **Valsalva** maneuver the murmur does not return immediately. (See page 306 for an explanation of the effect of the Valsalva maneuver on murmurs.)

5. Where is the humming murmur usually heard best?

ANS.: Although it is best heard between the apex and the left sternal border, it is surprising how widespread and difficult it is to localize this innocent murmur.

6. What suggests that it is a form of "flow" ejection murmur and is not due to obstruction?

ANS.: a) It becomes louder when the subject is supine and often disappears when the subject is upright.

b) The murmur is never louder than grade 3/6.

c) The murmur is usually short and reaches its peak early.

d) Children with this murmur tend to have shorter preejection periods than those without it [15]. (See page 407 for an explanation of a preejection period.)

e) It is often associated with a loud venous hum [9] (see p. 352).

f) It consists of low and medium frequencies, i.e., between 75 and 160 cycles per second. A murmur that is relatively low in pitch suggests that it is due mostly to flow with very little gradient.

Note: These humming murmurs may become as long as important murmurs in the presence of further increased blood flow, such as that occurring with high fever or severe anemia.

The Aortic Sclerosis Murmur

1. What percentage of patients over age 50 have an easily audible aortic ejection murmur without valvular stenosis?

ANS.: About 50 percent. Therefore, we have called this the "50 over 50" (50/50) murmur. However, if you eliminate patients with previous infarction or elevated blood pressure with ECG evidence of LV hypertrophy, then only about 30 percent will have an aortic sclerosis murmur [48].

2. What is the cause of this aortic ejection murmur?

ANS.: There are several theories:

a) It is due to fibrosis, thickening, and often some calcification involving the bases of the aortic cusps. They do not open fully because of stiffness (aortic valve sclerosis), but they do open enough to prevent any gradient across the orifice. However, there is enough narrowing to cause turbulence and an ejection murmur.

b) It is due to calcific spurs on the aortic ring, which may protrude into the bloodstream when calcium is laid down at the roots of the cusps.

c) It is due to atherosclerotic plaques in the ascending aorta that may cause turbulence as the aortic stream strikes the roughened endocardium.

Note: 1) The general condition alluded to by these theories is called aortic sclerosis.

2) If the calcification that caused the sclerosis murmur becomes excessive, severe aortic valve obstruction may occur; this is known as calcific aortic stenosis.

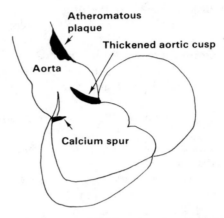

A slight but abrupt protuberance (e.g., a calcium spur) is capable of producing a murmur of considerable intensity.

3. What factors in the elderly are known to increase the incidence of the 50/50 murmur?

ANS.: a) Hypertension. The higher the blood pressure, the more likely the murmur.

Note: In one series of severely hypertensive patients, every one was found to have an ejection murmur [29].

b) Sex. The incidence of this murmur is almost twice as high in women as in men.

4. How loud can a murmur due to aortic sclerosis be?

ANS.: Up to grade 4/6.

5. What are the most important methods of distinguishing by physical examination a loud murmur of aortic sclerosis from that of AS?

ANS.: a) Palpation of the carotid will generally differentiate between the slow rise of AS and the normal rise of aortic sclerosis.

b) An early peak to the crescendo–decrescendo murmur denotes a small or absent gradient. (See page 416 for the use of ejection times in differentiating these two lesions, and page 41 for exceptions to the slow rates of rise seen with AS.)

AORTIC STENOSIS EJECTION MURMURS

Valvular Aortic Stenosis Murmurs

Murmur Shape, Duration, and Quality

1. How can you tell the severity of aortic stenosis by the shape and length of the murmur?

   ANS.: In general, the later the peak of the crescendo and the longer the murmur, the more severe the stenosis.

       * *Note:* Even though the peak of the crescendo in valvular AS extends only very slightly beyond midsystole no matter how severe the stenosis, a rough correlation can be found between the Q-peak interval and the presence of either mild or severe AS. If the Q-peak interval is less than 200 msec, severe stenosis (valve area less than 0.75 cm^2) is very unlikely. If the Q-peak interval is more than 240 msec, severe stenosis is likely [5]. In another study, a Q-peak interval of less than 220 msec excluded severe AS in the elderly [22]. If the patient is hypertensive, the peak may occur falsely early [24].

2. How may the pitch and quality of an aortic ejection murmur sound at the apex? Why is this confusing? What is this phenomenon called?

   ANS.: The high-frequency components tend to radiate to the apex and may even sound musical at this site. Therefore, a murmur of MR is suggested. This is called the Gallavardin phenomenon.

       Note: In the elderly patient, the murmur of calcific AS often sounds musical or cooing at the apex. Commissural fusion is commonly absent in these valves, allowing the cusps to vibrate and produce pure frequencies [51].

3. What is the characteristic quality of the loud murmur of moderate to severe AS?

   ANS.: It tends to be harsh, rasping, grunting, and coarse, sounding like a person clearing his throat. This murmur can be imitated by placing your palm on the diaphragm of a stethoscope and listening through the earpiece while you scratch the dorsal surface of the hand with your fingernail.

Loudness and Site

1. Where is the aortic systolic murmur of valvular AS heard loudest?

   ANS.: Anywhere in a straight line from the second right interspace to the apex. (If the patient is obese or has emphysema, the murmur may be loudest above or on the clavicle.)

2. Where is the classic *aortic area*? What is wrong with this term?

   ANS.: This area is in the second right interspace. All aortic valvular events can be best heard anywhere in a "sash" or "shoulder harness" area from the second right interspace to the apex.

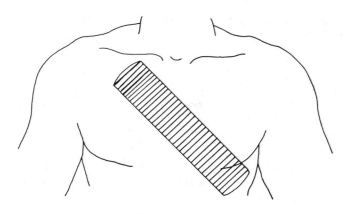

Aortic area

Since aortic ejection murmurs and clicks are often best heard at the apex area, and aortic regurgitation murmurs are usually best heard along the left lower sternal border or midsternum, it should no longer be taught that the "aortic area" is the second right interspace.

3. What term should we use instead of *aortic area*?

   ANS.: The second right interspace. It is confusing to a student to be told that aortic murmurs and ejection sounds are often best heard at the left sternal border or apex and then to hear the second right interspace called the aortic area.

4. What is characteristic of the upward radiation of an aortic murmur?

   ANS.: a) It tends to radiate into the neck bilaterally but often radiates well along the innominate vein, making the murmur slightly louder on the *left* (contrary to earlier impressions reported in the literature). If the murmur radiates better to the right carotid then to the left you should suspect supravalvular AS. (See p. 300.)

   b) It not only radiates well to the right clavicle but is usually amplified there. Because the aortic ejection murmur is usually louder over the right clavicle than over the right carotid, any murmur louder over the carotid than the clavicle should be considered a local arterial murmur [54].

   Note: a) Innocent aortic ejection murmurs are characteristically maximal along the left sternal border near the anatomical aortic valve area. With significant aortic valvular obstruction, however, the maximum turbulence occurs farther downstream from the orifice and tends to be loudest at the second right interspace [57].

   *b) Occasionally an aortic ejection murmur sounds louder near the carotid bifurcation than lower in the neck, presumably because the bifurcation is closer to the skin than the common carotid and subclavian arteries [35].

5. Is a loud ejection murmur (at least grade 4/6) ever associated with mild AS?

   ANS.: Yes. Although a loud murmur usually signifies severe AS, a small percentage of such murmurs occurs in moderate and even mild AS [2].

   Note: If a loud murmur is associated with an absent or very soft A$_2$, it almost always indicates severe AS because the soft A$_2$ implies heavy calcification [2].

6. How soft can the murmur of a severe AS become if heart failure develops with a resultant reduced stroke volume?

ANS.: It may almost disappear.

*Note: a) Concomitant mitral stenosis (MS) will also decrease the loudness of the AS murmur, but unless the MS is very severe, the AS murmur will dominate the picture and even cause the MS murmur to be absent because the loss of compliance caused by the left ventricular hypertrophy (LVH) can result in slow diastolic expansion of the LV, attenuating the MS murmur [61].

b) A low flow due to a cardiomyopathy may result in almost no murmur across a moderately obstructed aortic valve. This occurs because the physiological cross-sectional area of the aortic valve opening during systole is always smaller than the potential anatomical area, and the lower the flow, the smaller the physiological cross-sectional area used by the forward stream [59].

7. Why may the murmur of severe AS be soft in the elderly in the absence of heart failure?

ANS.: a) There is commonly an increased anteroposterior chest diameter in the elderly, especially at the base of the heart.

b) The stiff cusp bases and lack of commissural fusion may cause some of the blood to be ejected between the cusps and, therefore, to form a "spray" rather than a jet. This may make the murmur not only more musical but also less loud and harsh [51].

Summary of Auscultatory Clues to the Diagnosis of Severe Valvular Aortic Stenosis

The AS is probably severe, i.e., the gradient is at least 70 mm Hg, or, in the presence of congestive heart failure, at least 50 mm Hg, if:

1. An S_4 is present in a patient under age 40 [10].
2. The murmur is long, with its peak in midsystole, is at least grade 4/6, and is associated with a soft or absent A_2. (Such a murmur may be only grade 3/6 if the patient has a large, thick chest, heart failure, or significant MS or MR.)

Hypertrophic Subaortic Stenosis Murmurs

1. What causes the obstruction in **hypertrophic subaortic stenosis** (HSS)?

ANS.: The obstruction is caused by the combination of a hypertrophied septum, which bulges into the LV outflow tract during systole, and abnormal anterior motion of the anterior leaflet of the mitral valve. The outflow tract, which is the space between the septum and the anterior leaflet of the mitral valve, becomes narrow. This has been substantiated by two-dimensional echocardiography [30].

Note: *a) Some cardiologists believe that MR rather than LV outflow obstruction is the cause of the ejection type of murmur in patients with HSS. This theory ignores the finding of only trivial MR that is often seen on angiography in some HSS patients with a loud systolic murmur.

b) Another good term for HSS is hypertrophic obstructive cardiomyopathy (HOCM).
c) Not all patients with hypertrophic cardiomyopathy have outflow
   obstruction.

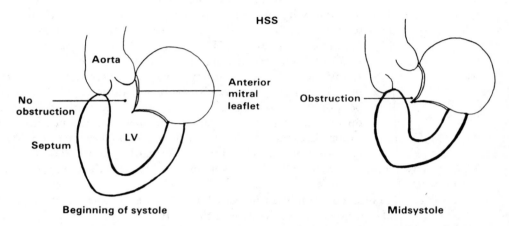

HSS

The asymmetric hypertrophy of the LV (sometimes shortened to ASH) causes no obstruction until the disproportionately hypertrophied septum meets the anterior mitral leaflet in midsystole.

2. When in systole does the obstruction begin in HSS?
   ANS.: Just prior to midsystole.
3. When does the ejection murmur begin in HSS?
   ANS.: The murmur usually begins at the same time as it does in valvular stenosis,
   i.e., at the beginning of systole. (This contrary to statements in the literature
   that are probably based either on very mild cases or on phonocardiograms
   that are too well filtered or too hastily examined.) The murmur usually
   begins early because even though the obstruction is delayed to slightly beyond the time of onset of aortic valve opening, the tremendously rapid early
   ejection characteristic of HSS can cause early turbulence. In the normal heart
   only about 50 percent of ventricular volume is ejected during the first half of
   systole, but in HSS 80 percent or more is ejected during this period [47].
   Even through a normal valve this rapid flow can produce a murmur in early
   systole. However, if the obstruction is mild, there may not be an early flow
   murmur, and only the delayed murmur due to the midsystolic obstruction
   may be present.
   *Note: Occasionally, a low-amplitude ejection sound can be seen on a
   phonocardiogram preceding the murmur. The rapid ejection in early
   systole can set up the necessary conditions for an ejection sound.
4. How can raising the blood pressure by a vasopressor agent or by having the patient
   squat help to differentiate between the ejection murmur of valvular AS and that of
   HSS?
   ANS.: In valvular AS, if an inotropic vasopressor such as metaraminol is used to
   raise the blood pressure, it will also stimulate contractility, increase the
   gradient, and make the murmur louder. Even if a noninotropic vasopressor
   agent produces a bradycardia by the vagal effect of suddenly raising the

blood pressure, there may be more time for diastolic filling, and in valvular AS the greater stroke volume may also increase the loudness of the murmur.

In patients with HSS, on the other hand, any vasopressor will decrease the murmur because the increased resistance to outflow tends to hold the outflow tract open by pushing the anterior mitral leaflet away from the septum.

Note: Maximum handgrip for 30 seconds, by raising the blood pressure, also causes the HSS murmur to diminish [1]. (You may ask the patient to squeeze steadily on a rolled-up towel.)

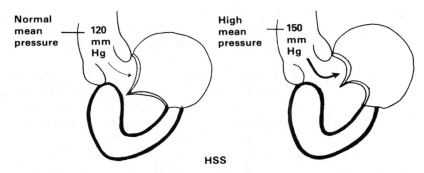

A high blood pressure during ejection pushes up on the mitral valve and spreads apart the LV outflow tract, which is made up of the septum and the anterior mitral leaflet.

5. What tends to make an HSS obstruction worse, making the LV cavity smaller, or making it larger? Why?

   ANS.: Making it smaller allows the hypertrophied septum to obliterate the outflow tract space more easily.

6. How can a **Valsalva maneuver** help to differentiate the ejection murmur of valvular AS from that of HSS?

   ANS.: During the Valsalva maneuver the venous return is decreased. Thus, the stroke volume is decreased, and the ejection murmur of valvular AS is decreased. However, in a patient with HSS, the decreased venous return produces a smaller LV and therefore more obstruction and a louder murmur.

   Note: a) The Valsalva maneuver may not always work because

   1) It may produce such a rise in systemic resistance and aortic pressure that it overcomes the effect of reducing heart size.

   2) It may produce such severe obstruction that there is too little flow across the outflow tract to make the murmur louder.

   *b) A **Mueller maneuver** will shift the septum to the left and could theoretically cause more obstruction [27].

*7. How can amyl nitrite inhalation differentiate the ejection murmur of valvular AS from that of HSS?

   ANS.: The blood pressure will drop immediately with amyl nitrite inhalation, but flow does not increase until about 20 sec later. Therefore, the murmur of valvular AS, which is dependent on flow, will not begin to increase for about 20 sec. The murmur of HSS, on the other hand, will become louder within a few beats after inhalation because as soon as the blood pressure drops (which occurs almost immediately), the loss of resistance to outflow causes a loss of support for the anterior leaflet of the mitral valve as the ventricle contracts. (See page 327 for the hemodynamic effects of amyl nitrite.)

8. How will squatting differentiate between the murmur of HSS and that of valvular AS?

ANS.: Squatting, especially for the first few beats, will diminish the murmur of HSS because it causes both increased venous return for a few beats and then a persistent increase in peripheral arterial resistance [45]. In the presence of valvular AS the increase in venous return will tend to increase the murmur.

*9. What is peculiar about the site of greatest loudness of the HSS murmur that may help to differentiate it from the murmur of valvular AS?

ANS.: It is usually loudest near the apex, but occasionally it is loudest at the left lower sternal border.

Note: a) When septal hypertrophy is so great that it also produces RV outflow (infundibular) obstruction (rare), the infundibular obstruction may cause the mumur to be louder at the base than elsewhere (as in other forms of pulmonic stenosis).

b) The term *asymmetric septal hypertrophy of the heart* is often used to describe the heart in HSS because the septum is disproportionately hypertrophied in relation to the hypertrophy of the free wall. The hypertrophied ventricle may so distort the mitral valve apparatus that it sometimes causes inflow obstruction of the LV and even of the RV, and can cause occasional mitral or tricuspid inflow gradients. The dominant obstruction, however, is almost always AS.

10. Why is an HSS murmur often mistaken for an MR murmur?

ANS.: Because the HSS murmur often tends to be loudest at the apex.

*Note: a) Some MR is usually present. Two explanations are offered for the presence of MR, which is usually trivial.

1) It is thought that the hypertrophied septum distorts the direction in which the papillary muscles pull on the valve cusps, so that a **Bernoulli effect** can pull an unsupported free edge of an anterior leaflet toward the septum. This could cause not only outflow obstruction but also some MR.

2) Mitral valve prolapse may occur in as much as 75 percent of patients with HSS. This may be due to the cavity obliteration that often occurs with HSS, causing the mitral ring to become too small for the area of valve tissue.

b) A pansystolic apical murmur of MR in a patient with HSS will probably not disappear after corrective surgery for HSS.

---

*Supravalvular Aortic Stenosis Murmurs

*1. Where in the aorta is the stenosis of supravalvular AS?

ANS.: Above the **sinuses of Valsalva**.

Note: It may be focal (hourglass), discrete membranous, or diffusely hypoplastic.

*2. At what unusual site might the murmur be loudest in supravalvular AS? Does this help differentiate it from valvular AS?

ANS.: It may be loudest in the suprasternal notch, the first right intercostal space, or over the manubrium sterni [4, 52A]. (However, it may also be loudest in the second right intercostal space, which is not an unusual best site for a valvular AS murmur.)

*3. What other murmurs are often found in patients with supravalvular AS?

ANS.: a) Those due to stenosis of the pulmonary arteries, termed *pulmonary branch stenosis.*

b) An AR murmur, because the aortic valve is frequently abnormal.

Note: The AR murmur is unusual in that often it is unexpectedly intensified with amyl nitrite [52A].

Summary of Clinical Findings in Supravalvular Aortic Sclerosis

1. Peculiar "elfin" facies in nonfamilial type. (See page 32 for facies of supravalvular AS.)
2. Pulse volume greater and murmur louder in the right than in the left carotid. (See page 53 for explanation.)
3. Blood pressure higher in the right arm.
4. No ejection sound.
5. Slight AR murmur.

*Discrete Subvalvular Aortic Stenosis

*1. Where may the obstructive ridge in discrete subvalvular AS be located, and of what may it consist?

ANS.: It is either a thin membrane on the ventricular septum just below the aortic valve or a fibrous ring about 1 cm below the aortic valve, and is associated with muscular hypertrophy of the outflow tract.

*2. What other murmur is common in patients with discrete subaortic stenosis?

ANS.: Aortic regurgitation may occur in as many as one-third of such patients [33].

Note: If the murmur is preceded by an ejection sound, it is not likely to be due to discrete subvalvular AS unless it happens to be associated with a bicuspid aortic valve.

PULMONARY STENOSIS EJECTION MURMURS

1. Where is the classic "pulmonary area"? What is wrong with this term?

ANS.: The classic pulmonary area is the second left interspace. Pulmonary events, however, may be best heard *anywhere* along the left sternal border (or even in the epigastrium in patients with chronic obstructive pulmonary disease).

2. Where is the best place for hearing the murmur of (a) valvular PS and (b) infundibular PS?

ANS.: a) The murmur of valvular PS is heard best at the second left interspace.

b) The murmur of infundibular PS is heard best at the third or fourth left interspace.

Note: The third left interspace parasternally has often been called Erb's point. This name seems unnecessary and confusing—first, because some authors include the fourth left interspace, and second, because medical dictionaries often do not give a definition of Erb's point on the chest but describe one on the neck over the brachial plexus.

3. What is the relation between the peak of the crescendo of the PS murmur and the severity of the obstruction?

ANS.: The later the peak, the more severe the obstruction. It may occur as late as four-fifths of the way through RV systole [63].

*Note: PS may be imitated by coarctation with a bicuspid aortic valve, because this combination may produce an ejection sound followed by a murmur with a late peak [7]. The murmur with the late peak in coarctation is probably due to flow through the intercostal collaterals or possibly through the coarcted segment itself.

4. Why is it that in AS the murmur rarely peaks much beyond midsystole, yet in PS it may easily go beyond midsystole?

ANS.: The RV is shaped like a teapot, with a main chamber, namely, the inflow tract (also known as the RV sinus), and a thick, high spout, which is the ouflow tract or **infundibulum**.

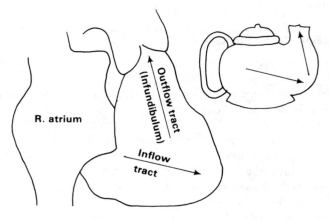

The outflow tract of the RV is a tubular structure made up mostly of muscle, called the crista supraventricularis, which separates the tricuspid from the pulmonary valves.

The inflow and outflow tract contract asynchronously in a peristaltic fashion, the inflow tract first, then the infundibulum or outflow tract. The worse the obstruction at the valve, the more hypertrophied is the muscle of the outflow tract and the later it contracts relative to the inflow tract. It is the late contraction of this RV outflow tract that apparently produces the late peak of the crescendo.

The LV, on the other hand, has no distinct muscular outflow tract. The anterior mitral leaflet and its chordae and papillary muscles form the posterolateral wall of a merely functional outflow tract, which is probably seldom anatomically independent enough to contract more than slightly late on the left side.

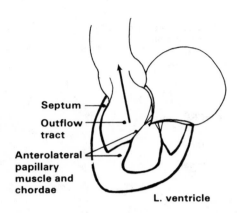

Septum

Outflow tract

Anterolateral papillary muscle and chordae

L. ventricle

There is no infundibulum in the LV because the mitral and aortic valves are in direct continuity.

*5. How does infundibular PS affect the length of the murmur? Why?

ANS.: If the stenosis is due to hypertrophy of the outflow tract (infundibulum), the murmur tends to be slightly longer than it is in valvular stenosis of similar severity [63]. In this type of pulmonic stenosis RV outflow is also reduced by the abnormal infundibulum contracting excessively during systole. The delay in contraction of the infundibulum is often so exaggerated that the infundibulum (and pulmonary artery) pressures are higher than those in the body of the RV for about 100 msec before the pulmonary valve closes [31]. This causes a wide splitting of the A_2–P_2 interval, even if the stenosis is mild.

Note: a) Infundibular stenosis can be imitated by a RV anomalous muscle bundle that traverses the RV cavity just below the infundibulum. It is most commonly found together with a VSD.

b) Pulmonary valve or branch stenosis can be imitated by a partially obstructing pulmonary embolus.

6. How can analysis of the phonocardiogram suggest the severity of the gradient across the pulmonary valve in PS with an intact septum?

ANS.: By the length of the murmur, the site of the peak of the crescendo, the presence or absence of an ejection click, and the width of the split of the S_2 [63].

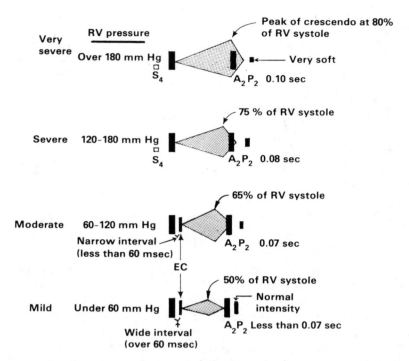

As the gradient across the pulmonary valve increases, the murmur peaks later and lasts longer, and the P₂ becomes further separated from the A₂ and softer. The ejection click (EC) may be absent above 60 mm of pressure in the RV, but may reappear on sitting or standing.

The Murmur in Pulmonary Stenosis With an Intact Ventricular Septum Versus the Murmur of Tetralogy of Fallot

1. In the absence of heart failure, when will there be severe PS but still a very short murmur?

   ANS.: If PS is accompanied by an aorta that straddles a VSD, i.e., **tetralogy of Fallot** is present. The more severe the PS, the shorter the murmur because the greater the obstruction at the pulmonary valve, the more the RV blood is diverted into the aorta, i.e., the right-to-left shunt increases, and so less blood goes through the pulmonary valve. This will make sense only if you know that the murmur of a tetralogy of Fallot with **cyanosis** is solely due to the PS. *Right-to-left shunts do not usually produce murmurs.*

   Note: This introduces the concept of two outlets for systole, which is important in the understanding of murmur changes with maneuvers and drugs. If a ventricle has two outlets for systole, increased resistance to flow through one of the outlets will cause more blood to go through the other outlet. If, on the other hand, resistance is *decreased* beyond an outlet, more blood will move through that outlet and less through the other. In tetralogy, the RV has two outlets, the pulmonary artery and the aorta that overrides the VSD. In cyanotic tetralogy you should think of the RV as pumping directly into the aorta and not into the LV first.

*2. Why will the degree of cyanosis tend to correlate with the softness of the murmur?

ANS.: a) Increased cyanosis means increased polycythemia, which in turn means increased blood viscosity. The greater the viscosity, the less the turbulence across an obstruction and therefore, the softer the murmur [23]. (See explanation of Reynolds number on page 282.)

b) The greater the right–to–left shunt, the softer the murmur, because less blood is flowing through the pulmonary valve.

Note: In a very severe tetralogy the systolic murmur is usually no louder than grade 2/6 [62].

*3. How can amyl nitrite differentiate between the murmur of PS in tetralogy and that occurring when the ventricular septum is intact?

ANS.: In tetralogy the immediate decrease in peripheral resistance, with no effect on pulmonary resistance, causes an increased flow into the overriding aorta and, therefore, decreased flow through the stenotic pulmonary valve, resulting in a softer murmur. If, on the other hand, there is PS with an intact ventricular septum, lowering the systemic resistance causes no change in the PS murmur, but the increase in venous return after about 20 sec causes the PS murmur to become louder.

*Note: a) The murmur of severe PS with a "muscle-bound" RV may also diminish with amyl nitrite, presumably by dilating the infundibulum due to the increase in venous return caused by the nitrite. Therefore, amyl nitrite cannot be used to distinguish *severe* PS from tetralogy [64]. It can still be used, however, to distinguish mild or moderate PS (which are never "muscle-bound") from tetralogy. A muscle-bound RV is one with such an excessive degree of outflow tract hypertrophy that RV systolic pressure fails to fall to less than 100 mm Hg immediately after valvotomy. It can be suspected by the paradoxical effect of amyl nitrite and by the jugular tracing, which shows a very slow and shallow Y descent (or no Y descent at all) in the absence of tachycardia, suggesting considerable loss of diastolic compliance.

b) In PS with an intact ventricular septum, the beta-stimulating effect of metaraminol may make the murmur louder because of its positive inotropic effect [6]. Methoxamine, however, is a pure alpha constrictor and will produce little change in a PS murmur if the septum is intact. However, it will increase the loudness of the PS murmur in tetralogy of Fallot because the increase in peripheral resistance will raise aortic systolic pressure and "force" more blood across the stenotic pulmonary valve.

*4. How does the effect of a long diastole following a premature beat help to distinguish pure PS from tetralogy of Fallot?

ANS.: If the postextrasystolic beat has a significantly louder murmur than the normal beats, the septum is probably intact. This reflects the fact that in pure PS the pressure in the RV for the beat ending the compensatory pause usually rises more than 15 mm Hg above its regular pressure, whereas in tetralogy of Fallot the pressure rises only slightly above control levels because the pressure in the aorta falls more than the pressure in the pulmonary artery during the long diastole [28].

THE EFFECT OF RESPIRATION ON EJECTION MURMURS

1. Which phase of respiration can increase a gradient across (a) a pulmonary valve and (b) an aortic valve? How should this affect their murmurs?

   ANS.: a) Inspiration increases the filling of the RV, which in turn increases flow across the pulmonary valve. Therefore, inspiration increases the gradient and the loudness of the murmur. A gradient increases by the square of the increased flow.

   b) Conversely, inspiration decreases flow into the LV and across the aortic valve and, therefore, decreases both the gradient and the murmur.

   Note: A pulmonary flow murmur, such as that heard in an ASD, in which there is only a slight gradient across the pulmonary valve, may not become louder on inspiration because the slight increase in velocity of flow due to inspiration is overcome by the increase in distance from the stethoscope caused by chest expansion. Even on intracardiac phonocardiograms, only two-thirds of ASDs show an increased amplitude of murmurs in the pulmonary artery on inspiration [21].

2. Why may a PS ejection murmur not always increase during inspiration?

   ANS.: a) Inspiration may place too much lung between the stethoscope and the heart, especially in the upper parasternal region (the basal area of the heart). Therefore, listen low on the chest or even posteriorly for the effect of inspiration.

   b) Sinus arrhythmia may cause shorter diastoles during inspiration. This will decrease stroke volume during inspiration and tend to soften the murmur.

   Note: If the murmur is due to hypertrophic cardiomyopathy with the septum bulging into the RV outflow tract, the murmur will actually increase on expiration because any maneuver that makes the RV smaller will cause more obstruction at the infundibulum [44].

3. Why does standing tend to exaggerate the increase in a PS murmur caused by inspiration?

   ANS.: The increase in pulmonary flow caused by inspiration is about 15 ml whether the subject is lying down or standing. The total stroke volume, however, is decreased on standing, so that the same 15-ml increase in stroke volume on inspiration comprises a proportionately larger amount of stroke volume ejected.

   For example, an increase on inspiration of 15 percent for a supine stroke volume of 100 ml is 15 ml. The stroke volume on standing can be decreased by 25 percent [40]. With a standing stroke volume of 75 ml, the 15-ml increase on inspiration is now a 20 percent increase. Therefore, on standing there is a proportionately greater increase in gradient across the pulmonary valve.

   Note: The increased sympathetic tone caused by standing may decrease the degree of sinus arrhythmia.

*4. How can a Valsalva maneuver distinguish a pulmonary ejection murmur from an aortic ejection murmur?

   ANS.: During the strain phase, the decreased venous return causes all ejection murmurs (with the rare exception of the HSS murmur) to diminish. When the strain is released, the maximum loudness of the pulmonary ejection murmur will return immediately, i.e., within two or three beats. The maximum loudness of the aortic murmur will, however, be delayed for about six to ten beats owing to the time needed for the dammed-up venous blood to pass through the lungs to the LV and aorta [3].

**Summary of How to Distinguish a Pulmonary
from an Aortic Stenosis Murmur by Auscultation**

1. The AS murmur decreases slightly on inspiration. The PS murmur increases on inspiration, especially on standing and if you listen low on the chest posteriorly.
2. An AS murmur may be maximal in the second right intercostal space or at the apex. The PS murmur will only be maximal somewhere along the left sternal border.
3. The post-Valsalva effect causes an immediate return of loudness of the PS murmur but a delay in the return of loudness of the AS murmur.
4. If an ejection click is present, it will decrease or disappear on inspiration only with PS.
5. A wide, normally moving split S_2 following the murmur usually indicates a murmur of PS rather than of AS.
6. A right-sided S_4, i.e., one that is heard at the left lower sternal border or epigastric area and increases on inspiration, is due to PS, whereas an S_4 that is heard only at the apex and increases or becomes audible only on expiration suggests that the murmur is due to AS.

THORACIC, SUBCLAVIAN, CAROTID, AND THYROID ARTERY FLOW MURMURS

1. What is characteristic of the timing and duration of a physiological (nonobstructive) vascular murmur?
   ANS.: When you can hear the heart sounds or, if not, when related to the pulse, they are early in systole and short.
   Note: Innocent vascular murmurs increase after sudden long diastoles, exercise, or the administration of amyl nitrite [34].
2. What are the characteristics of an arterial murmur due to obstruction?
   ANS.: If a pressure difference proximal and distal to the obstruction is present in both systole and diastole, the murmur will be continuous, and the systolic murmur is always louder than the diastolic. The murmurs will have either a midsystolic or a late systolic peak if the obstruction is severe.
3. What is the difference between a bruit and a murmur?
   ANS.: The word *bruit* (pronounced "brooee") is French for "noise" or "sound." In France, the first and second heart sounds are the first and second bruits. Our S_1 and S_2 are their B_1 and B_2. We tend to misuse the word to mean an arterial murmur. Because arterial murmurs sound the same as murmurs heard elsewhere, there seems to be no need for a change of terminology, especially since the word has even been used by some to mean a heart murmur [19].

4. Which arterial flow murmur may cause an ejection type of murmur at the second right or left interspace?

ANS.: Rapid flow through the proximal branches of the aorta in young people. This is often mistaken for an aortic ejection murmur.

Note: A carotid murmur is present in about 80 percent of children up to 4 years old but is found in only 10 percent of those in older age groups.

5. How can you differentiate the supraclavicular arterial murmur of childhood from a basal valvular murmur?

ANS.: a) If, as you inch gradually toward the supraclavicular area with your stethoscope, a short early murmur becomes louder, it is an arterial murmur unless it is louder over the clavicle than above it. Aortic valvular murmurs tend to be amplified over the clavicle.

b) If the arm flow is increased by hand-clenching exercise, the arterial murmur may become louder, but a valvular murmur will not.

c) If the arm is stretched downward and backward, the subclavian artery is compressed between the clavicle and the first rib. The arterial murmur will gradually diminish as the subclavian artery is compressed.

d) Compress the subclavian artery with your finger, and note how the murmur changes with varying degrees of obstruction.

Note: Listen also for a venous hum and an S_3 to confirm the presence of a hyperkinetic circulation [55]. (See page 352 for a method of eliciting a venous hum.)

6. What kind of peripheral arterial murmurs are heard in **coarctation?**

ANS.: Systolic flow murmurs with delayed onset (due to the time required for the systolic flow to reach the vessel and therefore continuing beyond the S_2) can be heard over the large collateral vessels of the back. These murmurs may become softer or disappear if the arteries are compressed.

Note: If the systolic delayed murmur is heard between the left scapula and spine, it is questionable whether it is caused by flow through the coarctation itself or through the collaterals. It has been heard there when there is complete occlusion of the coarcted segment. It has generally been taught that the more severe the coarctation, the longer the murmur over the coarcted site. Thus, if the narrowed segment is severely narrowed, the murmur will crescendo in late systole and go into diastole (continuous murmur). A mild coarctation is said to have a short, early murmur.

7. Why do patients with coarctation have murmurs over the intercostal arteries?

ANS.: When the intercostals are collaterals, they become tortuous. Tortuosity creates turbulence.

8. What kind of murmur over the thyroid is heard in hyperthyroid patients?

ANS.: The arterial murmur is systolic. If a continuous murmur is heard, it is a venous hum.

---

*Aorta-Coronary Artery Bypass Surgery Vascular Murmurs

*1. How common is a new vascular systolic murmur after coronary bypass graft surgery?

ANS.: Up to one-half of bypass procedures to the anterior descending artery have produced such a murmur.

* 2. What factors suggest that the systolic vascular murmur heard after coronary bypass surgery is indeed due to the bypass?

ANS.:
a) It is often noted in patients who did not have the murmur prior to surgery.
b) When it disappears, the bypass has often been found to be occluded.
c) In one study, when the murmur was present, the graft was invariably found to be patent [32].
d) It has been heard only when the anterior descending artery has been bypassed.

* 3. What suggests that the mechanism for the production of a coronary bypass graft murmur is probably retrograde flow across the native coronary artery stenosis that engendered the operation?

ANS.:
a) The bypass graft has no aortic valve covering it at its aortic junction as does the normal coronary ostium, i.e., the native coronary ostium is "protected" by the aortic valve leaflet in systole, whereas the graft ostium is open to the full pressure of systole. This mechanism also explains why the bypass graft murmur is louder in systole than in diastole, even though we know that coronary flow is greater in diastole.
b) In no patient with a completely occluded native stenosis has the murmur developed, and if the native stenosis was later found to be completely occluded, the murmur had disappeared.
c) The murmur does not occur with a right coronary artery bypass, presumably because the distal anastomotic site is well away from the chest wall.
d) The murmur has not been heard on or around the aorta with a stethoscope during open heart surgery.

4. What is the timing and intensity of the bypass murmur? How is it brought out?

ANS.: It is a short, early ejection murmur, not much more than grade 2/6 in loudness. It is best heard when the patient is sitting up and leaning forward with held expiration. It can be intensified by an injection of dipyridamole (at 0.14 mg/kg/min), which can even bring out a diastolic component of the murmur [46].

* 5. Where are bypass graft systolic murmurs best heard?

ANS.: They are usually localized to the second, third, or fourth left interspace parasternally [3].

* 6. What is the significance of (a) a disappearing and (b) a persistent bypass murmur?

ANS.:
a) A disappearing murmur has no significance because many become softer after a few months, and by one year, almost all either are soft or have disappeared.
b) A persistent murmur strongly suggests that the bypass graft is open.

---

* Pulmonary Artery Stenosis Murmurs

* 1. What types of pulmonary arterial stenosis are there?

ANS.:
a) Pulmonary branch stenosis, i.e., multiple peripheral stenosis or stenosis of only the right or left pulmonary artery.
b) Stenosis of the pulmonary trunk.

Note: a) With this there is commonly another congenital lesion present, such as pulmonary valve stenosis or supravalvular AS.

b) Pulmonary artery branch stenosis is commonly seen with the rubella syndrome, other features of which may be cataracts, deafness, mental retardation, or poor growth.

*2. What murmurs may be produced by peripheral pulmonary branch stenosis?

ANS.: If the stenosis is unilateral, an ejection murmur may be present. If it is bilateral, however, either an ejection murmur or a continuous murmur may be produced [16]. It requires bilateral pulmonary branch stenosis or some other cause of pulmonary hypertension to produce a continuous gradient and murmur.

Note: a) A pulmonary artery branch may be stenosed and produce no murmur at all if the distal segment is supplied by enough bronchial collaterals to reduce the gradient across the stenosed segment [43].

b) A pulmonary artery stenosis murmur begins, peaks, and ends later in systole than a proximal stenosis or flow murmur. It is rarely louder than grade 3/6.

*3. Where are the murmurs of unilateral pulmonary branch stenosis heard? What can mimic them?

ANS.: These murmurs are heard anywhere on the chest. Wide radiation with equal loudness throughout, i.e., to the axillae and back, is the hallmark of a pulmonary artery branch stenosis murmur. The pulmonary artery flow murmur found in some patients with an ASD can mimic this murmur; it can also be heard anywhere on the chest wall and will disappear with closure of the ASD.

Note: A partially obstructing pulmonary embolus can produce a similar murmur. These murmurs can even be continuous just as in pulmonary branch stenosis if there are repeated bilateral pulmonary emboli with pulmonary hypertension. The pulmonary embolus murmur will also increase with inspiration and may disappear with anticoagulation and resolution of the embolus [11].

REFERENCES

1. Aronow, W. S., and Prakash, R. Effect of isometric exercise on systolic murmur of patients with idiopathic hypertrophic subaortic stenosis. *Chest* 67:395, 1975.
2. Bergeron, J., et al. Aortic stenosis—Clinical manifestations and course of the disease. *Arch. Intern. Med.* 94:911, 1954.
3. Bertrand, C. A., Milne, I. G., and Hornick, R. A study of heart sounds and murmurs by direct heart recordings. *Circulation* 13:49, 1956.
4. Beuren, A. J., Apitz, J., and Harmjanz, D. Supravalvular aortic stenosis in association with mental retardation and certain facial appearance. *Circulation* 26:1235, 1962.
5. Bonner, A. J., Sacks, H. N., and Tavel, M. E. Assessing the severity of aortic stenosis by phonocardiography and external carotid pulse recordings. *Circulation* 48:247, 1973.
6. Bousvaros, G. A. Effect of norepinephrine on the phonocardiographic, auscultatory and hemodynamic features of congenital and acquired heart disease. *Am. J. Cardiol.* 8:328, 1961.
7. Bousvaros, G. A. Diagnostic auscultatory complex in coarctation of the aorta. *Br. Heart J.* 29:443, 1967.
8. Bruns, D. L. A general theory of the causes of murmurs in the cardiovascular system. *Am. J. Med.* 27:360, 1959. Classic article.

9. Bujack, W., Gioia, F., and Cayler, G. G. An innocent thrill. A common finding with an innocent murmur. *J.A.M.A.* 235:2417, 1976.

10. Caulfield, W. H., et al. The clinical significance of the fourth heart sound in aortic stenosis. *Am. J. Cardiol.* 28:179, 1971.

11. Cohen, S. I., et al. Flow murmur associated with partial occlusion of the right pulmonary artery. *Am. Heart J.* 90:376, 1975.

12. Cotter, L., Logan, R. L., and Poole, A. Innocent systolic murmurs in healthy 40-year-old men. *J. Royal Coll. Physicians* (London) 14:128, 1980.

13. Datey, K. K., et al. Straight back syndrome. *Br. Heart J.* 26:614, 1964.

14. Daves, M. L. Cardiovascular anachronisms. *J.A.M.A.* 224:879, 1973.

15. Dawson, A. A., and Palmer, K. N. V. The significance of cardiac murmurs in anemia. *Am. J. Med. Sci.* 25:554, 1966.

16. D'Cruz, I. A., et al. Stenotic lesions of the pulmonary arteries. *Am. J. Cardiol.* 13:441, 1964.

17. DeLeon, A. C., Jr., et al. The straight back syndrome. *Circulation* 32:193, 1965.

18. deMonchy, C., vanderHoeven, G. M. A., and Beneken, J. E. W. Studies on innocent praecordial vibratory murmurs in children. *Br. Heart J.* 35:685, 1973.

19. Dock, W. Examination of the chest: Advantages of conducting and reporting it in English. *Bull. N.Y. Acad. Med.* 49:576, 1973.

20. Feruglio, G. A. An intracardiac sound generator for the study of the transmission of heart murmurs in man. *Am. Heart J.* 63:232, 1962.

21. Feruglio, G. A., and Steenivasan, A. Intracardiac phonocardiogram in thirty cases of atrial septal defect. *Circulation* 20:1087, 1959.

22. Flohr, K. H., Weir, E. K., and Chesler, E. Diagnosis of aortic stenosis in older age groups using external carotid pulse recording and phonocardiography. *Br. Heart J.* 45:577, 1981.

23. Garb, S. The relationship of blood viscosity to the intensity of heart murmurs. *Am. Heart J.* 25:568, 1944.

24. Genovese, B., et al. Effect of hypertension on the clinical assessment of severity in aortic stenosis. *Circulation* (Suppl. III) 55 & 56:69, 1977.

25. Goldberg, L. M., and Unland, H. Heart murmurs in pregnancy. *Dis. Chest* 52:381, 1967.

26. Groom, D., et al. The normal systolic murmur. *Ann. Intern. Med.* 52:134, 1960.

27. Guzman, P. A., et al. Transseptal pressure gradient with leftward septal displacement during the Mueller manoeuvre in man. *Br. Heart J.* 46:657, 1981.

28. Hoffman, J. I. E., et al. Physiologic differentiation of pulmonic stenosis with and without an intact ventricular septum. *Circulation* 22:385, 1960.

29. Humerfelt, S. Bj. An epidemiological study of high blood pressure. *Acta Med. Scand.* (Suppl. 406) 173:64, 1963.

30. Jinnouchi, J., et al. Mechanism of outflow obstruction in hypertrophic cardiomyopathy with asymmetric septal hypertrophy: Two-dimensional echocardiographic study. *J. Cardiography* 7:23, 1977.

31. Johnson, A. M. Functional infundibular stenosis, its differentiation from structural stenosis and its importance in atrial septal defect. *Guys Hosp. Rep.* 108:373, 1959.

32. Karpman, L. The murmur of aortocoronary bypass. *Am. Heart J.* 83:179, 1972.

33. Kelly, D. T. Wulfberg, E., and Rowe, R. D. Discrete subaortic stenosis. *Circulation* 46:309, 1972.

34. Kesteloot, H., Sluyts, R., and Van Houte, O. A phonocardiographic study of physiological and pathological vascular murmurs. *Acta Belgica Arte Med.* 13:16, 1967.

35. Kistler, J. P., et al. The bruit of carotid stenosis versus radiated basal heart murmurs. *Circulation* 5:975, 1978.

36. Leatham, A. Systolic murmurs. *Circulation* 17:601, 1958.

37. Leatham, A., and Gray, I. Auscultatory and phonocardiographic signs of atrial septal defect. *Br. Heart J.* 18:193, 1956.

38. Lessof, M., and Brigden, W. Systolic murmurs in healthy children and in children with rheumatic fever. *Lancet* 2:673, 1967.

39. Lewis, K. B., et al. The upper limb-cardiovascular syndrome. *J.A.M.A.* 193:98, 1965.

40. Lewis, M. L., and Christianson, L. C. Effects of posture on lung blood volume in intact man. *Circulation* (Abstracts) (Suppl. III) 55 & 56:74, 1977.

41. Longo, T., and Santa, A. Investigations on the hemodynamic changes responsible for the auscultatory findings in arterial stenosis. *Cardiovasc. Comp.* 1:49, 1966.

42. Luisada, A. A., and DiBartolo, G. High frequency phonocardiography. *Am. J. Cardiol.* 8:51, 1961.
43. Massumi, R., et al. Acoustically silent stenosis of branch of pulmonary artery. *Am. J. Med.* 40:773, 1966.
44. Mills, P., et al. Non-invasive diagnosis of subpulmonary outflow tract obstruction. *Br. Heart J.* 43:276, 1980.
45. Nellen, M., et al. Effects of prompt squatting on the systolic murmur in idiopathic hypertrophic obstructive cardiomyopathy. *Br. Med. J.* 3:140, 1967.
46. Nozawa, T., et al. Two cases with the heart murmur originated from aortocoronary bypass: The diagnostic use of dipyridamole. *J. Cardiography* 11:825, 1981.
47. Pierce, G. E., Morrow, A. G., and Braunwald, E. Idiopathic hypertrophic subaortic stenosis. *Circulation (Suppl. 4)* 30:152, 1964.
48. Perez, G. L., et al. Incidence of murmurs in the aging heart. *J. Am. Geriatrics Soc.* 24:29, 1976.
49. Ranganathan, N., Sivaciyan, V., and Chisholm, R. Effects of postextrasystolic potentiation on systolic time intervals. *Am. J. Cardiol.* 41:14, 1978.
50. Rawlings, M. S. The "straight back" syndrome. A new cause of pseudoheart disease. *Am. J. Cardiol.* 5:333, 1960.
51. Roberts, W. C., Perloff, J. K., and Costantino, T. Severe valvular aortic stenosis in patients over 65 years of age. *Am. J. Cardiol.* 27:497, 1971.
52. Sabbah, H. N., Lee, T. G., and Stein, P. D. Role of blood viscosity in the production of innocent ejection murmurs. *Am. J. Cardiol.* 43:753, 1979.
52A. Sakamoto, T., et al. Auscultatory and phonocardiographic findings in supravalvular aortic stenosis. *Cardiovasc. Sound Bull.* 3:323, 1973.
53. Sakamoto, T., et al. Echocardiogram and phonocardiogram related to the movement of the pulmonary valve. *Jap. Heart J.* 16:107, 1975.
54. Spodick, D. H., et al. Clavicular auscultation; Preferential clavicular transmission and amplification of aortic valve murmurs. *Chest* 70:337, 1976.
55. Stapleton, J. F., and El-Hajj, M. M. Heart murmurs simulated by arterial bruits in the neck. *Am. Heart J.* 61:178, 1961.
56. Stefadouros, M. A., Mucha, E., and Frank, M. J. Paradoxic response of the murmur of idiopathic hypertrophic subaortic stenosis to the Valsalva maneuver. *Am. J. Cardiol.* 37:89, 1976.
57. Stein, P. D., and Sabbah, H. N. Aortic origin of innocent murmurs. *Am. J. Cardiol.* 39:665, 1977.
58. Stein, P. D., et al. Comparison of turbulence in the pulmonary artery and aorta of man. *Circulation* (Abstracts) (Suppl. III), 55 & 56:114, 1977.
59. Stein, P. D., and Munter, W. A. New functional concept of valvular mechanics in normal and diseased aortic valves. *Circulation* 44:101, 1971.
60. Sung, C-S., et al. Is postextrasystolic potentiation dependent on Starling's law? *Circulation* 62:1032, 1980.
61. Uricchio, J. F., et al. Combined mitral and aortic stenosis. *Am. J. Cardiol.* 4:479, 1959.
62. Vogelpoel, L., and Schrire, V. Auscultatory and phonocardiographic assessment of pulmonary stenosis with intact ventricular septum. *Circulation* 22:55, 1960.
63. Vogelpoel, L., and Schrire, V. Auscultatory and phonocardiographic assessment of Fallot's tetralogy. *Circulation* 22:73, 1960.
64. Vogelpoel, L., et al. The pre-operative recognition of the "muscle-bound" right ventricle in pulmonary stenosis with intact ventricular septum. *Br. Heart J.* 26:380, 1964.
65. Wennevold, A. The origin of the innocent "vibratory" murmur studied with intracardiac phonocardiography. *Acta. Med. Scand.* 181:1, 1967.

14. *Systolic Regurgitant Murmurs*

1. What is meant by a systolic regurgitant murmur?

    ANS.: This is a murmur produced by retrograde flow from a high pressure area of the heart through some abnormal opening into an area of lower pressure.

2. List the four usual abnormal openings that allow systolic regurgitation.

    ANS.: 1) Incompetent mitral valve (high-pressure area LV to low-pressure area left atrium).

    2) **Ventricular septal defect** (VSD) (high-pressure area left ventricle [LV] to low-pressure area right ventricle [RV]).

    3) Incompetent tricuspid valve (high-pressure area RV to low-pressure area right atrium).

    4) Arteriovenous communication such as **persistent ductus arteriosus** (PDA) (high-pressure area aorta to low-pressure area pulmonary artery).

3. What characteristics are common to all systolic regurgitant murmurs?

    ANS.: a) If there are early components, they start with the first heart sound. If there are late systolic components, they always extend to or beyond the second heart sound of the same side.

    b) When soft, they are predominantly high-pitched and blowing because the opening is probably very small, and there is a high **gradient** between a ventricle and any chamber into which retrograde flow occurs.

    c) They tend to remain the same after long diastoles. (For rare exceptions to this rule, see pages 315, 321.)

4. How can you imitate various kinds of high-pitched blowing murmurs?

    ANS.: a) Whisper a drawn-out "haaaa" or "hoo."

    b) Say a drawn-out "shsh."

    c) Hold the diaphragm of the stethoscope against the palm of your hand and listen through the earpieces while you run the pads of your fingers across the back of your hand.

5. What are regurgitant murmurs called if they stretch from the S_1 to or beyond the S_2?

    ANS.: Pansystolic or holosystolic murmurs.

6. What are the advantages and disadvantages of each of these terms?

    ANS.: *Holos* is a Greek word meaning "wholly," "complete," "entire," or "all." *Pan* is a Greek work meaning "each" and "every," as well as "all." Therefore, holosystolic has only one meaning, which fits the timing of the murmur (from S_1 to S_2) well. However, *pan* is such a universally used prefix, with such a well-understood meaning, "all," that there is no point in teaching an unfamiliar prefix such as *holo* for the sake of pedantic purism. *Holo* has probably become popular in English-speaking countries because it means the same as "wholly," which sounds enough like *holo* to be easily remembered.

    Note: If a regurgitant murmur extends far enough beyond the S_2 to be

Boldface type indicates that the term is explained in the Glossary.

recognized as reaching into diastole by auscultation, it is called a continuous murmur.

THE EFFECT OF A LONG DIASTOLE ON LEFT-SIDED REGURGITANT MURMURS

1. What will happen to the loudness of a left-sided regurgitant murmur, such as that heard in mitral regurgitation (MR) or VSD, after a sudden long diastole?

   ANS.: The loudness usually remains about the same. (Listening for the effect of a long diastole is one of the best ways to differentiate an ejection from a regurgitant murmur.)

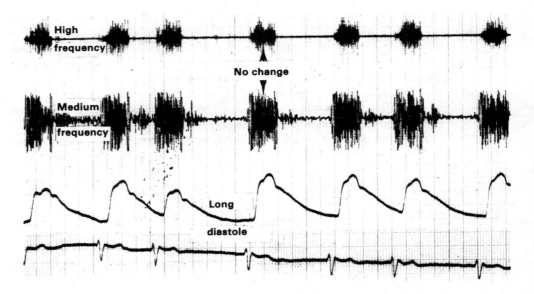

A high- and medium-frequency phonocardiogram taken at the apex together with an external carotid tracing from a 45-year-old woman with moderately severe chronic rheumatic MR, with few symptoms on digitalis alone. Because of atrial fibrillation, short and long diastoles are present, demonstrating that the murmur does not grow louder after long diastoles than after short or average diastoles.

   Note: If the pause is caused by a premature ventricular contraction (PVC), compare the postextrasystolic beat not with the PVC but with the normal cycle following the postextrasystolic beat. A PVC may be so premature that there is no time for any significant ventricular filling. Therefore, the loudness of a murmur produced by the PVC itself is of no significance.

2. Why does the left-sided regurgitant murmur not usually become louder despite a larger volume in the ventricle after a long diastole?

   ANS.: In MR, VSD, and PDA, the LV has two outlets during systole. The amount ejected through each outlet depends on the relative resistance beyond each outlet. During the PVC, the aortic pressure is less than normal because of the small stroke volume. During the long diastole after the PVC, the pressure beyond the aortic outlet falls still more, owing to continued long runoff into the periphery. Thus, by the time of the next systole, the resistance at the aortic valve has dropped so low that blood is preferentially ejected into the aorta, and relatively less is regurgitated through the other orifice. One would think at first that this would make the murmur softer. However, because there is more volume in the LV at the end of a long diastole, the absolute quantity of blood regurgitated remains about the same as that after short diastoles.

* *Note:* The quantity of retrograde flow in MR and in a VSD actually does increase during isovolumic contraction in the beat after the long pause, but this does not affect the loudness of the murmur during the major part of systole, when the amount regurgitated is not increased [68].

3. When may the MR murmur become softer after a long diastole?

   ANS.: a) In the prolapsed mitral valve syndrome. (See page 334 for explanation.)

   b) In some papillary muscle dysfunction murmurs, when myocardial ischemia rather than fibrosis causes the MR. The long diastole may decrease myocardial ischemia by allowing more time for coronary filling and by decreasing the afterload due to the increased time allowed for aortic pressure to fall [2, 22].

   c) When a larger LV produces more regurgitation, as it does when MR results from the types of papillary dysfunction in which the papillary muscle is either abnormally short, due to scarring, or displaced downward and laterally, due to LV dilatation.

   Note: In Wolff-Parkinson-White (W-P-W) pre-excitation, type B, in which RV contraction precedes LB contraction, the MR murmur is made louder after a long diastole, but the reason for this is unknown [13]. This type of pre-excitation has also brought out a tricuspid regurgitation and an innocent ejection murmur [13].

MITRAL REGURGITATION MURMURS

Terminology

1. Why may it be preferable to use the term *mitral regurgitation* rather than *mitral incompetence* or *mitral insufficiency,* even though cardiologists are about equally divided as to the preferred usage?

   ANS.: The abbreviation for mitral incompetence or insufficiency is MI, which is also used as an abbreviation for myocardial infarction. There is no confusion when MR is used.

   Note: Regurgitation describes the direction of flow, whereas *incompetence* or *insufficiency* describes the condition of the valve. For the sake of consistency, we shall use the terms *aortic, pulmonary,* and *tricuspid regurgitation,* instead of *incompetence* or *insufficiency.*

---

* Material marked with an asterisk is for reference and for advanced students in cardiology.

Causes

1. List the four commonest causes of MR murmurs in the adult.

   ANS.: Prolapse of the mitral leaflet into the left atrium, papillary muscle dysfunction, rheumatic valve damage, and ruptured chordae.

*2. List some rare causes of MR in the adult.

   ANS.: Left atrial myxoma, calcified mitral annulus, and endocardial cushion defects with a cleft anterior leaflet.

   Note: a) About 10 percent of patients with mitral annulus calcification have severe MR [46].

   b) A cleft mitral valve can also occur with a secundum ASD, but this is rare [51, 116].

*3. What are the likely causes of a MR murmur at the apex in an infant?

   ANS.: a) Papillary muscle dysfunction secondary to either an anomalous left coronary artery arising from the pulmonary artery or to endocardial fibroelastosis.

   b) Acute myocarditis.

   c) Endocardial cushion defect with cleft mitral valve.

   d) Myxomatous degeneration of the mitral valve with or without Marfan's syndrome.

   Note: About 50 percent of patients with Marfan's syndrome have MR [103].

   e) Ebstein's anomaly of the left atrioventricular (AV) valve (actually a tricuspid valve) in corrected transposition of the great vessels.

4. What suggests that mitral annular dilatation is in itself a rare cause of MR?

   ANS.: a) Many patients with grossly dilated hearts due to such conditions as aortic regurgitation (AR) or **cardiomyopathies** have no MR.

   b) The surface area of the billowing mitral leaflets is more than twice the area of the mitral orifice.

   c) Severe LV dilatation may occur without any dilatation of the annulus— i.e., the midportion between the apex and the base expands most.

   d) The fibromuscular portion of the annulus contracts during systole and produces a sphincterlike action.

   *Note: The mitral ring decreases in area by about 10–50 percent in systole Annular calcification prevents normal contraction during systole and can cause almost any degree of MR. (Since it also prevents dilatation, a moderate degree of mitral stenosis may also be produced [102].)

*5. When will corrected transposition produce a murmur that mimics MR?

   ANS.: Corrected transposition means that both the great vessels and the ventricles are transposed. Therefore, an anatomical RV on the left side of the heart feeds the aorta but receives blood through a tricuspid valve. (It should be easy to remember that the valves stay with the appropriate ventricle rather than with the atrium because the chordae tendineae and papillary muscles are attached to the valves.) If the tricuspid valve becomes regurgitant, as with an Ebstein's anomaly (downward displacement of a deformed tricuspid valve), it will *seem* to be MR. There is a high incidence of left AV (tricuspid) valve regurgitation in patients with corrected transposition [12]. Anomalous insertion of chordae into the left AV valve has been found to be the cause when no Ebstein's deformity is present.

6. What are the usual causes of papillary muscle dysfunction murmurs?

ANS.: a) Myocardial infarction, recent or old, with or without a ventricular **aneurysm** and with or without papillary muscle fibrosis. Infarction of the ventricle at the base of the papillary muscles or ischemia of that area of the ventricle that may occur with an attack of angina may cause marked MR even with a normal papillary muscle. An anomalous coronary artery arising from the pulmonary artery can cause MR in an infant, probably due to infarction of both the papillary muscle and the ventricle at the base of the papillary muscle.

   Note: Many patients with papillary muscle fibrosis do not have MR at all. In experiments on dogs, it has not been possible to produce MR by causing papillary muscle ischemia unless it is combined with infarction of the LV at the base of the papillary muscle [90].

*b) Congenital MR can occur when a poorly developed, small papillary muscle arises at a higher-than-normal point on the LV wall.

c) **Hypertrophic subaortic stenosis** (HSS) can cause MR because

   1) The anterior leaflet may be pulled down in systole toward the septum and away from the posterior leaflet. This movement of the leaflet toward the septum is due either to the abnormal angle at which the anterolateral papillary muscle is attached to the grossly hypertrophied septum or to the **Bernoulli effect** of the high-velocity stream being ejected past the anterior mitral leaflet.

   2) The obliteration of the cavity that takes place during systole in HSS can cause the mitral orifice to become small to a degree that makes much of the mitral leaflets redundant and, therefore, causes them to prolapse into the left atrium.

7. When acute infarction causes MR due to papillary muscle dysfunction, what happens to the murmur during the course of the acute infarction?

ANS.: About 10 percent of papillary muscle dysfunction murmurs that are due to acute infarction will disappear before the patient leaves the hospital [56].

Loudness, Sites, and Radiation of Mitral Regurgitation Murmurs

1. Where are MR murmurs loudest?

ANS.: At the apex area or slightly lateral to the site of the apex impulse.

   *Note: There is at least one report of an MR murmur that was loudest at the second right interspace. This patient has only moderate MR, probably from some unusual cause [120]. Another article reports 2 patients with probable rheumatic MR in whom the murmur was just as loud at the second right interspace as at the apex area [134]. These patients also had only mild to moderate MR. The jet in these unusual cases probably was directed anteriorly against the aortic root, which lies against the anterior atrial wall. (See page 323 for diagram.)

2. When may an MR murmur seem to be louder at the left sternal border than at the apex area? ·

ANS.: In very long chests in which the apex area is very medially placed—i.e., the LV impulse is actually near the left sternal border. You must try to shift the apex laterally either by turning the patient to the **left lateral decubitus position** or by having him sit up with his legs on the bed. (In the standing position the apex area moves even more medially.)

3. Where is the best radiation zone of the usual MR murmur?

ANS.: It usually radiates best to the axilla and the left posterior intrascapular area of the chest. However, if loud enough it will radiate to the right, but to a lesser degree.

Note: When the murmur is due to ruptured chordae, it may have an unusual radiation zone (see page 323).

* 4. Besides an obese or emphysematous chest, what can cause silent, severe MR?

ANS.: a) Concomitant mitral stenosis (MS) can apparently direct the MR stream in such as way that the murmur is inaudible [6].

b) Prosthetic mitral valve MR due to suture breakdown may also be silent.

Note: a) Almost all adults with silent MR who have been reported had severe regurgitation, and most had paroxysmal nocturnal dyspnea or were in atrial fibrillation [122]. A widely split S_2 in the presence of a large LV and unexpectedly large left atrium were the only clues.

b) MR may become severe and a murmur may be heard only when myocardial ischemia develops due to an attack of angina. This MR may become so severe that the patient may even develop pulmonary edema [82].

Shape, Pitch, and Duration of Mitral Regurgitation Murmurs

1. What are all the possible shapes of an MR murmur?

ANS.:

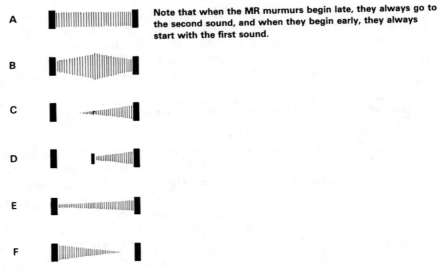

Note that when the MR murmurs begin late, they always go to the second sound, and when they begin early, they always start with the first sound.

2. What shape are the loudest MR murmurs?

ANS.: Pansystolic crescendo–decrescendo murmurs are usually the loudest. The crescendo–decrescendo shape in these patients is very slight and is better described as a spindle shape on a phonocardiogram.

3. How does the pitch of a murmur correlate with gradient and flow?

ANS.: High gradients and little flow produce high-pitched murmurs. High flow and low gradients produce low–pitched murmurs. Combined high flow and high gradients produce murmurs with mixed frequencies, which when loud become harsh.

4. Which MR murmurs are always associated with almost pure high frequencies, i.e., only a blowing sound?

ANS.: All soft murmurs with small volume flows and high gradients, e.g., those due to trivial MR.

Note: The gradient between the left atrium and LV usually reaches more than 100 mm Hg during the peak of systole.

5. Why does the MR murmur extend slightly beyond the S_2?

ANS.: Because LV pressure is higher than left atrial pressure even after the aortic valve closes.

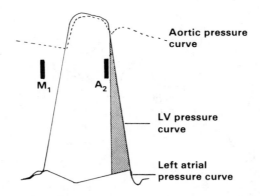

Note that the LV pressure is above left atrial pressure even after the A_2.

6. Is an MR murmur louder on inspiration or expiration?

ANS.: It is usually louder on expiration because that is when blood is pushed into the LV from the lungs.

*Note: Unusual rotations caused by inspiration may bring the heart closer to the stethoscope and cause the murmur paradoxically to sound louder on inspiration. This can often be counteracted by placing the stethoscope lateral to the apex beat. If the heart sounds also become louder on inspiration, rotation may be the cause. Unusual cardiac rotations with respiration are common after cardiac surgery.

PAPILLARY MUSCLE DYSFUNCTION MURMURS

1. How can different kinds of papillary muscle dysfunction produce MR murmurs of different shapes?

ANS.: a) Disproportionate lengths of papillary muscle due to lack of contraction will cause MR murmurs by the following mechanism. If one papillary muscle is unable to contract or is attached to infarcted muscle at its base, its muscles plus chordae will be longer than the opposite contracting papillary muscle plus chordae when the ventricle and normal papillary muscle contract [14]. As the pressure rises and the LV cavity decreases in size, the portion of the mitral leaflets with the relatively long papillary muscle plus chordae will project more and more into the left atrium, producing a crescendo murmur to the S_2.

b) Fixed shortening of a papillary muscle may also cause MR. If a papillary muscle is shortened by marked fibrosis or is attached to an aneurysmal or dilated akinetic area, then regurgitation will be pansystolic. The shape of the murmur may be decrescendo if dilatation was the major cause of the regurgitation. If a piece of mitral valve attached to the normal muscle loses support of the opposite leaflet in midsystole owing to too short a papillary muscle-to-opposite leaflet length, it may suddenly flip upward, producing a midsystolic nonejection click or a late systolic murmur.

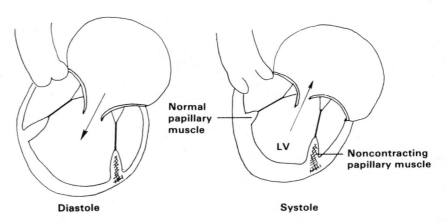

A noncontracting papillary muscle may make its chordae plus papillary muscle relatively longer as the ventricle becomes smaller. This is most likely to produce a murmur that becomes progressively louder as systole proceeds (crescendo murmur to the S_2).

2. How can the shape or loudness of the MR murmur tell you whether its etiology is rheumatic fever or papillary muscle dysfunction?

ANS.: a) If the murmur is crescendo to the S_2, it is more likely to be due to papillary muscle dysfunction. Rheumatic MR is rarely crescendo to the S_2 except during the healing phase of acute rheumatic fever, usually in a patient under age 20, who has had an acute attack of rheumatic fever within a few months, during which there was also a pansystolic murmur [137].

*Note: Because papillary muscle dysfunction due to HSS almost always produces a decrescendo murmur, if a pansystolic murmur is heard at the apex in a patient with HSS, coincidental rheumatic MR should be suspected. This murmur will probably become louder with squatting and persist after surgery for the HSS [77].

b) If the murmur becomes louder as the heart becomes smaller when the patient compensates for failure, fixed rheumatic MR is suggested. Papillary muscle dysfunction murmurs tend to become softer as the heart becomes smaller with improvement of heart failure.

c) If an S_4 is present, it strongly suggests papillary muscle dysfunction secondary to a cardiomyopathy. Rheumatic MR is rarely associated with an S_4.

d) Papillary muscle dysfunction murmurs due to coronary disease often become softer after long diastoles [21] (see p. 315 for explanation).

e) Papillary muscle rupture is a sequel of myocardial infarction and produces the physical findings of sudden, severe MR, mimicking the most severe case of ruptured chordae. However, the MR is so severe that, together with the myocardial damage of the myocardial infarction, the murmur of papillary muscle rupture is rarely ever louder than grade 3/6, i.e., it is rare to feel a thrill with it. This finding helps to distinguish this murmur from that of ventricular septal rupture, in which 50 percent of patients have murmurs of grade 4/6 or louder.

3. What is characteristic of the S_1 with papillary muscle dysfunction murmurs?
ANS.: The S_1 tends to be louder than normal. The cause is unknown [22].

MITRAL REGURGITATION DUE TO RUPTURED CHORDAE

1. How many chordae are capable of rupture?
ANS.: There are about 120 chordae attached to both mitral leaflets. There are about 12 chordae attached to each of about six heads of each papillary muscle, and these chordae divide about three times before they attach to their leaflets [109].

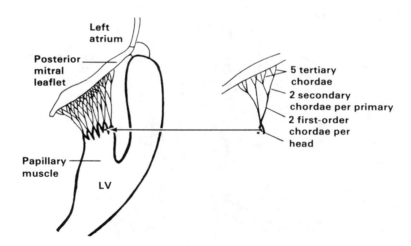

Note: Spontaneous ruptures usually occur in one of the 25 major chordae closer to the papillary muscles than in those attached to the leaflets, thus involving at least four or five small terminal branches [106]. If only a few terminal branches are torn off, infective endocarditis has probably caused the rupture.

2. How can you tell if an MR murmur is due to papillary muscle dysfunction rather than to ruptured chordae?
ANS.: a) Ruptured chordae superimposed on rheumatic heart disease produce a sudden onset of severe MR and failure (a loud S_3, a murmur of grade 3/6 or more, and an increase in symptoms). The usual papillary muscle dysfunction produces signs only of mild to moderate MR, with a mur-

mur that is rarely more than grade 3/6 and is usually crescendo to the S_2. Exceptionally, however, papillary muscle dysfunction due to a large infarcted area at the base of the papillary muscle can produce severe MR. Also, rupture of only a few unimportant posterior chordae superimposed on a normal heart may produce few symptoms.

b) A decrescendo, mixed-frequency murmur associated with symptoms of high left atrial pressure (orthopnea or paroxysmal nocturnal dyspnea) suggests ruptured chordae of recent onset. This is because the left atrium does not enlarge much with acute severe MR, probably because of the non-distensible pericardium around the atria. This poor left atrial compliance may raise the V wave pressure to a very high peak in systole. The rise in left atrial pressure plus a precipitous fall in LV pressure toward the end of systole decrease the gradient and murmur toward the end of systole.

*Note: a) Chordal rupture of the posterior leaflet may cause only moderate MR. Two chordae, larger and thicker than the rest, insert into the anterior leaflets. Rupture of one of these two so-called strut chordae often results in severe MR and a flail anterior leaflet [106].

b) Left atrial pressures as high as 70 mm Hg have been recorded toward the end of systole in patients with ruptured chordae.

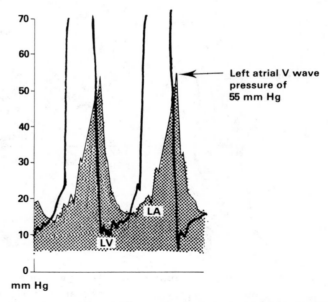

This is a left atrial (wedge) and LV pressure tracing from a 23-year-old woman with ruptured mitral chordae. The shaded area is under the left atrial (wedge) pressure curve. The slight delay in the peak wedge pressure is due to the fact that wedge pressures (taken by a catheter wedged into the distal pulmonary arterial branches) always show a delay in comparison with direct left atrial pressure tracings. The rapid increase in V wave pressure during systole rapidly decreases the gradient across the mitral valve and will tend to cause both a decrescendo gradient and murmur. The decompressing effect on the LV of the massive loss of blood into the left atrium causes a late systolic fall in LV pressure. This end-systolic decrease in LV pressure further decreases the gradient across the mitral valve toward the end of systole.

3. Why may ruptured chordae imitate aortic stenosis (AS)?
   ANS.: If posterior chordae rupture, producing a flail posterior cusp, the stream of regurgitation may strike the atrial septum in such a way that murmurs with the shape and radiation into the carotids that are typical of those seen with AS murmurs are produced [117]. To further confuse the picture, the murmur at the second right interspace may even be shorter than the one at the apex. However, only about half of posterior rupture murmurs radiate into the neck [117].
   *Note: a) Radiation of a posterior rupture murmur may sometimes be better into the lower back than into the neck. The reason is unknown.
   b) Despite good radiation into the second right interspace and neck, the murmur of a posterior chordae rupture is still usually loudest at the apex [64].

4. What is the characteristic radiation of an MR murmur caused by a rupture of the anterior chordae?
   ANS.: It may radiate along the spine and if loud, even to the top of the head [48, 89].
   Note: There have been rare reports of patients with anterior chordal rupture who had murmurs that also imitated AS [125]. The reason is unknown, but such murmurs have mixed findings, such as the good transmission to the back that is also characteristic of an anterior flail leaflet.

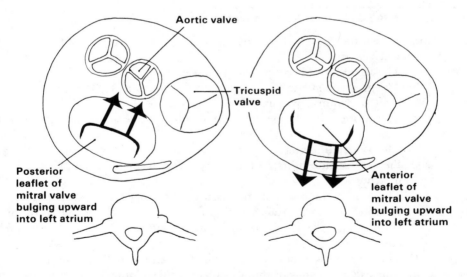

These views of the valve rings from above show how posterior ruptured chordae (on left) can direct the regurgitant stream against the aorta and cause the murmur to be transmitted like an aortic ejection murmur. The diagram at right shows how ruptured anterior chordae can direct the regurgitant stream posteriorly against the spine.

5. How do diastolic sounds tell you that a loud MR murmur is due to ruptured chordae rather than to rheumatic heart disease?

ANS.: The healthy atrial wall resists dilatation in patients with ruptured chordae. It responds to the stretch produced by the massive regurgitant stream with a **Starling effect.** By contracting strongly, it often produces an S_4, which is rare in rheumatic MR.

6. What is the commonest cause of ruptured chordae?

ANS.: The commonest cause is **infective endocarditis** on an abnormal valve such as that found in patients with rheumatic heart disease or myxomatous transformation. The next most common cause is idiopathic [117].

　　　Note: a) It is probable that most "idiopathic" ruptures occur on the basis of a prolapsed mitral valve with some myxomatous degeneration [50]. Often a murmur of prolapse has been present for years before the rupture but has not been recognized as such [7]. A cleft in the posterior cusp, with billowing, voluminous leaflets has sometimes been associated with idiopathic ruptures, suggesting that an unusual strain is placed on at least one chorda [81].

　　　　　　b) Most patients with ruptured chordae on previously "normal" valves are males [7].

7. What most closely imitates the auscultatory findings of ruptured chordae?

ANS.: Severe myxomatous degeneration of the mitral valves. This is often known as the "floppy valve syndrome."

Quantitating the Degree of Mitral Regurgitation

1. How can you tell the degree of MR by physical examination?

ANS.: The MR is greater

　　a) The larger the LV by palpation (see p. 127).

　　b) The greater and later the left parasternal movement. (This may represent the left atrium expanding during systole.)

　　c) The more palpable the early rapid filling wave at the apex. (See page 325.)

　　d) The louder and longer the apical systolic murmur (with the exception of the decrescendo murmur caused by a very high left atrial pressure heard in acute MR).

　　e) The louder the S_3, since this is roughly proportional to the torrential diastolic flow, with the exception of sudden severe MR due to ruptured chordae on a previously normal mitral valve. The S_3 here is either soft or absent [7].

　　f) The longer and louder the diastolic flow murmur following the S_3.

　　g) The wider the split of the S_2, unless the development of severe pulmonary hypertension narrows the split.

　　Note: Although ruptured chordae murmurs may be decrescendo, they are almost always at least grade 4/6 in loudness [7].

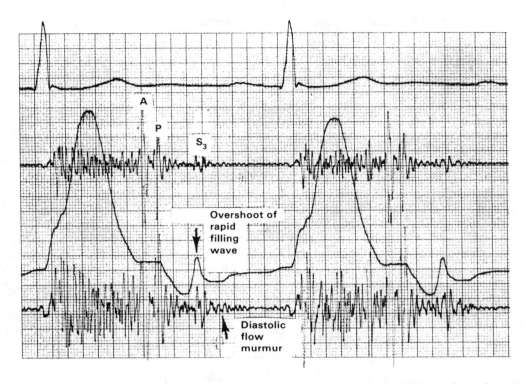

A

P

S₃

Overshoot of
rapid
filling
wave

Diastolic
flow
murmur

This phonocardiogram and apical pulse tracing is from the same 15-year-old girl with severe rheumatic MR as in the figure on page 254. The pulse tracing was taken over the LV impulse in the supine position and is therefore an apex precordiogram instead of an apex cardiogram, which is taken in the left lateral decubitus position. The phonocardiograms are from the third left parasternal interspace. The upper one is taken at medium frequency; the lower one is a logarithmic tracing that brings out low and medium frequencies. Note the following signs of severe MR: (1) the widely split S₂ of 50 msec; (2) the diastolic flow murmur after the S₃, both of which are so loud that they can be recorded at the left sternal border (see figure on p. 254 for the same S₃ and diastolic flow murmur at the apex of this patient); (3) the exaggerated early rapid filling peak of the apical impulse (this would be palpable in the left lateral decubitus position).

*2. How can you determine the degree of MR by a left parasternal precordiogram?

ANS.: In the presence of MR, the initial left parasternal movement is due mostly to the RV, and the late movement is due mostly to left atrial expansion with the regurgitant volume. Therefore, a ratio of late to early outward movement correlates with regurgitant volume [10]. If you draw a horizontal line at the onset of the initial outward movement, the amplitude of the early and late movements above this line comprises a ratio of late outward movement over early outward movement. As the regurgitant volume increases, the ratio becomes larger, with an r value of 0.93 when correlated with angiographically determined regurgitation. The ratio is nullified by mixed mitral stenosis and MR or anything that causes RV movement such as an atrial septal defect or tricuspid regurgitation. (The time constant of the equipment may have to be at least 650 msec.) The regression equation for pure MR is

$$\text{Regurgitant volume (in ml)} = \left(32 \times \frac{\text{late}}{\text{early}}\right) + 34$$

EFFECTS OF DRUGS AND MANEUVERS ON REGURGITANT MURMURS

Raising Peripheral Resistance

1. What happens to left-sided regurgitant murmurs if the peripheral resistance is increased? Why?

   ANS.: They become louder, because with regurgitation there are two outlets for systole, and an increased resistance at the aortic outlet promotes more outflow through the other outlet.

2. How will raising the blood pressure with handgrip, squatting, or phenylephrine help you to determine whether a long systolic murmur at the apex is due to AS or MR?

   ANS.: With increased peripheral resistance, aortic ejection murmurs will either be unchanged or become softer, but MR murmurs will become louder [87].

   *Note: a) A vasopressor drug with a strong positive inotropic effect, such as norepinephrine, will only add a confusing variable. Phenylephrine has only weak inotropic effects. The dose of phenylephrine is 0.4–0.7 mg, given by slow intravenous infusion until a rise of about 20 mm Hg in systolic pressure is achieved [11].

   b) Handgrip has little effect on the peripheral resistance of normal subjects or on most patients with either labile or fixed hypertension unless they have evidence of left ventricular hypertrophy or enlargement on ECG or x-ray [38]. If patients are in failure, however, they cannot increase their cardiac output adequately in response to handgrip and will instead increase the blood pressure by an increase in peripheral resistance [24].

   Although at least 30 percent of maximum voluntary contraction is necessary to produce circulatory changes, 50 percent of maximum voluntary contraction will often produce a greater elevation of blood pressure. A contraction that is 75 percent of maximum will achieve a peak response in 1 minute [38].

   c) Standing to increase peripheral resistance will not necessarily increase the loudness of the murmur of MR. If the MR murmur is primarily dependent on dilatation, the smaller heart caused by the pooling effect brought about by standing may even make the murmur softer. If dilatation is not a factor, the increased peripheral resistance caused by standing should make the murmur become louder, but the decreased volume of regurgitation due to the diminution of venous return on standing causes the murmur to stay about the same. (The MR murmur of the prolapsed valve syndrome becomes louder on standing. See page 334 for details.)

   d) You can bring out the type of MR murmur of papillary muscle dysfunction that is transient and is associated only with episodes of coronary insufficiency and angina by passive leg-raising to increase the LV volume [78].

Decreasing Peripheral Resistance with Nitrites

1. How does amyl nitrite affect blood pressure and cardiac output? How do its effects differ from those of nitroglycerin?

   ANS.: Amyl nitrite causes an immediate and *marked* drop in blood pressure. After about 20 sec the cardiac output is *increased*. Nitroglycerin causes a *mild* drop in blood pressure and a *fall* in cardiac output.

2. Why does amyl nitrite cause an increase in cardiac output whereas nitroglycerin causes a fall in cardiac output?

   ANS.: The rapid and profound drop in blood pressure produced by amyl nitrite results in a strong reflex sympathetic outflow that constricts the veins [83]. Amyl nitrite is a volatile substance that is dissipated in the capillary system and therefore never reaches the veins. The direct effect of amyl nitrite on the capillaries may open up shunts between the dilated arterioles and venules. The increased venous return, together with the reflex tachycardia, increases the cardiac output.

   Nitroglycerin, on the other hand, does affect the veins and reduces venous return by causing venous pooling. The mild drop in blood pressure produced by nitroglycerin is not strong enough to result in sufficient sympathetic outflow to cause venous constriction.

3. How will amyl nitrite help to separate an aortic ejection murmur from an MR murmur at the apex?

   ANS.: By decreasing the peripheral resistance, it makes the MR murmur softer. By causing an increased velocity of ejection through the aortic valve, it makes the aortic ejection murmur louder.

   Note: A marked effect may be achieved with only three inhalations of amyl nitrite. The following precautions are helpful when using amyl nitrite:

   a) Wear rubber gloves, or the odor may remain on your fingers for days. After use, flush the used capsule down the toilet, or it will impart its odor to your examining room for hours.

   b) Never use it unless the patient is supine, or you may produce syncope.

   c) Warn the patient that he will feel flushed and that his heart will pound for about 30 sec. Reassure the nervous patient by telling him that the drug was formerly used to take away "heart pain" but is no longer used because of its lingering odor.

   d) An assistant should call out the systolic blood pressures throughout the entire procedure so that you will know whether and to what degree the blood pressure is affected.

THE BALLOONED OR PROLAPSED MITRAL VALVE

Definitions and Terminology

1. What is meant by a ballooned or prolapsed mitral valve? What auscultatory findings does it cause?

   ANS.: This term refers to the bulging or buckling of one or both mitral valve leaflets into the left atrium during systole, so that one or more crisp systolic sounds or clicks and a later systolic MR murmur are commonly heard. The systolic murmur goes to the A_2.

Note: a) Although a redundant posterior leaflet is the one that most commonly balloons into the atrium, the anterior leaflet may also be involved.

b) About 6 percent of women between the ages of 17 and 54 in one study had either a midsystolic nonejection click, a late systolic murmur, or both. About 60 percent of these women had both the click and the murmur, 5 percent had only the late systolic murmur, and the remainder had only the click [105]. In another series of patients with prolapse, only 25 percent had both a click and a murmur, and 30 percent had only a murmur. The rest had only clicks [79]. In a two-dimensional echocardiographic screening study of 100 asymptomatic women aged 18 to 35, only 2 percent had prolapse [151].

2. What are the names given to the prolapsed mitral valve click and murmur complex?

ANS.: a) Prolapsed mitral valve syndrome (the commonest term).

b) Ballooned valve syndrome.

c) Systolic click-murmur syndrome.

d) Barlow's syndrome.

e) Click, late-systolic murmur syndrome.

f) Billowing mitral valve syndrome.

Note: a) The word *syndrome* is applied because in this condition there are often symptoms of nonspecific chest pain, an ECG showing T-wave abnormalities (negative T in aVF or the left precordium or abnormally notched T waves), and ventricular arrhythmias, which occasionally lead to sudden death. However, T inversion in the inferior leads usually occurs in patients with a cardiomyopathy or coronary disease [4].

b) It is unfortunate that *prolapsed valve* rather than *ballooned valve* became the most common term because *prolapse* suggests to the novice a downward movement into the LV when actually it is a backward and upward movement into the left atrium.

c) *Billowing* suggests that the normal valve does not billow, which is not true. *Barlow's syndrome* is not descriptive for the beginner. *Click, late systolic murmur* syndrome ignores those patients with only the click or only the murmur.

The term *floppy valve syndrome* has been applied by some as a synonym for the prolapsed valve syndrome. This is unfortunate because this term was originally meant to describe the most marked degree of myxomatous degeneration with elongated chordae, causing severe MR [107, 120]. In the usual prolapsed valve syndrome, the MR is at most only moderate.

3. What can we call the click or sound that often precedes the delayed systolic murmur?

ANS.: A nonejection click or sound. It cannot be called midsystolic because at times it may come as early as an ejection click and as late as a widely split S_2.

Note: a) The click often comes slightly after the onset of the murmur.

b) Multiple clicks are common.

c) If the etiology is primarily myocardial infarction and papillary muscle dysfunction, it is not so likely to sound like a click.

Etiology, Pathology, and Physiology of the Prolapsed Valve Syndrome

1. What is the usual mitral valve abnormality seen at surgey or necropsy when a prolapsed mitral valve is examined?

ANS.: Myxomatous transformation. This may be recognized only on careful inspection, since the valve may appear grossly normal to casual examination by the surgeon or pathologist.

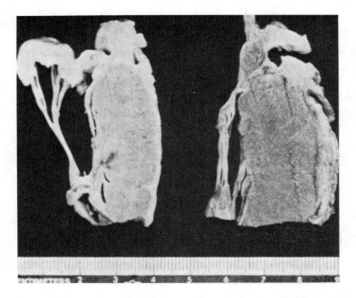

On the left is a cross section of the abnormal middle scallop of the posterior leaflet. On the right is the same area from a woman with left ventricular hypertrophy but no MR. (From J. K. Trent, A. G. Adelman, E. D. Wigle, and M. D. Silver. *Am. Heart J.* 79:539, 1970.)

Note: a) **Marfan's syndrome** is commonly associated with myxomatous valves, and about 20–30 percent of patients with prolapsed valves have joint laxity, high arched palates, or other skeletal abnormalities such as scoliosis, **pectus excavatum,** and straight backs— i.e., it may be occasionally a **forme fruste** of Marfan's syndrome.

*b) Ehlers-Danlos syndrome is commonly associated with prolapsed mitral valves (9 of 11 patients in one series [16A]).

c) The tricuspid valve has also been found to prolapse in about 15 percent of patients with clicks and late systolic murmurs at the left lower sternal edge [80, 98].

2. List the suspected causes of mitral valve prolapse.

ANS.: a) Congenital myxomatous transformation with elongated chordae.

Note: Because a significant percentage of patients have abnormal ventricular wall motion, a myocardial component may be important in many of them.

      b) Papillary muscle dysfunction or ventricular asynergy due to myocardial infarction or ischemia [136A, 147].

     *c) Dysfunction of muscle adjacent to the posterior leaflet, as in myocardial infarction or congenital absence of the left circumflex coronary artery.

     *d) Effects of mitral valve surgery, probably due to unequal length of the chordae [9].

     *e) Hypertrophic subaortic stenosis, probably because of unequal length of the chordae due to asymmetrical hypertrophy as well as the hyperkinetic contraction that obliterates the cavity and contracts the mitral valve orifice, making the mitral leaflets too large for the orifice [31].

     *f) The occasional patient with mitral stenosis has enough free unfibrosed leaflet to buckle up into the left atrium and produce a nonejection click [25].

     *g) There are some who believe that rheumatic fever can cause a prolapsed mitral valve, even proposing that all patients with prolapse should have rheumatic fever prophylaxis unless T-wave abnormalities are present, because then the prolapse is not due to rheumatic fever [138].

3. Which congenital cardiac condition has been found to be commonly associated with the prolapsed valve syndrome?

  ANS.: Atrial septal defect.

     Note: a) In one series about 50 percent of patients with ASD had mitral valve prolapse that decreased or disappeared after surgery [100]. With ASD closure the LV enlarges and with it the mitral orifice [121]. However, if the MR is due to some other cause, such as a cleft mitral valve, closure of the ASD will increase the MR [74].

      *b) In the past it was thought that MR was present only in the primum or endocardial cushion type of ASD and that it was always due to cleft mitral valves. Now it is conceded that MR can occur in secundum ASD due not only to a cleft mitral valve (very rare) but also to myxomatous degeneration of the valve with prolapse [88]. Occasionally, the MR is due to an abnormally high insertion of the chordae near the top of the ventricular septum.

4. What is the cause of the nonejection click preceding the delayed systolic murmur?

  ANS.: The "chordal snap" theory contends that the click is due to a sudden stretch of chordae as they give way with the peak pressure in midsystole [28]. However, because the papillary muscles contract early, the chordae are under too much tension from the beginning of systole to "snap" during ventricular ejection [115]. Therefore, this theory has been challenged by another theory that suggests that the click is a *valvular* sound produced by the loss of support of one leaflet by its opposing leaflet due to redundant valve tissue or to an abnormality of chordal length. Thus, a small piece of unsupported leaflet may suddenly flip upward to its full extent to produce a click [32].

    Note: a) Some reports claim that the click always occurs at the point of maximum ballooning, but this is controversial [37].

      b) Although on auscultation the click usually seems to initiate the murmur, on the phonocardiogram in many patients it may actually follow shortly after the onset of the murmur.

*5. What is the "contraction ring" theory of the cause of the nonejection click?

ANS.: Often there is a posteroinferior area in the LV in which there is excessive contraction during midsystole. This area is attached mainly to the posterior papillary muscle. Since this part of the LV contracts excessively, it pushes up the posterior papillary muscle and causes the chordae to become slack. Further systole then pulls the chordae taut, producing the click [34]. However, this type of contraction abnormality is not seen in a majority of patients with the prolapsed valve syndrome.

Note: To support further the theory that prolapse of the mitral valve may sometimes be due to a primary myocardial abnormality, the following findings may be listed:

a) Angiograms have shown that at least 80 percent of patients with prolapsed mitral valves have LV asynergy (abnormal areas of contraction or absence of contraction). At least six types of asynergy have been described [119].

1) "Ballerina foot" pattern in right anterior oblique views (vigorous posteromedial contraction and anterior convexity).
2) Reduction of the extent of shortening of the inflow tract area around the mitral valve ring [76].
3) "Hourglass," ringlike contraction of the middle of the ventricle.
4) Inadequate shortening of the long axis.
5) Posterior akinesis.
6) Cavity obliteration.

b) Late systolic clicks have been heard for the first time in patients during the course of their infarction [136A].

c) A late systolic murmur and click developed in one patient after radiopaque dye was inadvertently injected directly beneath the posterior leaflet.

d) Patients with coronary disease are sometimes found to have a click and a late systolic murmur on squatting [21]. This is the opposite to what happens in the usual young patient with the prolapsed valve syndrome.

6. How much MR is present if a delayed murmur to the S_2 is present?

ANS.: Since there is little or no regurgitation at the beginning of systole in these patients, only a mild to moderate amount of MR is likely to be present with this kind of murmur.

*7. What can cause the development of heart failure in a patient with mild MR secondary to the prolapsed valve syndrome?

ANS.: a) Occasionally, chordae will rupture and produce severe MR [50, 81, 135].
b) Gradual progression from mild to severe MR can also occur, but this is rare [67].
c) Infective endocarditis on the mitral valve can occur.

*8. What are the noncardiac causes of midsystolic clicks?

ANS.: a) A small left-sided pneumothorax. When loud, it may be heard at some distance from the patient. It lasts an average of 1½ days [58]. One theory claims that these clicks are produced by the heart flipping the lingula against the thoracic wall [41]. Another theory is that these clicks are produced by the cardiac movement displacing air bubbles between the visceral and parietal pleura. They often disappear with a change of position and reappear with a deep breath [58]. (The fact that they often occur in diastole as well as in systole helps to rule out a valvular etiology.)

b) Pleural-pericardial adhesions.

Note: During the first half of this century all midsystolic clicks were considered to be due to pleural-pericardial adhesions, probably because

a) Gallavardin described 4 cases in which autopsy evidence showed pleural-pericardial adhesions [52].

b) When multiple clicks are heard with prolapsed valves, they may mimic a pericardial friction rub [67].

c) A very uncommon cause of a midsystolic click is the to-and-fro snapping of a floating balloon cathether against the septum in the RV. A diastolic sound will also be heard in such a case and is more common than a systolic click [63].

d) Complete absence of the pericardium has caused the complete syndrome of click and late systolic murmur with no prolapse on either echocardiography or angiography. It increases on inspiration [85].

e) An isolated bicuspid pulmonary valve, especially with right bundle branch block (RBBB) (*very rare*).

f) An aneurysm of the atrial septum may produce a midsystolic click at the time of maximal bulging of the atrial septum into the right atrium. (The atrial septum bulges first into the left atrium in early systole and then suddenly back into the right atrium in midsystole [3].)

g) In patients with aortic regurgitation a midsystolic sound has been recorded that is simultaneous with the dip in the associated bisferiens pulse. The cause is unknown [45, 110].

Prolapsed Valve Auscultatory Findings

Shape and Loudness of Click and Murmur

1. What is the usual shape of delayed systolic murmurs in the prolapsed valve syndrome?

ANS.: To the ear, they often sound crescendo to the second sound.

Note: Most of these murmurs actually are crescendo-decrescendo on a fast-paper-speed phonocardiogram [8].

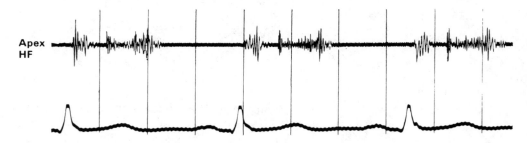

Apex
HF

The midsystolic sound was a click heard loudest at the apex in this 45-year-old woman. The murmur following it is crescendo to the S_2. This is the classic ballooned valve click-murmur complex by auscultation.

3. What is the loudest grade of murmur in the prolapsed valve syndrome?

ANS.: If it is not a whoop or a honk, which can be grade 6, it is almost never more than grade 3/6.

Note: a) Systolic musical honks or whoops are not an uncommon sign of a prolapsed valve [40]. They are usually transient and disappear with different phases of respiration; when they have disappeared, a regurgitant murmur is almost always present. (The word honk refers to the similarity of this sound to the honking of a goose.) These musical honks or whoops are the loudest murmurs heard in cardiologic practice. Many of these patients can hear their own murmurs, and some murmurs can be heard by others, even across the room [40].

*b) Much more rarely, a loud, musical systolic murmur may be present in the left chest when an anomalous fibrous band or cord stretches across the ventricular cavity like the string of a musical instrument. When this is stretched by cardiac dilatation, it may become taut enough to produce a murmur [108].

c) Musical MR murmurs or honks are probably due to vibrations of the valves themselves [44]. Simultaneous echo-phono-cardiography shows regular valve leaflet flutter at a frequency identical to that of the musical murmur [146A]. The usual murmur is caused by turbulence around the valve rather than by the vibrations of the valves themselves. Honks and whoops may sometimes be caused by the vibration of an elongated papillary muscle [61]. A tricuspid whoop in one report was associated at autopsy with two extremely long, thin chordae that were thought to be responsible for the murmur [23]. In two echocardiographic studies, a tricuspid honk was associated with tricuspid valve flutter, and in one study, the undulations of the flutter were at the same frequency as the honk [129, 143].

d) There are several reports of tricuspid whoops in patients with pulmonary hypertension, one with mild TR secondary to an idiopathic cardiomyopathy [145]. The whoop or honk usually disappears if the pulmonary hypertension is relieved [70].

Tricuspid valve prolapse with the click and murmur of TR without a honk has been reported in patients with right ventricular hypertrophy and dilatation secondary to pulmonary hypertension [132].

Changing the Click and Murmur with Maneuvers or Drugs

1. What happens to the nonejection click and murmur when blood volume to the LV is decreased, as occurs with standing, inspiration, or a Valsalva strain? Why?

ANS.: They both occur earlier and they often become louder. Indeed, they may only be heard on sitting or standing. The click may actually occur so early on standing that it may fuse with the first heart sound and may seem to disappear altogether [8].

Note: a) The click may also become louder in the left lateral decubitus position, perhaps because of the change in blood pressure that occurs in some patients in that position.

*b) A PAC or PVC can cause more severe and earlier prolapse because of the contraction that occurs with a smaller volume than normal.

c) After the release of a Valsalva maneuver, the click may become louder because of the overshoot of blood pressure.

2. Why does the prolapsed valve murmur become louder and begin earlier on standing or with any maneuver that makes the heart smaller?

ANS.: Angiograms have shown that an increase in prolapse occurs in the upright position. This may occur because the redundant tissue acts like the dome of a parachute whose diameter is decreased if the edges are held down and pulled toward each other. That is, when the ventricle becomes smaller and the diameter is reduced, the center of the "parachute" is pushed up, owing to the fixed length of chordae and papillary muscles in the smaller ventricle.

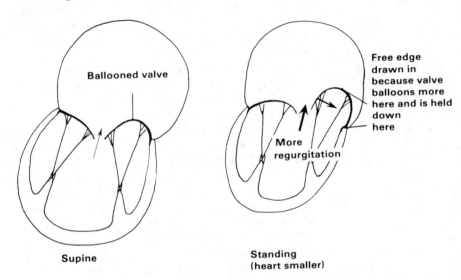

One of the diagnostic characteristics of the ballooned valve murmur is that it becomes louder and begins earlier when the heart is made smaller.

3. What maneuver can tell you that a crescendo systolic murmur to the S_2 is due to papillary muscle dysfunction rather than to the prolapsed valve syndrome if the latter happens to have no click?

ANS.: Only the prolapsed valve murmur will become louder and longer on sitting or standing.

*4. What happens to the (a) click and (b) murmur position and loudness with amyl nitrite?

ANS.: a) The click occurs earlier and usually becomes softer and may even disappear. The smaller end–diastolic volume causes the click to come earlier, and the low systolic pressure makes it softer [114].

b) Usually the murmur immediately becomes softer and occurs earlier, and then after about 30 sec it may become louder owing to the overshoot of blood pressure. If the control murmur is only late systolic, amyl nitrite may cause it to become pansystolic.

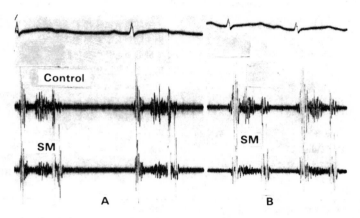

(A) A late systolic murmur moved toward early systole and (B) became pansystolic after amyl nitrite inhalation decreased heart size.

*5. What is the effect of increasing blood pressure with phenylephrine or methoxamine on the position and loudness of the (a) click and (b) murmur?

ANS.: a) The click takes variable positions and usually becomes louder because of the greater force exerted on the mitral valve structure.

b) The murmur becomes louder, and you may even bring out a late systolic murmur if only a click is present.

Note: a) Occasionally only a vasopressor agent can bring out any clicks or murmurs at all. Presumably a critical systolic pressure is necessary to cause prolapse and may account for the increased incidence of these clicks and murmurs with age [114].

b) In one study, in subjects with an isolated systolic nonejection click, a late systolic murmur developed with a vasopressor agent in one-third of the patients, with amyl nitrite in 4 percent, with standing in 10 percent, and during and after a Valsalva maneuver, in about one-third [111].

c) If the heart is made larger by slowing the rate with propranolol, both the click and the murmur may diminish or disappear.

d) When the prolapse is due to the floppy valve syndrome with severe myxomatous transformation and loud pansystolic MR, the response to maneuvers that make the heart smaller is the same as that seen with nonprolapsed causes of MR [84].

*6. How do nonejection clicks following mitral valvotomy differ from other nonejection clicks?

ANS.: These clicks are

a) Louder but lower in frequency and therefore have less of a clicking quality.

b) Usually earlier in systole (more easily confused with an ejection sound) but occasionally situated late in the murmur or even at the end of an early systolic murmur.

       c) Not constant in terms of the effect of maneuvers on them.

       d) Likely to become single or multiple spontaneously.

7. How can you differentiate the late systolic murmur of papillary muscle dysfunction from the late systolic murmur of a prolapsed mitral valve without a click by auscultation?

    ANS.: Papillary muscle dysfunction murmurs are usually associated with an S_4 and a loud S_1, often become softer after a sudden long diastole, and increase with squatting or amyl nitrite [21, 22]. Prolapsed valve murmurs have no characteristic S_1, do not usually feature an S_4, and may become softer with squatting or amyl nitrite.

       Note: With severe prolapse and a pansystolic murmur, the S_1 is louder than average; with ruptured chordae the S_1 is either softer than normal or absent [143]. When a late systolic murmur is made pansystolic by a Valsalva strain, the S_1 becomes louder and the click may disappear.

---

*The Apex Cardiogram with Prolapsed Valves

*1. How can the apex cardiogram (see p. 141) help to diagnose the prolapsed valve syndrome?

    ANS.: A midsystolic dip or retraction occurs at about the time of the nonejection click in about two-thirds of patients with the prolapsed valve syndrome. The timing of the dip changes with maneuvers and keeps a constant relationship with the click. If the retraction is absent or slight, it can often be accentuated with standing or amyl nitrite.

       Note: Kinetocardiograms (see p. 141) have shown that the late systolic movement may peak at the time of the click.

*2. What degree of MR is found with midsystolic retraction on the apex cardiogram?

    ANS.: It is associated with mild degrees of MR.

       Note: The retraction may be due to a sudden rotation of the heart as the mitral leaflet bulges upward.

TRICUSPID REGURGITATION MURMURS

Site, Loudness, and Shape

1. Where is the murmur of TR usually heard best? In what other places may it occasionally be heard best?

    ANS.: It is usually heard best at the left lower sternal border. It is occasionally heard best in the epigastrium, at the right sternal border, or, if the RV is very large, over the mid-left thorax at the site of the usual LV apex area, which may be taken over by the RV.

      Note: In chronic obstructive pulmonary disease, the TR murmur may be heard over the free edge of the liver, presumably because the diaphragm pushes the RV hard against the liver on inspiration.

2. What is the classic method of diagnosing TR by auscultation?

    ANS.: Listen for a pansystolic murmur that becomes louder with inspiration at the left lower sternal border (or wherever a palpable RV lift is felt). This has been called the Carvallo sign of TR [107A].

3. Why does the TR murmur usually increase in loudness on inspiration?

ANS.: Because more blood is drawn into the RV and becomes available for regurgitation. Since the net pulmonary artery pressure rises slightly on inspiration, there is increased resistance in that direction. (If the intrathoracic pressure drop on inspiration is not subtracted from the pulmonary artery pressure as taken with a manometer in the pulmonary artery, the pulmonary artery pressure will give a false impression of falling with inspiration.)

Note: a) The murmur of TR remains louder on held inspiration (inspiratory apnea), i.e., it does not require moving respiration, as when one is looking for movement in the S_2 split. As long as intrathoracic pressure is kept low by an expanded lung, more blood will be brought into the RV than on expiration.

b) Occasionally the TR murmur will not increase with inspiration. This may be because

1) The regurgitation may be so severe that the slight increase in regurgitant volume on inspiration is unnoticeable.

2) Inspiration may not bring much more blood into the RV because of the decreased vital capacity caused by pulmonary congestion or hypertension.

3) Inspiration may so lower pulmonary vascular resistance that the extra blood drawn in on inspiration is ejected into the pulmonary artery rather than regurgitated.

4) The RV may be so damaged that it is functioning on a plateau of the **Starling** curve, so that an increased volume and pressure in the RV cause little change in the strength of contraction.

4. How, besides by inspiration, can you increase venous return in order to bring out a TR murmur?

ANS.: a) By exercise

b) By having someone hold the patient's legs up or having the patient bend his knees up toward his chest.

c) By amyl nitrite inhalation.

d) By pressure over or just below the liver [20, 49A].

Note: Pressure over or below the liver plus deep inspiration may work better than either maneuver alone.

*5. When is a TR murmur decrescendo?

ANS.: In acute, severe TR due to rupture of tricuspid chordae. (See page 322 for an explanation of a similar effect on the left side.)

Note: Occasionally *no* murmur at all may be heard if free TR is present, causing the atrium and ventricle to form almost one chamber in systole. (This can also occur with a ruptured papillary muscle in the LV.)

Differential Diagnosis of Tricuspid and Mitral Regurgitation by Auscultation

1. Why is it often difficult to tell tricuspid regurgitation (TR) from MR?

ANS.: a) The MR murmur transmitted to the left sternal border may sometimes increase on inspiration, thus mimicking TR. This is presumably due to some rotational phenomenon, which should be suspected if the heart sounds also increase with inspiration.

b) The TR murmur may be loud at the usual apex area, which may be usurped by an enlarged RV.

2. How can a Valsalva maneuver help to distinguish TR from MR on auscultation if the site of maximal loudness and the effect of respiration are questionable?

ANS.: Upon release of the strain the TR murmur returns to the pre-Valsalva level of loudness within about 1 sec [92]. An MR murmur should not return for at least about 3 sec.

* 3. How can vasopressors and vasodilators help you distinguish between MR and TR?

ANS.: a) A pure vasopressor will increase the murmur of MR without affecting a TR murmur. (Norepinephrine cannot be used for this purpose because it may raise pulmonary resistance in subjects with pulmonary hypertension [36].

b) The administration of amyl nitrite is even more useful, because it has the opposite effect on the TR and MR murmurs—i.e., it usually makes the TR murmur louder by increasing venous return and the MR murmur softer by lowering peripheral resistance.

Note: a) If the amyl nitrite causes a fall in pulmonary artery pressure because the pulmonary arteriolar constriction was vasoactive rather than fixed, the RV will eject more blood into the pulmonary artery, and therefore the TR murmur will not increase despite the increase in venous return.

b) Serotonin (2 mg administered over 1 minute) will increase only pulmonary resistance and the TR murmur without affecting the MR murmur. It has not been used often enough, however, to know whether or not it has dangerous side effects.

Causes of Tricuspid Regurgitation

1. Does a hypertrophied RV, due to high pressure within it (as in severe pulmonary stenosis or pulmonary hypertension) usually cause TR by itself?
ANS.: No.

2. Does a large RV volume alone (as in ASD) usually cause TR?
ANS.: No.

3. What is necessary before secondary TR can be expected to occur, i.e., in the absence of primary tricuspid valve deformities?

ANS.: *Both* a high pressure and a large volume in the RV. The TR thus caused is *secondary* TR.

Note: Primary TR means TR occurring without pulmonary hypertension, such as that due to trauma, to **Ebstein's anomaly,** or to infective endocarditis; the last of these is seen primarily in heroin addicts.

4. What is the commonest cause of both a high pressure and a large volume in the RV, so that TR is expected?

ANS.: Any cause of severe pulmonary hypertension, e.g., primary pulmonary hypertension or secondary pulmonary hypertension, as with MS, **atrial septal defect,** or severe LV failure.

* *Note:* TR secondary to chronic obstructive pulmonary disease is nearly always trivial [131].

*5. When can a TR murmur be produced by primary tricuspid valve abnormalities other than **Ebstein's anomaly,** trauma, or endocarditis?

ANS.: a) With a prolapsed tricuspid valve.

b) With papillary muscle dysfunction due to RV infarction [86].

c) When a pacemaker wire distorts a tricuspid valve.

Note: Late systolic scratchy murmurs that increase with inspiration have been reported with RV pacemakers. Occasionally, only a systolic murmur is produced by a pacemaker through the tricuspid valve, usually only when the pacemaker is not on. This murmur does not increase with inspiration, is crescendo–decrescendo, and is very early. The cause is unknown [133].

THE CARDIORESPIRATORY MURMUR

1. What is meant by a cardiorespiratory (or cardiopulmonary) murmur?

ANS.: It is an extracardiac murmur, probably produced when the systolic motion of the heart compresses an expanded lung segment between the pericardium and the pleura.

2. What is the pitch and timing of this murmur?

ANS.: It is high-pitched, usually short, and may occur anywhere in systole and even in early diastole. It is heard best during deep inspiration. It tends to disappear near the end of expiration and during held inspiration.

3. What are the most important differential diagnoses of the cardiorespiratory murmur?

ANS.: A late systolic MR murmur, a short aortic regurgitation (AR) murmur, and a TR murmur.

VENTRICULAR SEPTAL DEFECT MURMURS

Shapes and Length

1. Where is the usual ventricular septal defect (VSD) situated?

ANS.: In the membranous septum, i.e., in a small translucent area, extending about 1 or 2 cm below the aortic valve.

* *Note:* The attachment of the septal leaflet of the tricuspid valve bisects the membranous septum, so that the usual VSD is below the attachment, but if the VSD is above this attachment, it may shunt blood directly into the right atrium.

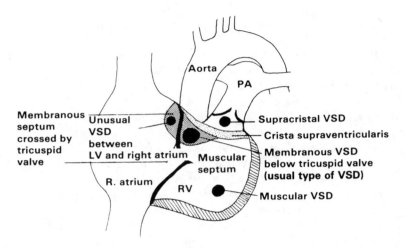

Defects in the membranous septum below the tricuspid valve are the most common.

2. What are the various shapes of VSD murmurs?
   ANS.:

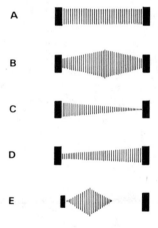

A

B

C

D

E

Unlike some MR murmurs, VSD murmurs probably always begin with the M₁.

3. What is the usual shape of the murmur of a moderate to large VSD on the phonocardiogram when the pulmonary artery pressure is less than 50 mm Hg?
   ANS.: It is usually a pansystolic plateau (rectangular) murmur [57].

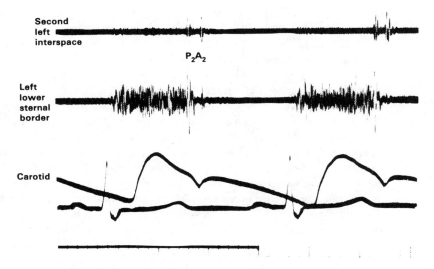

Second
left
interspace

P_2A_2

Left
lower
sternal
border

Carotid

This murmur is plateau in the first cycle, suggesting a pulmonary artery pressure less than 50 mm Hg. The crescendo in the second cycle suggests that the VSD is not large, because small VSDs are the usual cause of murmurs that are crescendo to the S_2.

*4. When is the VSD murmur mostly decrescendo?

ANS.: a) If it is of the muscular type, i.e., in the muscular part of the septum. Muscular contraction of the septum can close the VSD off toward the end of systole.

Note: On a phonocardiogram these murmurs may have a marked crescendo–decrescendo in the first third of systole, and careful scrutiny will usually show that they actually extend as far as the S_2 [148].

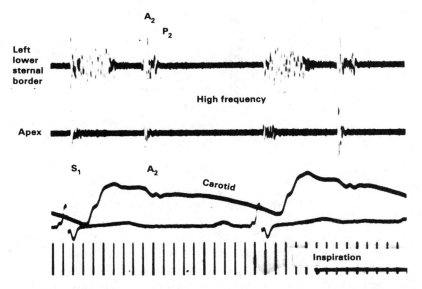

Phonocardiogram from a child with a muscular VSD. The murmur ends well before the S_2. Note the normally moving split of S_2 on inspiration.

b) If moderate pulmonary hypertension is present with a large VSD, the murmur may end before the S_2 and may be decrescendo. (One must, however, avoid the area of the pulmonary ejection murmur that is due to the excess flow into the pulmonary artery.)

* 5. How can you make the short decrescendo of a muscular VSD obviously pansystolic?

ANS.: By using a vasopressor agent, which by raising the peripheral resistance to outflow, causes more left-to-right shunt even during the end of systole.

Note: The murmur of a very small VSD as recorded in the RV can also be crescendo-decrescendo [149]. It is as if a small VSD acts like a valvular obstruction in that it produces almost the same shape as an ejection murmur. If the crescendo-decrescendo murmur is preceded by an early nonejection click, the VSD will be found on angiography to be at the apex of a membranous septum aneurysm that protrudes into the RV outflow tract [104]. However, most VSDs associated with an aneurysm of the ventricular septum produce a crescendo murmur to the S_2 [42].

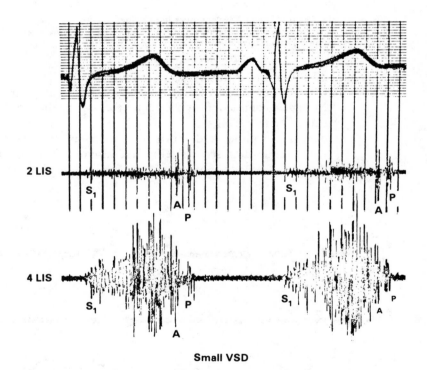

Small VSD

The crescendo-decrescendo effect of this small VSD is best recorded at the fourth left interspace (4 LIS), where the A_2 is obscured by the long murmur.

6. Why may a very large VSD produce a short ejection murmur or no murmur at all?

ANS.: It may create, in effect, a single ventricle, with the same systolic pressure in both RV and LV. When this pressure is transmitted to the pulmonary arterioles, the latter constrict reflexly in response. The raised resistance in the pulmonary circuit prevents much left-to-right flow through the VSD, and the shunt murmur may be soft or may even disappear. Thus, the systolic murmur that you hear may be only an ejection murmur due to flow into a slightly dilated pulmonary artery.

Note: The syndrome of a VSD with pulmonary hypertension severe enough to cause a right–to–left shunt is called Eisenmenger's complex, because this is what Eisenmenger originally described. If the right–to–left shunt is at PDA or ASD levels, it is often called **Eisenmenger's syndrome,** or an Eisenmenger reaction.

Factors Controlling Loudness of VSD Murmurs

1. What is the relationship between the size of the VSD and the loudness of the murmur?

   ANS.: If it is very small (pinhole VSD), the murmur may be very soft. If it is very large, so that there are almost equal pressures in the RV and the LV, the murmur may also be very soft. If, however, it is moderately large, there is usually a very loud murmur. (Some of the loudest murmurs observed in cardiological practice, next to prolapsed valve honks, are caused by moderately large VSDs.)

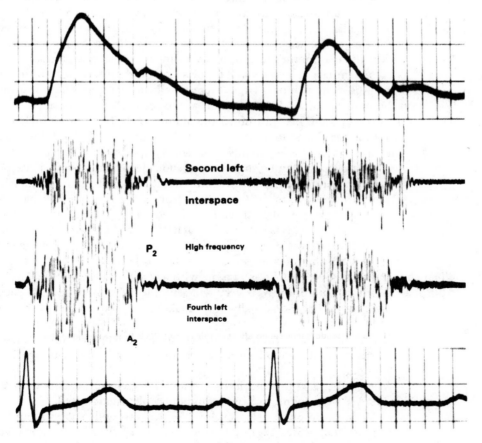

Loud pansystolic harsh murmur found in a patient with a large VSD.

2. What auscultatory clues indicate that a soft VSD murmur is due to a large VSD with severe pulmonary hypertension?

ANS.: a) The murmur is often preceded by an ejection sound when pulmonary artery pressure is high.

b) The murmur will be followed by a loud single S_2 that in turn may be followed by an early diastolic blow of pulmonary regurgitation (Graham Steell murmur).

c) If a large flow is still present (the pulmonary hypertension is then said to be hyperkinetic, vasoactive, or vasospastic), a mitral diastolic murmur due to excess flow through the mitral valve may be heard.

Factors Controlling Sites of Loudness

1. What is the usual site of maximal loudness of the VSD murmur?

ANS.: The left lower sternal border.

2. When may a VSD murmur be louder between the apex and the left lower sternal border than at the left sternal border?

ANS.: Only very rarely,

a) When a large RV has displaced the LV to the left.

b) When the VSD is in the muscular part of the septum near the apex. This is not an unusual site for a ruptured septum secondary to infarction [9].

*c) When a large VSD shunts directly into the right atrium [57]. (Clockwise rotation of the heart (viewed from below) by the large right atrium may shift the maximum murmur away from the left sternal edges, although the murmur may radiate well to the second right interspace. (If the shunt into the right atrium is large, there may be a tricuspid inflow murmur.)

*3. When can the murmur of a VSD be loudest at the second left interspace?

ANS.: If it is supracristal, i.e., just under the pulmonary valve. The site where this murmur is heard next loudest is the first rather than the third left interspace.

Note: a) Because these patients have widely split second sounds and their murmur may be slightly crescendo-decrescendo with a late peak, their murmurs may be confused with the murmur of PS [30, 138].

b) It is easy to tell a PS murmur from a VSD murmur if the patient has complete RBBB and a delayed T_1, e.g., after surgery for tetralogy. This is because with RBBB on a phonocardiogram, right-sided events such as PS start late, i.e., with the T_1, whereas with a VSD the murmur starts with the M_1 [11].

*4. When should you suspect that PS is present with a VSD on auscultation?

ANS.: a) When the split of the S_2 is very wide and the pulmonary component (P_2) is very soft. The P_2 is usually of normal or increased loudness with a pure VSD.

b) When there is an area low on the chest near the epigastrium where the murmur becomes louder on inspiration especially when the patient is standing.

c) When AR is also present; in one series 50 percent of patients with VSD plus AR were found to have infundibular obstruction [69].

Note: Very commonly, AR develops in patients with subpulmonic (supracristal) VSDs because the right coronary cusp of the aortic valve prolapses through the defect.

*5. What hemodynamic problem should you suspect if a large VSD is suggested by x-ray signs of pulmonary plethora (shunt vascularity) and cardiomegaly, yet the murmur is less than grade 4/6?

ANS.: a) Another source of shunt flow through a PDA or an ASD.

b) Pulmonary hypertension.

c) Multiple VSDs.

Note: The patient with multiple VSDs (Swiss cheese defect) usually has a softer murmur than expected, i.e., grade 3/6 or less, even though such patients usually have a large shunt [43]. This softer murmur may result because

1) These are muscular defects and thus tend to close off during the end of systole.

2) Each individual hole may produce a moderately loud murmur, but two moderately loud murmurs may not necessarily combine to make a louder murmur, because each one may transmit its second to a different place on the chest wall or be maximally loud at a different frequency.

6. What is meant by "maladie de Roger"?

ANS.: In 1861 the French pediatrician Henri Roger presented the first comprehensive description of an *asymptomatic* VSD and described the murmur through the defect as loud and long, with its maximum intensity over the upper third of the medial precordial area [153]. The expression is now used to refer to a small VSD with a loud murmur at the left lower sternal border. Roger, however, neither specified the size of the VSD nor placed the murmur at the lower sternal border.

The Ventricular Septal Defect Murmur Versus the Mitral Regurgitation Murmur

*1. When does the effect of amyl nitrite on the VSD murmur differ from that on the MR murmur?

ANS.: Amyl nitrite causes all MR and uncomplicated VSD murmurs to become softer. In the presence of hyperkinetic or vasospastic pulmonary hypertension, however, a VSD murmur may become louder. Amyl nitrite usually does not affect pulmonary artery pressure unless there is vasospastic constriction. In the presence of pulmonary artery constriction amyl nitrite may dilate the pulmonary arterioles and diminish pulmonary resistance *even more than systemic resistance*. The murmur will therefore then become louder or stay the same. This may be used as a test for fixed pulmonary resistance with VSDs, because severe pulmonary hypertension fixed by hypertrophy or obliteration will not be affected by amyl nitrite and the murmur will become softer due to the fall in systemic resistance [149].

Note: a) The combination of a VSD and MR is so rare that when it is found, you should strongly suspect the presence of a corrected transposition in which the left AV valve (tricuspid valve) is incompetent [94].

b) Hypoxia can elevate pulmonary artery pressure without affecting aortic pressure. Ten percent oxygen plus 90 percent nitrogen can decrease the VSD murmur within 5–15 minutes. Little effect should occur on the murmur of MR [29].

2. When may a VSD murmur be loudest near the apex?

ANS.: When the ventricular septum ruptures because of infarction, it may do so in the muscle near the apex and mimic the site of murmur of MR.

* *Note:* The murmur of a VSD due to a rupture is not loudest exactly at the apex; with careful attention, it will be found to be louder slightly medial to the apex. Furthermore, papillary muscle ruptures rarely ever have a grade 4/6 murmur, but VSD murmurs commonly have this loud a murmur (about 50 percent). Also, a VSD due to a ruptured septum commonly has a presystolic murmur that is of medium to high frequency [53].

CONTINUOUS MURMURS

Definitions and Causes

1. What are the two definitions of a continuous murmur?
   ANS.: a) The murmur never stops; i.e., it is truly continuous throughout systole and diastole.
   b) The murmur can be heard to go beyond the S_2 but stops before the next S_1; i.e., it is not truly continuous but does envelop the second sound and go more than slightly beyond it.

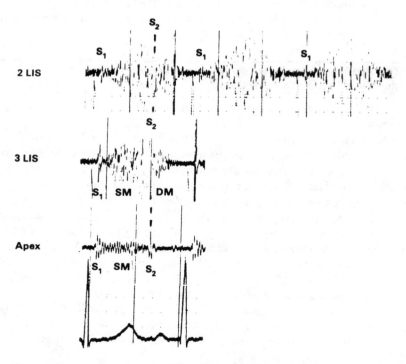

Phonocardiograms from a patient with a PDA. The S_2 at the apex marks the beginning of diastole for the tracings of the continuous murmur, which envelops and obliterates the second sound at the left sternal border. This murmur did not sound truly continuous at the third left interspace (3 LIS) since it seemed to end in mid-diastole. The pulmonary artery systolic pressure was 35 mm Hg. The pulmonary flow was slightly more than twice the systemic flow.

2. What is a systolic and diastolic murmur heard in the same area called if it is not continuous?

ANS.: A to-and-fro murmur. This implies that the systolic component is due to blood flowing in one direction and the diastolic murmur is due to flow in the opposite direction, e.g., an AS ejection murmur plus an AR murmur. (See figure on page 385.) A continuous murmur, on the other hand, implies a murmur that is due to continuous flow in the same direction in both systole and diastole.

Note: The systolic murmurs of a VSD or MR plus an AR diastolic murmur are also to-and-fro murmurs, i.e., the forward and backward flow does not have to be through the same orifice.

*3. Are all continuous murmurs regurgitant?

ANS.: No. Continuous murmurs may be caused by

a) Partial obstruction to a vessel, as in bilateral peripheral pulmonary artery stenosis.

b) Excessively rapid flow through tortuous vessels, as in collateral circulation secondary to a coarctation of the aorta.

c) Extracardiac arterial or venous turbulence:

1) The mammary souffle (see p. 359).

*2) Bilateral pulmonary artery branch stenosis.

*3) Bronchial collateral circulation in cyanotic congenital heart disease with severe obstruction to pulmonary arterial flow.

*4) An arteriovenous fistula, either pulmonary artery to pulmonary vein or internal mammary to adjacent vein [152].

*5) Total anomalous pulmonary venous connection into a left vertical vein (sometimes referred to as a left superior vena cava) [66].

4. List the causes of continuous murmurs primarily in or transmitted to the chest.

ANS.: Those due to transmission from above the clavicle:

a) The venous hum in children (see p. 352).

*b) An arteriovenous fistula in the neck, either congenital or acquired (usually by trauma).

*c) A partial subclavian artery obstruction due to atherosclerosis, with poor collateral circulation beyond the obstruction [127].

Those involving the thoracic aorta:

a) A PDA.

b) Coarctation of the aorta with large subcostal collaterals.

*c) An aortic-pulmonary septal defect (see p. 351).

*d) A rupture of a **sinus of Valsalva** into the pulmonary artery, right atrium, or ventricle.

*e) An internal mammary to pulmonary vein fistula.

Intracardiac:

*a) Through a small ASD in the presence of a high left atrial pressure due to MS. (An ASD with rheumatic MS is called Lutembacher's syndrome.)

*b) Coronary artery to right heart fistula (see p. 356).

*c) A **cor triatriatum.** A continuous murmur high in the left axilla has been noted in one such patient [65].

*Note: The descent of the base (mitral valve ring) during ventricular systole probably causes the systolic component of the murmur in cor triatriation. i.e., from a "suction effect" by the decrease in pressure between the accessory chamber and the true left atrial chamber. This murmur is intermediate in frequency between that of an MS diastolic rumble and an aortic regurgitation high-frequency murmur [142].

5. Why should you search for a continuous murmur in the arms, legs, or abdomen in any patient in congestive failure of obscure etiology?

   ANS.: A search must be made for an arteriovenous fistula, congenital or traumatic. If such a fistula is large (1 cm or more in diameter), signs and symptoms of failure may occur over a period of years.

   *Note: This is a high output type of failure without actual myocardial insufficiency. The arteriovenous shunt causes a low peripheral resistance for which the body tries to compensate by increasing blood volume and **filling pressure** [96]. The sympathetic outflow that causes the high venous pressure may increase peripheral resistance. This in turn creates more shunt flow, causing a vicious cycle of more increase in blood volume and venous pressure until peripheral edema occurs. A high left atrial pressure also results and can cause pulmonary congestion and dyspnea despite a normal cardiac output.

6. What is the commonest cause of a continuous murmur?

   ANS.: Persistent ductus arteriosus (usually called patent ductus arteriosus or PDA).

THE PERSISTENT DUCTUS ARTERIOSUS

Shape and Duration

1. What are some of the other names for the continuous murmur of PDA when it is truly continuous?

   ANS.: a) Machinery murmur.
   b) Gibson murmur [47].

2. Why is a PDA murmur continuous?

   ANS.: Because there is a continuous aortic-pulmonary pressure gradient throughout both systole and diastole (if the pulmonary artery pressure is not far from normal).

3. When is the continuous murmur of PDA not "machinery" in quality or duration?

   ANS.: When it is not truly continuous, i.e., when it begins slightly after the S_1 and crescendos to the S_2, ending after a short decrescendo in early or mid-diastole.

   *Note: a) About half of PDA murmurs in children are not truly continuous, and many are merely pansystolic, exactly mimicking a VSD murmur. This is because with the pulmonary vasoconstriction secondary to the shunt, there is often moderate pulmonary hypertension, which decreases the aortic-pulmonary artery gradient more in diastole than in systole. The low aortic pressures of infants and children, plus the reflex low diastolic pressure caused by the effect of a large volume of blood on the carotid sinus, tends to decrease the gradient further. When only a long systolic murmur is present, differentiation from a VSD is difficult [49]. In any child with a VSD type of pansystolic murmur, a bounding pulse with a pulse pressure of more than 50 should make you strongly suspect either only a PDA or a PDA in addition to a VSD [118].

b) Raising the aortic pressure with methoxamine or ephedrine is an excellent way of bringing out the continuous nature of the murmurs. However, if norepinephrine is used, the murmurs may disappear altogether because the pulmonary artery pressure may increase more than the systemic pressure, presumably because the reactive pulmonary hypertensive arterioles are extremely sensitive to norepinephrine.

c) The combination of clenched fists, overlapping fingers, rocker-bottom feet, and excessively wrinkled skin in infants with trisomy 16-18 suggests that both a PDA and a VSD are present.

*4. Until what age is the aortic-pulmonary gradient usually small enough to prevent the diastolic component of the PDA murmur, so that only a VSD-like pansystolic murmur is heard?

ANS.: Up to the age of 1 year, the thick fetal pulmonary arterioles may not have involuted enough to keep the pulmonary artery pressure normal as it tries to accommodate the increased shunt flow. Despite this, about a third of newborns with PDA are said to have a continuous murmur (with a short diastolic component) for at least a few hours while the fetal ductus is still patent (it normally remains patent for about a week), and many typical PDA murmurs begin at age 6 weeks [15].

Note: A right-to-left shunt occurs in about 12 percent of newborns for a few hours, especially when they are crying [96].

5. Where in systole does the typical PDA murmur reach its maximum intensity?

ANS.: It is crescendo to a peak at or slightly before the S_2, and then is decrescendo to beyond the S_2.

*Note: a) The aortic-pulmonary gradient does not accurately reflect the shape of the murmur because the gradient is maximum in midsystole and the murmur is maximum in late systole. A murmur shape is more related to the acceleration of flow than it is to gradient. The earlier the systolic peak, the greater the caliber of the ductus, as shown by the finding that when the shunt is large, the peak of the murmur occurs well before the A_2.

b) If the PDA is in the low pressure area distal to the site of an aortic coarctation, a continuous murmur may still be present because, despite the low pulse pressure, the mean pressure beyond the coarctation is almost the same as normal aortic mean pressure [27].

Loudness and Site

1. Where is a PDA murmur heard (a) loudest and (b) next loudest?

ANS.: a) Loudest in the second left interspace.

b) Next loudest in the first left interspace.

*Note: a) With a right-sided aortic arch, the PDA murmur may be best heard in the first or second *right* interspace.

b) If the cause of the continuous murmur is not a PDA but some other cause in the chest or heart, the next loudest area will be the third left interspace.

*2. What can make a PDA murmur disappear transiently without any change in pulmonary artery pressure?

ANS.: Some ducti are thought to kink and so close off. One such ductus murmur paradoxically diminished with methoxamine [14]. Another one intermittently disappeared with no constant maneuver; a slightly angulated course was found at surgery [128]. In another case a valvelike structure was found inside the ductus [71].

Note: a) Permanent closure of PDAs can occur with endarteritis due to infective endocarditis and with atheromatous thrombosis.

b) A PDA murmur may be masked by an unimportant aortic stenosis and regurgitation to-and-fro murmur [1].

*3. What is the most difficult differential diagnosis between a to-and-fro murmur and a continuous PDA murmur?

ANS.: A small VSD with a crescendo murmur to the A_2, together with AR and its decrescendo murmur after the A_2. If the harsh quality of the VSD murmur suddenly gives way to the breathy blow of the AR murmur it is unlike the PDA murmur, which does not suddenly change character in diastole.

OTHER AUSCULTATORY SIGNS OF PATENT DUCTUS ARTERIOSUS

*1. Explain the effect on the typical PDA murmur of (a) a vasopressor agent such as methoxamine and (b) a vasodilator such as amyl nitrite.

ANS.: a) A vasopressor increases the murmur because it increases the aortic-pulmonary gradient.

b) Amyl nitrite decreases the murmur because it decreases the gradient.

Note: In the presence of hyperkinetic pulmonary hypertension, amyl nitrite may increase a PDA murmur because it may relax the hyperactive pulmonary arterioles more than it diminishes the peripheral systemic resistance.

*2. List the auscultatory signs of a large PDA shunt flow besides the continuous murmur.

ANS.: a) A paradoxically split S_2.

b) A diastolic mitral murmur or even an opening snap due to an excess flow through the mitral valve.

c) Multiple systolic clicks or crackles (sometimes called "eddy sounds"), especially in the second half of systole and in early diastole.

Note: Eddy sounds have been theorized to be due to a "head-on" collision of streams from the ductus and the pulmonary artery. They are usually heard only in large flow ducti and may be present even if the diastolic component of the murmur is absent or very short [60].

PERSISTENT DUCTUS ARTERIOSUS WITH HIGH PULMONARY ARTERY PRESSURE

1. By inspection alone, how can you tell that a reversed shunt flows through a PDA rather than at the atrial or ventricular level, i.e., how can you differentiate between the Eisenmenger syndromes?

    ANS.: The feet may be more cyanotic and clubbed than the hands. This is known as "differential **cyanosis** and **clubbing**."

    Note: The differential cyanosis can be brought out by raising the pulmonary artery pressure still more with exercise.

2. What causes differential cyanosis in a PDA Eisenmenger situation, and why may the left hand be more cyanotic and clubbed than the right hand?

    ANS.: The ductus often joins the pulmonary artery to the aorta just beyond the left subclavian artery. Unsaturated pulmonary artery blood will then pass beyond the left subclavian artery, and both hands will be less clubbed and cyanotic than the feet. (With pulmonary hypertension, unsaturated blood flows through a ductus from the pulmonary artery to the aorta.) If, however, the ductus is at the junction of the aorta and the left subclavian artery, this artery may also receive unsaturated blood, and the left hand will be as cyanotic and clubbed as the feet.

3. Which component of the continuous murmur is the first to disappear as pulmonary artery pressure rises owing to pulmonary hypertension?

    ANS.: The diastolic component disappears first because the diastolic gradient disappears first.

    * *Note:* a) There is a report of one adult patient whose systolic murmur disappeared with hyperkinetic pulmonary hypertension and a large left-to-right shunt. Only a pandiastolic murmur remained [99].

4. When will a right-to-left shunt (reversed ductus flow due to pulmonary hypertension) produce a murmur?

    ANS.: It is a general rule that right-to-left shunts do not produce murmurs.

---

*Ductus Arteriosus Versus Aortic-Pulmonary Septal Defect Murmurs

*1. What is meant by an aortic-pulmonary septal defect (sometimes called "aortic-pulmonary window")?

    ANS.: It is an opening between the ascending aorta and the pulmonary artery about 1 cm above the pulmonary valves.

*2. What auscultatory clues are there to differentiate a PDA from an aortic-pulmonary septal defect murmur?

    ANS.: Although the site of maximum loudness may be at the second left interspace in both, the next loudest site in PDA is usually one interspace higher, whereas the aortic-pulmonary septal defect murmur is more likely to be second loudest one interspace lower.

    Note: There is more likely to be a continuous murmur in a PDA than in an aortic-pulmonary septal defect, because only about 15 percent of aortic-pulmonary septal defects are small enough to have pulmonary artery pressures that are sufficiently low to allow a continuous murmur [95].

THE VENOUS HUM

1. Where is a venous hum best heard?

   ANS.: Just above the clavicle either medial to the sternocleidomastoid or between its insertions. It is best heard on the right side of the neck.

   Note: A venous hum is more likely to be heard on the right side because the right jugular is larger than the left since it must carry about two–thirds of the intracranial venous drainage.

2. What does a venous hum sound like?

   ANS.: Sometimes it is like a continuous roar; at other times it is like "the sound of the sea" heard by putting a seashell to the ear. Sometimes it is a whining sound. The diastolic component is often higher pitched and louder than the systolic. Probably the only quality that is *never* present is that of an actual hum.

3. What causes the venous hum?

   ANS.: Two theories have been proposed:

   a) Turbulence caused by a confluence of flow through the internal jugular and subclavian veins as they pour into the superior vena cava.

   b) Anterior angulation of the internal jugular vein by the transverse process of the atlas [30]. (This angulation and also the murmur can be shown to increase by turning the head away from the side of the hum.)

4. How can you elicit a venous hum if you cannot hear it by merely placing the stethoscope on the neck?

   ANS.: a) Ask the patient to sit up with his feet on the bed to bring maximum blood volume to the heart from both the lower body and head.

   b) Apply the bell lightly to the right side of the neck, as closely as possible to the clavicle and anterior border of the sternocleidomastoid muscle or between its insertions. A small bell may be necessary in order to maintain a good air seal without excess pressure. Too much pressure will eliminate the hum.

   c) Turn the patient's head away. When maximum rotation is reached, raise the chin as high as possible.

   d) When a continuous roar or whine is heard, test for the presence of a hum by applying moderate pressure with the fingers a few inches above the stethoscope. A venous hum will disappear with moderate pressure on the internal jugular vein.

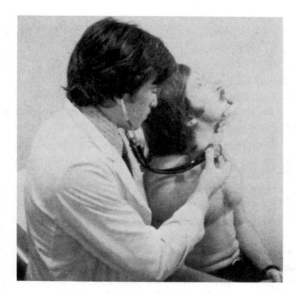

A small bell is invaluable in enabling you to apply airtight light pressure anterior to the sternomastoid muscle.

5. What is the significance of a venous hum that can be elicited without much head turning?

ANS.: It suggests that the circulation time is at least normal and may even be faster than normal.

Note: a) An unelicited venous hum is commonly found in young children but only in about 10 percent of normal subjects over age 50. However, in about half of subjects over age 50, it can be elicited by rotating and raising the head. The unelicited venous hum is of most help in confirming the presence of hyperthyroidism in the young and in suggesting the diagnosis of apathetic hyperthyroidism in the elderly, i.e., hyperthyroidism with no apparent symptoms or signs of thyrotoxicosis and often with atrial fibrillation [33]. The nonelicited venous hum is also common in patients with severe uremia with a low hematocrit and also in pregnant women.

b) If a venous hum is not only unelicited but actually difficult to obliterate, it is almost pathognomonic of a very rapid circulation time, as in thyrotoxicosis. A venous hum (continuous murmur) can also be heard over the femoral veins if the circulation is hyperkinetic [139].

c) Although a venous hum should always be expected if you are diagnosing hyperthyroidism, the hum may disappear if the patient goes into enough heart failure to slow venous flow.

6. What are the methods of eliminating the venous hum besides applying pressure above or with the stethoscope?

ANS.: a) Turn the patient's head toward the side of the hum.

b) Decrease venous return from the jugular veins by placing the patient in a supine position.

Note: a) When the diastolic component of a venous hum is high-pitched, it can be transmitted to the upper chest and may minic AR. This hum is especially likely to be mistaken for AR because only the diastolic component of the hum may be transmitted downward. Such false AR can be elicited in approximately 10 percent of subjects with severe uremia and anemia who have a venous hum.

b) Anemia alone may also cause a loud venous hum. One patient with a hematocrit of 30 percent had a venous hum that was heard by the patient himself as a loud roaring in both ears [52A].

c) A venous hum is common in the inguinal area in normal subjects in the supine position [42A].

7. What besides the venous hum might cause a supraclavicular continuous murmur?

ANS.: a) A traumatic or congenital arteriovenous fistula.

b) Partial obstruction of any of the arteries arising from the aorta (aortic arch syndromes).

Note: A continuous murmur due to aortic branch stenosis means that there is poor collateral circulation distal to the obstruction. (Good collateral circulation would raise the pressure distal to the obstruction enough to prevent a continuous gradient across the obstruction.)

8. When does a venous hum mimic a PDA?

ANS.: In some children the venous hum is transmitted downward to the upper chest, and since it sounds like a continuous murmur, it has been mistaken for the murmur of PDA.

Note: *a) The continuous murmur in some small tortuous PDAs may disappear in a sitting position. This should cause no confusion with a venous hum, which responds in the opposite way to changes in posture [144].

*b) In patients with total anomalous pulmonary venous connection with a left vertical vein (which in turn drains into the innominate vein), the torrential flow may produce a continuous murmur like a venous hum that may be loudest slightly lower than the second left interspace [19]. This may be due to partial obstruction of the vertical vein between the pulmonary artery and the left main bronchus [66].

*CONTINUOUS MURMURS OF PULMONARY ARTERY AND PULMONARY ARTERY BRANCH STENOSIS

*1. What is necessary before a pulmonary artery stenosis can produce a continuous murmur? (This does not refer to pulmonary *valve* stenosis.)

ANS.: The pulmonary artery stenosis must be multiple, causing pulmonary hypertension proximal to the obstruction. Experimentally, a continuous murmur can be produced by stenosis in a pulmonary artery only if the opposite artery is clamped [35].

Note: a) You should suspect multiple pulmonary artery branch stenosis if you diagnose severe pulmonary hypertension with or without cyanosis and hear a continuous murmur over the posterior chest as well as anteriorly, especially if there is a normal pulmonary artery on the roentgenogram [127].

b) If there is severe multiple pulmonary artery stenosis, the continuous murmur may be due to enlarged, tortuous bronchial arteries supplying the lungs [75].

*2. Where is a continuous murmur sometimes heard if a large pulmonary embolus causes partial obstruction of a left pulmonary artery?

ANS.: Under the left scapula.

Note: It may increase with inspiration.

*3. How can a thoracic aortic aneurysm cause a continuous pulmonary arterial murmur?

ANS: An aneurysm can compress a pulmonary artery so that there is a gradient across the narrowed area in both systole and diastole.

PULMONARY ARTERIOVENOUS FISTULAS

1. What is meant by a pulmonary arteriovenous fistula?

ANS.: This is a right-to-left shunt from the pulmonary artery to the pulmonary vein. It is usually congenital.

*2. What is the effect of respiration and body position on the continuous murmur of a pulmonary arteriovenous fistula?

ANS.: Inspiration usually makes the murmur louder because it increases the pulmonary artery–pulmonary vein pressure gradient. Compression of the fistula brought about by lying on the side of the malformation or by elevating the diaphragm by lying supine may attenuate or eliminate the murmur [54].

Note: A continuous murmur is heard in only about two-thirds of patients with this fistula.

3. By inspection alone, what clues indicate that the continuous murmur is due to a pulmonary arteriovenous fistula?

ANS.: a) Cyanosis and clubbing.

b) Telangiectasis on the skin or mucous membranes.

---

*CONTINUOUS MURMURS OF BRONCHOPULMONARY ANASTOMOSES

*1. What should you suspect as a cause of a continuous murmur that is heard bilaterally in a patient with cyanosis and a roentgenogram that suggests no pulmonary artery at all?

ANS.: Large bronchial arteries supplying the lungs in a patient with

a) A persistent truncus arteriosus with small pulmonary arteries, or

b) A solitary arterial trunk with pulmonary atresia.

Note: Pulmonary plethora (shunt vascularity) on chest x-ray examination in a cyanotic patient does not exclude the possibility that a continuous murmur is due to bronchial artery collateral circulation because bronchial collaterals can produce excessive flow to the lungs.

*2. What is suggested as a cause of a unilateral continuous murmur in a cyanotic patient with a PS murmur?

ANS.: A tetralogy of Fallot with
   a) An absent pulmonary artery on one side. The continuous murmur may then be due to bronchial collateral circulation on that side.
   b) One pulmonary artery arising from the aorta.
   c) A PDA. However, a continuous murmur with uncomplicated tetralogy of Fallot is more likely to be due to the bronchial collateral circulation associated with pulmonary atresia because a PDA with an uncomplicated tetralogy of Fallot is very rare [17, 101].
   Note: A continuous murmur in a cyanotic newborn may be due to mitral atresia with a forced left-to-right flow through a small ASD or stretched foramen ovale.

CONTINUOUS MURMURS OF CORONARY ARTERY OR AORTA TO RIGHT HEART FISTULAS

1. What besides an aortic-pulmonary septal defect can cause a continuous murmur that has either the maximum intensity or the second loudest area lower than the second left interspace?
   ANS.: a) A left or right coronary artery (usually dilated) that communicates with the coronary vein, right atrium, RV, or pulmonary artery.
   b) Rupture of a sinus of Valsalva into the right atrium or RV.
   * *Note:* Both these lesions will tend to produce diastolic accentuation of the murmur. But the murmur due to rupture of the sinus of Valsalva tends to be much louder than the coronary artery murmur and often has a cooing or musical quality. Look for a dicrotic pulse (see p. 50), which is very common in subjects with rupture of a sinus of Valsalva [94].

* 2. Why will the anomalous coronary artery to right heart fistula usually produce diastolic accentuation of the continuous murmur?
   ANS.: Because there is more coronary flow in diastole than in systole.
   Note: *a) An anomalous left coronary artery originating from the pulmonary artery may occasionally produce a to-and-fro murmur in the adult, which is best heard at the fourth left interspace. If a vasopressor agent such as methoxamine causes the diastolic component to decrease, it suggests that most of the collaterals are passing through the ventricular septum and are squeezed off [154].
   *b) A right coronary artery fistula to the LV may produce only a diastolic murmur that may be maximal at the apex [136] or over the lower sternal border [69]. It may, however, produce a to-and-fro murmur in which the diastolic component is dominant and maximal in the epigastrium [97].
   *c) If the continuous murmur is soft and is due to a left coronary artery to pulmonary artery fistula, only the diastolic components may be heard, and it may mimic AR except that its site of maximal loudness will be lower, i.e., at the third or fourth interspace [62].

*3. Which abnormal drainage areas of the coronary artery are suggested by a continuous murmur that is loudest at the (a) second or third right interspace, (b) second left interspace, (c) left lower sternal border, (d) upper sternum, (e) apex, (f) third or fourth right interspace, or (g) lower sternum? (This question is for reference purposes and not for memorization.)

ANS.: a) Right coronary artery to right atrium [55, 73, 75].

b) Left coronary artery to pulmonary artery [73]. Right coronary artery to PA [59].

c) Left coronary or circumflex artery to coronary sinus [73]. Left coronary artery or circumflex artery to RV [93]. Right coronary artery to pulmonary artery [93, 150], or left coronary artery to left atrium [5].

d) Right coronary artery to RV [73].

e) Circumflex artery to coronary sinus [72]. Left coronary artery to pulmonary artery or to apex of RV [73].

f) Right coronary artery to coronary sinus or to right atrium [72, 91].

g) Left coronary artery to RV [91].

Note: Even if the murmur is loudest at the left lower sternal border, if it transmits well to the *right* lower sternal border, or if only the diastolic component is louder to the right of the sternum, it should still suggest a shunt from the right coronary artery to the right atrium or ventricle [18, 55].

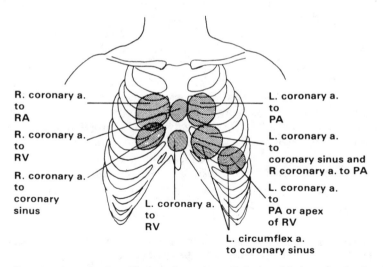

R. coronary a. to RA

R. coronary a. to RV

R. coronary a. to coronary sinus

L. coronary a. to RV

L. coronary a. to PA

L. coronary a. to coronary sinus and R coronary a. to PA

L. coronary a. to PA or apex of RV

L. circumflex a. to coronary sinus

Coronary artery fistulas will often give a clue to their site of drainage by the site of the loudest murmur.

*4. Why may a rupture of a sinus of Valsalva into the RV produce diastolic accentuation of the continuous murmur?

ANS.: The muscular walls encircling the orifice of the communication may relax in diastole allowing more regurgitation [16].

Note: Because a continuous murmur that has a louder diastolic component than a systolic component is an important differentiation point from PDA, it is occasionally useful to use a maneuver that will make the diastolic component louder than the systolic if the murmur is not due to a PDA. Raising the systemic pressure by a post-Valsalva effect or isometric handgrip will increase all diastolic components of a continuous murmur if the murmur is due to a sinus of Valsalva that has ruptured into the RV [14]. If the diastolic components decrease with these maneuvers, suspect a coronary artery-to-right-heart fistula with collaterals passing through the ventricular septum.

*5. Where is the continuous murmur loudest if a sinus of Valsalva ruptures into (a) the RV or (b) the right atrium?

ANS.: a) If the rupture is into the RV, the murmur is loudest at the third left or right interspace or at the left sternal border.

b) If it is into the right atrium, the murmur is loudest in the lower left or right sternal border or in the epigastrium [124].

Note: If on turning the patient into the right lateral decubitus position, the murmur is directed into the right chest, a communication with the right atrium is likely.

*CONTINUOUS MURMURS OF TOTAL ANOMALOUS PULMONARY VENOUS CONNECTION AND ATRIAL SEPTAL DEFECT

*1. Why will total anomalous pulmonary venous drainage into the right atrium occasionally produce a continuous murmur? Where is this murmur heard?

ANS.: a) Torrential flow from a persistent left superior vena cava into a dilated right superior vena cava may produce a continuous murmur under the right clavicle.

b) The venous return from a persistent left superior vena cava may be compressed between the pulmonary artery and the left main bronchus [19, 66]. This murmur is heard around the second left interspace.

*2. Under what conditions besides the presence of total anomalous pulmonary venous drainage will there be a continuous murmur in a patient with an ASD?

ANS.: When MS or severe MR is also present, bringing about an elevation in left atrial pressure that causes a persistent gradient across a small ASD. An ASD plus rheumatic MS is known as Lutembacher's syndrome.

CONTINUOUS MURMURS OF COARCTATION

1. What causes the continuous murmur in coarctation?

ANS.: Although the systolic and diastolic pressure gradient across a severe coarctation has been shown by intra-aortic phonocardiography to produce a continuous murmur, collateral intercostal vessel flow is probably the most likely cause of a continuous murmur heard in coarctation. In mild or moderate coarctation, there is only a systolic murmur over the area of actual coarctation.

*2. What is the clue for differentiating a PDA murmur from a coarctation murmur by auscultation of the posterior chest?

ANS.: If the murmur is heard just as easily or even more easily over the posterior chest, it is much more likely to be due to coarctation, i.e., either to the collateral circulation on the chest wall or to the coarctation itself.

Note: If a continuous murmur is heard only over the lower two or three ribs posteriorly, you should suspect an abdominal coarctation [127].

THE MAMMARY SOUFFLE

1. What is the cause of the mammary souffle?

   ANS.: It is an arterial murmur due to a large flow of blood into the breast during pregnancy and lactation in a minority of pregnant women.

   Note: That the murmur arises in the superficial arteries of the breast is shown by the observation that firm pressure with the stethoscope or manual pressure lateral to the stethoscope can abolish the murmur. Palpable arterial pulsations in the relevant intercostal spaces are present in most cases. Its high pitch, systolic accentuation, and absence of any effect of a Valsalva maneuver suggest further that it is an arterial rather than a venous murmur [123].

2. What is the usual site and loudness of the mammary souffle?

   ANS.: It is usually heard along the left sternal border, and it is rarely more than grade 4/6.

   Note: It may disappear when the patients sits up.

3. In which trimester of pregnancy does the mammary souffle begin, and how long does it last postpartem?

   ANS.: Although it usually begins in the second or third trimester, it may not begin until the first postpartem week. It usually lasts from several weeks to 2 months postpartem.

4. What is characteristic of the timing of the mammary souffle?

   ANS.: There is a delay between the S_1 and the murmur, which often spills over the S_2 into early diastole [140]. Therefore, it must be distinguished from other causes of continuous murmurs.

REFERENCES

1. Abbott, J. A., and Shively, H. H. Auscultatorily silent patent ductus arteriosus. *Chest* 63:371, 1973.
2. Agarwal, A. K. A new observation on papillary muscle dysfunction. *Chest* 82:130, 1982.
3. Alexander, M. D., et al. Atrial septal aneurysm: A cause for midsystolic click. *Circulation* 63:1186, 1981.
4. Allen, H., Harris, A., and Leatham, A. Significance and prognosis of an isolated late systolic murmur: a 9- to 22-year follow-up. *Br. Heart J.* 36:525, 1974.
5. Arani, D. T., Greene, D. G., and Klocke, F. J. Coronary artery fistulas emptying into left heart chambers. *Am. Heart J.* 96:438, 1978.
6. Aravanis, C. Silent mitral insufficiency. *Am. Heart J.* 70:620, 1965.
7. Auger, P., and Wigle, E. D. Sudden, severe mitral insufficiency. *Can. Med. Assoc. J.* 96:1493, 1967.
8. Barlow, J. B., et al. Late systolic murmurs and nonejection ("mid-late") systolic clicks. *Br. Heart J.* 30:203, 1968.

9. Barnard, P. M., and Kennedy, J. H. Postinfarction ventricular septal defect. *Circulation* 32:76, 1965.

10. Basta, L. L., et al. The value of left parasternal impulse recordings in the assessment of mitral regurgitation. *Circulation* 48:1055, 1973.

11. Beck, W., et al. Hemodynamic effects of amyl nitrite and phenylephrine on the normal human circulation and their relation to changes in cardiac murmurs. *Am. J. Cardiol.* 8:341, 1961.

12. Beck, W., Schrire, V., and Vogelpoel, L. The value of phonocardiography in the assessment of the surgical closure of ventricular septal defect. *Am. Heart J.* 67:742, 1964.

13. Bergland, J. M., et al. Pre-excitation as a cause of appearance and increased intensity of systolic murmurs. *Circulation* 33:131, 1966.

14. Burch, G. E., DePasquale, N. P., and Phillips, J. H. Clinical manifestations of papillary muscle dysfunction. *Arch. Intern. Med.* 112:158, 1963.

15. Burnard, E. D. A murmur from the ductus arteriosus in the newborn baby. *Br. Med. J.* 1:806, 1958.

16. Buzzi, A. Evaluation of a precordial continuous murmur. *Am. J. Cardiol.* 4:551, 1959.

16A. Call, T., Leier, C., and Wooley, C. Cardiac defects in the Ehlers-Danlos syndrome. *Circulation* (Abstracts) (Suppl. III) (Abstracts) 55:69, 1977.

17. Campbell, M., and Deuchar, D. C. Continuous murmurs in cyanotic congenital heart disease. *Br. Heart J.* 12:173, 1961.

18. Carmichael, D. B., and Davison, D. G. Congenital coronary arteriovenous fistula. *Am. J. Cardiol.* 8:846, 1961.

19. Carter, R. E. B., Capriles, M., and Noe, Y. Total anomalous pulmonary venous drainage. *Br. Heart J.* 31:45, 1969.

20. Cha, S. D., Gooch, A. S., and Maranhao, V. Intracardiac phonocardiography in tricuspid regurgitation: Relation to clinical and angiographic findings. *Am. J. Cardiol.* 48:578, 1981.

21. Cheng, T. O. Late systolic murmur in coronary artery disease. *Chest* 61:346, 1972.

22. Cheng, T. O. Characterization of late systolic murmur associated with coronary artery disease. *Circulation* (Abstracts) (Suppl. II) 43:31, 1971.

23. Cho, K., et al. Tricuspid whoop—an autopsied case. *Cardiovasc. Sound Bull.* 4:655, 1974.

24. Chrysant, S. G., and Frohlich, E. D. Autonomic sympathetic adjustments in patients with labile and fixed essential hypertension. World Congress Cardiology, Tokyo, 1978. P. 0982.

25. Chun, P. K. C. Nonejection systolic click in mitral stenosis. *Am. Heart J.* 3:463, 1981.

26. Cohen, E. M., Loew, D. E., and Messer, J. V. Internal mammary arteriovenous malformation with communication to the pulmonary vessels. *Am. J. Cardiol.* 35:103, 1975.

27. Crevasse, L. E., and Logue, R. B. Atypical patent ductus arteriosus. *Circulation* 19:332, 1959.

28. Criley, J. M., et al. Prolapse of mitral valve. *Br. Heart J.* 28:488, 1966.

29. Curiel, R. The cardiovascular effects of acute hypoxemia as a diagnostic aid. *Chest* 81:159, 1982.

30. Cutforth, R., Wiseman, J., and Sutherland, R. D. The genesis of the cervical venous hum. *Am. Heart J.* 80:488, 1970.

31. Desser, K. B., and Benchimol, A. The apexcardiogram in patients with the syndrome of midsystolic click and late systolic murmur. *Chest* 62:739, 1972.

32. Dock, W. Production mode of systolic clicks due to mitral cusp prolapse. *Arch. Intern. Med.* 132:118, 1973.

33. Dougherty, M. J., and Craige, E. Apathetic hyperthyroidism presenting as tricuspid regurgitation. *Chest* 63:767, 1973.

34. Ehlers, K. H., et al. Left ventricular abnormality with late mitral insufficiency and abnormal electrocardiogram. *Am. J. Cardiol.* 26:333, 1970.

35. Eldridge, F., Selzer, A., and Hultgren, H. Stenosis of a branch of the pulmonary artery. *Circulation* 15:865, 1957.

36. Endrys, J., and Bartova, A. Pharmacological methods in the phonocardiographic diagnosis of regurgitant murmurs. *Br. Heart J.* 24:207, 1962.

37. Engle, M. A. The syndrome of apical systolic click, late systolic murmur, and abnormal T waves. *Circulation* 39:1, 1969.

38. Ewing, D. J., et al. Static exercise in untreated systemic hypertension. *Br. Heart J.* 35:413, 1973.

39. Farru, O., Duffau, G., and Rodriguez, R. Auscultatory and phonocardiographic characteristics of supracristal ventricular septal defect. *Br. Heart J.* 33:238, 1971.
40. Felner, J. M., et al. Systolic honks in young children. *Am. J. Cardiol.* 40:206, 1977.
41. Fox, M. B. Clicking pneumothorax. *Lancet* 1:210, 1948.
42. Freedom, R. M., et al. The natural history of the so-called aneurysm of the membranous ventricular septum in childhood. *Circulation* 49:375, 1974.
43. Friedman, W. F., Mehrizi, A., and Pusch, A. L. Multiple muscular ventricular septal defects. *Circulation* 32:35, 1965.
44. Fujii, J., et al. Echocardiographic and phonocardiographic study on the genesis of the musical murmur. *J. Cardiography* 6:385, 1976.
45. Fukuda, N., et al. Studies on the genesis of the aortic thudding sound in patients with aortic insufficiency, with special reference to the aortic flow pattern. *J. Cardiography* 11:747, 1981.
46. Fulkerson, P. K., et al. Calcification of the mitral annulus: Etiology, clinical associations, complications and therapy. *Am. J. Med.* 66:967, 1979.
47. Gibson, G. A. Clinical lectures on circulatory affections. *Edin. Med. J.* 8:1, 1900.
48. Giuliani, E. R. Mitral valve incompetence due to flail anterior leaflet. *Am. J. Cardiol.* 20:784, 1967.
49. Gonzalez-Cerna, J. L., and Lillehei, C. W. Patent ductus arteriosus with pulmonary hypertension simulating ventricular septal defect. *Circulation* 18:871, 1958.
49A. Gooch, A. S., Cha, S. D., and Maranhao, V. The use of the hepatic pressure maneuver to identify the murmur of tricuspid regurgitation. *Clin. Cardiol.* 6:277, 1983.
50. Goodman, D., Kimbiris, D., and Linhart, J. W. Chordae tendeae rupture complicating the systolic click-late systolic murmur syndrome. *Am. J. Cardiol.* 33:681, 1974.
51. Goodman, D. J., and Hancock, E. W. Secundum atrial septal defect associated with a cleft mitral valve. *Br. Heart J.* 35:1315, 1973.
52. Hancock, E. W., and Cohn, K. The syndrome associated with midsystolic click and late systolic murmur. *Am. J. Med.* 41:183, 1966.
52A. Hardison, J. E., et al. Self-heard venous hums. *J.A.M.A.* 245:1146, 1981.
53. Haze, K., et al. Interventricular septal perforation secondary to acute myocardial infarction: Phonocardiographic appraisal of thirteen cases. *Cardiovasc. Sound Bull.* 5:593, 1975.
54. Hazlett, D. R., and Medina, J. Postural effects on the bruit and right-to-left shunt of pulmonary arteriovenous fistula. *Chest* 60:89, 1971.
55. Heidenreich, R. P., Leon, D. F., and Shaver, J. A. A case of anomalous right coronary artery to right atrial fistula presenting as atypical aortic insufficiency. *Am. J. Cardiol.* 23:453, 1969.
56. Heikkila, J. Mitral incompetence complicating acute myocardial infarction. *Br. Heart J.* 29:162, 1967.
57. Hollman, A., et al. Auscultatory and phonocardiographic findings in ventricular septal defects. *Circulation* 28:94, 1963.
58. Honda, M., et al. Observations of tapping sounds in pneumothorax. *J. Cardiography* 7:07, 1977.
59. Huang, M. T. C., Goodman, M. A. and Delaney, T. B. Left and right coronary artery-pulmonary artery fistula. *N.Y. State J. Med.* 79:1774, 1979.
60. Hubbard, T. F., and Neis, D. D. The sounds at the base of the heart in cases of patent ductus arteriosus. *Am. Heart J.* 59:807, 1960.
61. Iemoto, T., et al. An autopsied case of papillary muscle dysfunction with mid-systolic click and late systolic honk—with a special reference to its pathophysiology. *Cardiovasc. Sound Bull.* 4:633, 1974.
62. Ishikawa, T., et al. A case of coronary artery-pulmonary artery fistula presented diastolic blowing murmur. *J. Cardiogr.* 6:169, 1976.
63. Isner, J. M., Horton, J., and Ronan, J. A., Jr. Systolic click from a Swan-Ganz catheter: phonoechocardiographic depiction of the underlying mechanism. *Am. J. Cardiol.* 43:1046, 1979.
64. January, L. E., Fisher, J. M., and Ehrenhaft, J. L. Mitral insufficiency resulting from rupture of normal chordae tendineae. *Circulation* 26:1329, 1962.
65. Jegier, W., Gibbons, J. E., and Wigglesworth, F. W. Cor triatriatum: Clinical hemodynamic and pathological studies. Surgical correction in early life. *Pediatrics* 31:255, 1963.
66. Jensen, J. B. Total anomalous pulmonary venous return. *Am. Heart J.* 82:387, 1971.
67. Jeresaty, R. M. Mitral valve prolapse-click syndrome. *Progr. Cardiovasc. Dis.* 15:623, 1973.

68. Karliner, J. S., et al. Haemodynamic explanation of why the murmur of mitral regurgitation is independent of cycle length. *Br. Heart J.* 35:397, 1973.
69. Kawasaki, S., et al. A phonocardiographic study on two cases of congenital coronary artery fistula. *Cardiovasc. Sound Bull.* 4:603, 1974.
70. Keenan, T. J., and Schwartz, M. J. Tricuspid whoop. *Am. J. Cardiol.* 31:642, 1973.
71. Keith, T. R., and Sagarminaga, J. Spontaneously disappearing murmur of patent ductus arteriosus. *Circulation* 24:1235, 1961.
72. Kimbiris, D., et al. Coronary artery-coronary sinus fistula. *Am. J. Cardiol.* 26:532, 1970.
73. Koops, B., et al. Congenital coronary artery anomalies. *J.A.M.A.* 226:1425, 1973.
74. Kubota, K., et al. Echocardiographic follow-up of mitral valve prolapse associated with secundum atrial septal defect after its surgical repair. *J. Cardiography* 9:123, 1979.
75. Lees, M. H., and Dotter, C. T. Bronchial circulation in severe multiple peripheral pulmonary artery stenosis. *Circulation* 31:759, 1965.
76. Liedtke, A. J., and Gault, J. H. Systolic click syndrome. *Circulation* 58:453, 1973.
77. Lindgren, K. M., and Epstein, S. E. Idiopathic hypertrophic subaortic stenosis with and without mitral regurgitation. *Br. Heart J.* 34:191, 1972.
78. Lipp, H., et al. Intermittent pansystolic murmur and presumed mitral regurgitation after acute myocardial infarction. *Am. J. Cardiol.* 30:690, 1972.
79. Malcolm, A. D., et al. Clinical features and investigative findings in presence of mitral leaflet prolapse. Study of 85 consecutive patients. *Br. Heart J.* 38:244, 1976.
80. Maranhao, V., et al. Prolapse of the tricuspid leaflets in the systolic murmur-click syndrome. *Cath. Cardiovasc. Diagn.* 1:81, 1975.
81. Marchand, P., et al. Mitral regurgitation with rupture of normal chordae tendineae. *Br. Heart J.* 28:746, 1966.
82. Markiewicz, W., et al. Changing hemodynamics in patients with papillary muscle dysfunction. *Br. Heart J.* 37:445, 1975.
83. Mason, D. T., and Braunwald, E. The effects of nitroglycerin and amyl nitrite on arteriolar and venous tone in the human forearm. *Circulation* 32:755, 1965.
84. Matsue, T., et al. Anterior mitral leaflet prolapse with mitral opening snap: Report of a surgical case. *J. Cardiography* 7:243, 1977.
85. Matsuhisa, M., et al. Midsystolic click and late systolic murmur during inspiration (cardio-pulmonary murmur) in congenital absence of the pericardium or open heart surgical case. *J. Cardiography* 11:1009, 1981.
86. McAllister, R. G., Jr., Friesinger, G. C., and Sinclair-Smith, B. C. Tricuspid regurgitation following inferior myocardial infarction. *Arch. Intern. Med.* 95:99, 1976.
87. McCraw, D. B., et al. Response of heart murmur intensity to isometric (handgrip) exercise. *Br. Heart J.* 34:605, 1972.
88. McDonald, A., et al. Association of prolapse of posterior cusp of mitral valve and atrial septal defect. *Br. Heart J.* 33:383, 1971.
89. Merendino, K. A., and Hessel, E. A. The "murmur on top of the head" in acquired mitral insufficiency. *J.A.M.A.* 199:142, 1967.
90. Mittal, A. K., et al. Combined papillary muscle and left ventricular wall dysfunction as a cause of mitral regurgitation. *Circulation* 44:174, 1971.
91. Morgan, J., et al. Anomalies of the aorta and pulmonary arteries complicating ventricular septal defect. *Br. Heart J.* 24:279, 1962.
92. Morgan, J. R., and Forker, A. D. Isolated tricuspid insufficiency. *Circulation* 43:559, 1971.
93. Morgan, J. R., et al. Coronary arterial fistulas. *Am. J. Cardiol.* 30:433, 1972.
94. Morgan, J. R., Rogers, A. K., and Fosburg, R. G. Ruptured aneurysms of the sinus of Valsalva. *Chest* 61:640, 1972.
95. Morrow, A. G., Greenfield, L. J., and Braunwald, E. Congenital aortopulmonary septal defect. *Circulation* 25:463, 1962.
96. Moss, A. J., Emmanouilides, G., and Duffie, E. R., Jr. Closure of the ductus arteriosus in the newborn infant. *Pediatrics* 32:25, 1963.
97. Muraki, H., and Uozumi, Z. A case of congenital fistula of right coronary artery to left ventricle. *Cardiovasc. Sound Bull.* 5:159, 1975.
98. Nakano, T., et al. An autopsy case of tricuspid valve prolapse with special reference to the phonocardiographic and echocardiographic findings. *J. Cardiography* 9:133, 1979.
99. Nichimura, M., et al. Loud holodiastolic murmur in patent ductus arteriosus: A case report. *J. Cardiography* 6:419, 1976.

100. Nishiya, Y., et al. Mitral valve prolapse in atrial septal defect. *J. Cardiography* 10:33, 1980.
101. Ongley, P. A., et al. Continuous murmurs in tetralogy of Fallot and pulmonary atresia with ventricular septal defect. *Am. J. Cardiol.* 18:821, 1966.
102. Osterberger, L. E., et al. Functional mitral stenosis in patients with massive mitral annular calcification. *Circulation* 64:472, 1981.
103. Phornphutkul, C., et al. Cardiac manifestations of Marfan syndrome in infancy and childhood. *Circulation* 45:596, 1973.
104. Pombo, E., Pilapil, V. R., and Lehan, P. H. Aneurysm of the membranous ventricular septum. *Am. Heart J.* 79:188, 1970.
105. Procacci, P. M., et al. Prevalence of clinical mitral-valve prolapse in 1169 young women. *N. Engl. J. Med.* 294:1086, 1976.
106. Ranganathan, N., et al. Morphology of the human mitral valve. *Circulation* 41:459, 1970.
107. Read, R. C., Thai, A. P., and Wendt, V. S. Symptomatic valvular myxomatous transformation (the floppy valve syndrome). *Circulation* 32:897, 1965.
107A. Rivero-Carvallo, J. M. Signo para el diagnostico de las insuffiencias tricuspidias. *Arch. Inst. Cardiol. Mexico* 16:531, 1946.
108. Roberts, W. C. Anomalous left ventricular band. *Am. J. Cardiol.* 23:735, 1969.
109. Roberts, W. C., and Perloff, J. K. Mitral valvular disease. *Ann. Intern. Med.* 77:939, 1972.
110. Robertson, W. S., and Tavel, M. E. Mid-systolic sound associated with aortic insufficiency and bisferiens pulse. *Chest* 83:141, 1983.
111. Ronan, J. A., Jr., Waters, T. J., and Escorcia, E. Effect of simple bedside maneuvers on the isolated systolic click. *Circulation* (Suppl. II) 43:105, 1971.
112. Rotem, C. E., and Hultgren, H. N. Corrected transposition of the great vessels without associated defects. *Am. Heart J.* 70:305, 1965.
113. Sakamoto, T., et al. Clinical, electro- phono- mechano-, and echocardiographic observations of "click syndrome." *Cardiovasc. Sound Bull.* 4:507, 1974.
114. Sakamoto, T., et al. Atypical response of intermittent continuous murmur of patent ductus arteriosus to vasoactive agents, with particular reference to the external and intracardiac phonocardiography. *Jap. Heart J.* 8:318, 1967.
115. Salisbury, P. F., Cross, C. E., and Rieben, P. A. Chordae tendineae tension. *Am. J. Physiol.* 205:385, 1963.
116. Salomon, J., Augen, M., and Levy, M. J. Secundum type atrial septal defect with cleft mitral valve. *Chest* 58:540, 1970.
117. Sanders, C. A., et al. Severe mitral regurgitation secondary to ruptured chordae tendineae. *Circulation* 31:506, 1965.
118. Sasahara, A. A., et al. Ventricular septal defect with patent ductus arteriosus. *Circulation* 22:254, 1960.
119. Scampardonis, G., et al. Left ventricular abnormalities in prolapsed mitral leaflet syndrome. *Circulation* 48:287, 1973.
120. Schlesinger, Z., et al. An unusual form of mitral valve insufficiency simulating aortic stenosis. *Chest* 58:385, 1970.
121. Schreiber, T. L., Feigenbaum, H., and Weyman, A. E. Effect of atrial septal defect repair on left ventricular geometry and degree of mitral valve prolapse. *Circulation* 61:888, 1980.
122. Schrire, V., et al. Silent mitral incompetence. *Am. Heart J.* 61:723, 1961.
123. Scott, J. T., and Murphy, E. A. Mammary souffle of pregnancy. *Circulation* 18:1038, 1958.
124. Segal, B. L., Likoff, W., and Novack, P. Rupture of a sinus of Valsalva Aneurysm. *Am. J. Cardiol.* 12:544, 1963.
125. Shapiro, H. A., and Weiss, D. R. Mitral insufficiency due to ruptured chordae tendineae simulating aortic stenosis. *N. Engl. J. Med.* 261:272, 1959.
126. Shapiro, M. J. Coarctation of the abdominal aorta. *Am. J. Cardiol.* 4:547, 1959.
127. Shapiro, W. Unusual experiences with precordial continuous murmurs. *Am. J. Cardiol.* 7:511, 1961.
128. Shapiro, W., Said, S. I., and Nova, P. L. Intermittent disappearance of the murmur of patent ductus arteriosus. *Circulation* 22:226, 1960.
129. Sheikh, M. U., and Ali, N. Systolic honk in heart failure: Its origin and mechanism of production. *Clin. Cardiol.* 2:52, 1979.
130. Sherman, E. B., et al. Myxomatous transformation of the mitral valve producing insufficiency. *Am. J. Dis. Child.* 119:171, 1970.

131. Sherman, W. T., Ferrer, I., and Harvey, R. M. Competence of the tricuspid valve in pulmonary heart disease (cor pulmonale). *Circulation* 31:517, 1965.
132. Shimada, E., et al. Tricuspid valve prolapse associated with cor pulmonale: Report of 2 cases. *J. Cardiography* 10:163, 1980.
133. Chirato, C., and Ishikawa, K. Newly developed systolic murmur in patients with a transvenous pacemaker. *Am. Heart J.* 99:722, 1980.
134. Sleeper, J. C., Orgain, E. S., and McIntosh, H. D. Mitral insufficiency simulating aortic stenosis. *Circulation* 26:428, 1962.
135. Sloman, G., et al. Prolapse of the posterior leaflet of the mitral valve. *Isr. J. Med. Sci.* 5:727, 1969.
136. Sonotani, N., et al. A case of right coronary artery fistula to the left ventricle. *J. Cardiography* 6:573, 1976.
137. Steinfeld, L., Dimich, I., and Park, S. C. The late systolic murmur of rheumatic mitral regurgitation (MR). *Circulation* 44:106, 1971.
138. Steinfeld, L., et al. Clinical diagnosis of isolated subpulmonic (supracristal) ventricular septal defect. *Am. J. Cardiol.* 30:19, 1972.
139. Strano, A., DiRenzi, L., and Pennetti, V. On the peripheral venous murmurs of the circulatory hyperkinetic syndrome. *Angiology* 17:213, 1966.
140. Tabatznik, B., Randall, T. W., and Hersch, C. The mammary souffle of pregnancy and lactation. *Circulation* 22:1069, 1960.
141. Takahashi, M., et al. A case of ruptured aneurysm of Valsalva sinus, especially change in diastolic murmur. *J. Cardiography* 6:193, 1976.
142. Tanaka, M., et al. Acoustic characteristics and genesis of the heart murmur in classic form of cor triatriatum. *Cardiovasc. Sound Bull.* 4:457, 1974.
142A. Tashima, C. K. Femoral venous hum. *N.Y. State J. Med.* 65:2797, 1965.
143. Tei, C., Shah, P. M., and Tanaka, H. Phonographic-echographic documentation of systolic honk in tricuspid prolapse. *Am. Heart J.* 2:294, 1982.
144. Thapar, M. K., et al. Changing murmur of patent ductus arteriosus. *J. Pediatr.* 92:939, 1978.
145. Upshaw, C. B. Precordial honk due to tricuspid regurgitation. *Am. J. Cardiol.* 35:85, 1975.
146. Van der Hauwaert, L., and Nadas, A. S. Auscultatory findings in patients with a small ventricular septal defect. *Circulation* 23:886, 1961.
146A. Venkataraman, K., et al. Musical murmurs: An echo-phonocardiographic study. *Am. J. Cardiol.* 41:952, 1978.
147. Verani, M. S., Carroll, R. J., and Falsetti, H. Mitral valve prolapse in coronary artery disease. *Am. J. Cardiol.* 37:1, 1976.
148. Vogelpoel, L., et al. The atypical systolic murmur of minute ventricular septal defect and its recognition by amyl nitrite and phenylephrine. *Am. Heart J.* 62:101, 1961.
149. Vogelpoel, L., et al. Variations in the response of the systolic murmur to vasoactive drugs in ventricular septal defect, with special reference to the paradoxical response in large defects with pulmonary hypertension. *Am. Heart J.* 64:169, 1962.
150. Wald, S., et al. Anomalous origin of the right coronary artery from the pulmonary artery. *Am. J. Cardiol.* 27:677, 1971.
151. Wann, L. S., et al. Prevalence of mitral prolapse by two dimensional echocardiography in healthy young women. *Br. Heart J.* 39:334, 1983.
152. Wells, B. G., and Hurt, R. L. Congenital arteriovenous fistula of the internal mammary vessels. *Br. Heart J.* 19:135, 1957.
153. Willius, F. A., and Keys, T. E. *Cardiac Classics.* St. Louis: Mosby, 1941. P. 623–638.
154. Yanagihara, K., et al. Phonocardiographic features of anomalous left coronary artery originating from the pulmonary artery: Report of two cases. *J. Cardiography* 8:147, 1978.

15. *Diastolic Murmurs*

DIASTOLIC ATRIOVENTRICULAR VALVE MURMURS

Mitral Stenosis Murmurs

Timing and Shape

1. When in the cycle does the diastolic murmur of mitral stenosis (MS) begin? How does it relate to the S_2?

   ANS.: It begins just after the opening snap (OS). This means that there must be a pause between the A_2 and the diastolic murmur. This pause is due to isovolumic relaxation of the left ventricle (LV).

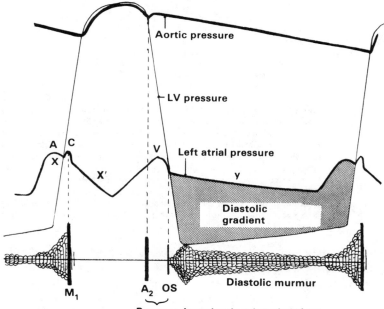

There should be no mitral murmurs between the A_2 and the OS because this is isovolumic relaxation time. Note the slow Y descent of the left atrium due to the difficulty in emptying the left atrium through the stenotic valve. This accounts for the pressure gradient and murmur, both of which are decrescendo except for the very beginning and end.

   * Note: There often seems to be a slight pause between the OS and the diastolic murmur of MS when listening with the stethoscope. Although inflow into the LV begins as soon as the mitral valve opens, the **gradient** and flow increase for a short period because the LV is still

* Material marked with an asterisk is for reference and for advanced students in cardiology.
Boldface type indicates that the term is defined in the Glossary.

rapidly expanding. This increase in gradient often shows on a phonocardiogram as a short, early crescendo-decrescendo. We hear the OS and then the peak of the crescendo as if there were a pause between the OS and the beginning of the murmur.

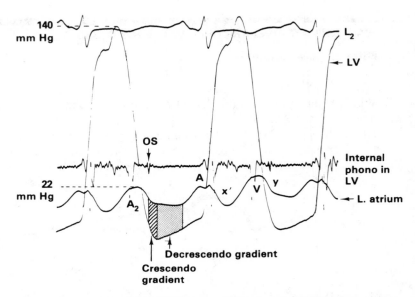

Phonocardiogram, left atrial and LV pressure tracings from a slightly hypertensive 50-year-old man with a mitral valve that was not calcified, but which barely admitted the surgeon's finger. These tracings were taken with equisensitive micromanometers at the tips of the catheters to eliminate any time delays due to tubing. The diastolic murmur (not shown here) follows the gradient and therefore should have a short early crescendo before the decrescendo. This gives a rhythm of "one---two-du huuu" to the heart sounds, opening snap and murmur. The distance between the "two" and the "du" is the time for isovolumic relaxation. The distance between the "du" and the "huuu" is the time to the peak of the early crescendo. The long 2–OS interval of about 90 msec (0.09 sec) in this patient is probably due to his hypertension (see p. 234 for explanation).

2. How do the rate and quantity of early rapid diastolic filling in moderate to severe MS differ from that in normal hearts?

   ANS.: Although there is more rapid filling in early than in later diastole even in significant MS, the rate of filling is often slower than normal and the quantity is less than normal.

   *Note: An apex cardiogram may show that the quantity of LV filling during the early filling phase is usually less than normal in MS because the early filling phase either has a slower slope than normal or is shorter than normal.

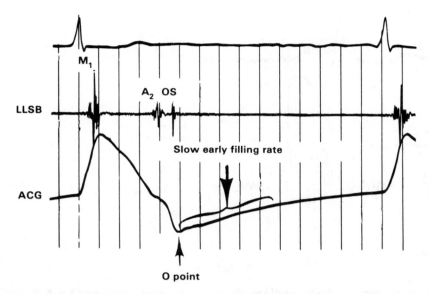

On an apex cardiogram (ACG), the mitral valve opens at the 0 point and is followed by an early, steep rapid filling wave. In MS, the rapid early filling wave is usually replaced by a slowly rising wave. Occasionally, a steep, early rapid filling rise is present, but it is shorter than normal. Note that the 0 point here follows the OS. The relation between the OS and the 0 point depends on the time constant of the pulse unit; the shorter the time constant, the earlier the 0 point. That this is from a patient with severe MS is shown by the lateness of the M_1 on the upstroke of the apex cardiogram, and because with the A_2–OS interval about 70 msec and the Q–M_1 interval 110 msec, the Q–1 minus 2–OS = 40 msec, which signifies severe MS (see p. 241).

3. What is the typical shape of the diastolic murmur of MS on auscultation? Why?
   ANS.: After a very short crescendo, there is a decrescendo rumble that ends with a late crescendo to the M_1. The decrescendo reflects the decrescendo gradient and flow between the left atrium and the LV. The late crescendo has a more complicated explanation (see following section).

The Crescendo Murmur to the M_1 in Mitral Stenosis (the "Presystolic" Murmur)

1. What is the appearance of a murmur that is produced by atrial contraction forcing blood through a stenotic mitral valve?
   ANS.: It should follow the curve of atrial pressure rise and fall—i.e., it should be crescendo–decrescendo.
2. What is the actual shape of the diastolic murmur produced by atrial contraction at the end of diastole in MS?
   ANS.: It is crescendo to the first sound. This murmur is often called "late diastolic" or "presystolic."
3. Does the presystolic crescendo murmur of MS extend to the M_1?
   ANS.: Yes.

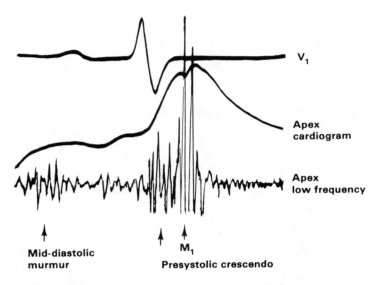

V_1

Apex
cardiogram

Apex
low frequency

Mid-diastolic
murmur

M_1

Presystolic crescendo

The "presystolic" murmur in this 45-year-old woman with moderately severe MS begins with the onset of ventricular contraction, as shown by the simultaneous apex cardiogram tracing taken at very fast speed. However, blood is still flowing from the left atrium to the LV until mitral valve closure (M_1). Therefore, cardiologists prefer to consider this period as part of diastole.

4. What may we call the time between ventricular contraction and closure of the mitral valve or M_1?

ANS.: The preisovolumic contraction period.

   Note: This period is prolonged in MS because both the high left atrial pressure and the stiffness of the mitral valve have to be overcome before the mitral valve can be closed.

5. If the presystolic crescendo murmur actually occurs during LV contraction, i.e., during the preisovolumic LV contraction period, is it really presystolic?

ANS.: If systole is defined as beginning with ventricular contraction (physiologists's systole), then only the first part of the murmur in sinus rhythm is presystolic because it begins at the time of peak atrial contraction before the ventricle contracts. Most of the murmur, however, is actually an early systolic murmur, because it occurs during the preisovolumic contraction period of LV contraction. This is apparent from the observation that most of the crescendo murmur to the M_1 occurs after the QRS. Also, if LV pressure or apex cardiograms are taken simultaneously with phonocardiograms, most of the murmur occurs with the onset of the LV pressure rise.

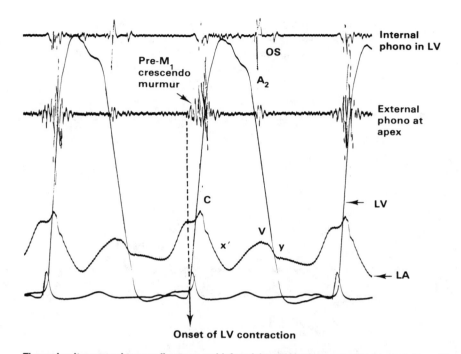

Pre-M₁ crescendo murmur (in figure)

OS (in figure)

A₂ (in figure)

C (in figure)

x′ (in figure)

V (in figure)

y (in figure)

Internal phono in LV (in figure)

External phono at apex (in figure)

LV (in figure)

LA (in figure)

Onset of LV contraction

These simultaneous phonocardiograms and left atrial and LV pressure tracings were taken with catheter-tip micromanometer pressure transducers to eliminate any time delays due to tubing. Note that the "presystolic" crescendo of the MS murmur occurs during ventricular systole. This is from a 43-year-old man, mildly symptomatic, with severe MS, but only a small amount of calcium in his mitral valve. His left atrial A wave was 32 mm Hg, but his cardiac index was 2.7, which is low-normal. He had a grade 3/6 diastolic rumble at the apex, of which only the presystolic component is seen well in these phonocardiograms.

However, because the auscultator's systole begins with the S_1, it is not necessary to change the traditional terminology of *presystolic* murmur. By a *presystolic* murmur, then, the auscultator means "immediately before the first heart sound."

* *Note:* Late diastolic mitral regurgitation (MR) has been proposed as the cause of the presystolic murmur [95]. But this is impossible because left atrial pressure is higher than LV pressure during much of preisovolumic LV contraction [89].

* 6. If blood is entering the LV during early (preisovolumic) ventricular contraction, how can a murmur become gradually louder (crescendo) when the pressure gradient, as well as the volume of the flow across the orifice, is being rapidly reduced?

ANS.: As the mitral orifice is reduced by LV contraction, the velocity of flow increases as long as the pressure is higher in the left atrium than in the LV [17]. Several studies have shown that even the slightest closing motion of a stenotic mitral valve during diastole can produce a diastolic murmur [30, 90].

Because the intensity of a sound is proportional to the fourth power of its velocity, a small change in blood velocity may cause marked changes in the intensity of a murmur. The increase in the loudness of a murmur as the mitral valve is closed by ventricular contraction can be compared to the effect of very rapid narrowing of the nozzle of a hose, whereas the decreasing gradient is analogous to turning the tap off.

Note: a) Angiograms or echocardiograms of the LV, together with simultaneous phonocardiograms, show that the valve is moving into a closed position at the time of the presystolic murmur [91].

b) Doppler studies in MS have shown a steady increase in velocity of flow during the QRS complex, reaching a peak 80–100 msec after the onset of the QRS [18].

*7. Is atrial contraction required to produce the presystolic crescendo murmur?

ANS.: No. In atrial fibrillation the late crescendo occurs during short diastoles [17, 91].

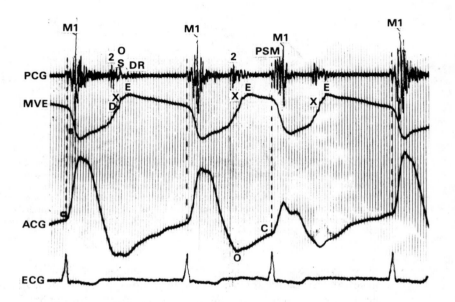

Presystolic murmur in a patient with mitral stenosis and atrial fibrillation. The best presystolic crescendo to the M_1, occurring at the end of a short diastole, begins with the start of mitral valve closure on the mitral valve "gated" echocardiogram (MVE) and with the start of LV contraction, point C of the apex cardiogram (ACG). The presystolic murmur occurs during preisovolumic LV contraction. (From P. Toutouzas et al. Mechanism of diastolic rumble and presystolic murmur in mitral stenosis. *Br. Heart J.* 36:1096, 1974.)

Note: The presystolic crescendo occurs only during short diastoles in atrial fibrillation because only during short diastoles is the left atrial pressure high enough to maintain high-velocity flow during preisovolumic ventricular contraction. It requires a gradient of more than 10 mm Hg at the onset of LV contraction to create a crescendo murmur to the M_1 [17].

This also explains why atrial contraction helps to produce the pre-M_1 crescendo. Atrial contraction can elevate left atrial pressure sufficiently to create the necessary increased velocity of forward flow as the mitral valve orifice is being reduced by ventricular contraction.

*8. What does the presence of a crescendo murmur to the M_1 tell you about the mitral valve in MS?

ANS.: The valve must be sufficiently flexible to change the size of the orifice, i.e., it must not be rigidly calcified (although it may be too fibrosed or calcified for a valvotomy) [50].

Note: Important MR complicating MS can eliminate this pre-M_1 accentuation even in sinus rhythm [99]. The loss of presystolic accentuation may be due to a poorly contracting left atrium secondary to both the dilatation and the greater rheumatic damage of the atrium associated with the combined lesion.

Pitch and Quality

1. Is the MS diastolic murmur high or low in pitch? Why?

ANS.: Low, because a murmur that is produced more by flow than by gradient produces low frequencies. The gradient across the mitral valve in diastole is relatively low as gradients go, no matter how severe the stenosis is; i.e., in the usual case of severe MS, the maximum diastolic gradient is about 30 mm Hg at the beginning of diastole and about 10 mm Hg at the end. In aortic or pulmonary stenosis peak systolic gradients with moderate to severe obstructions during systole are at least 50 mm Hg and may exceed 100 mm Hg.

2. What are some of the descriptions of the MS diastolic murmur that help to symbolize the low frequencies?

ANS.: a) Rumbling.
b) Like distant thunder.
c) Like a ball rolling down a bowling alley.
d) Blubbering (Austin Flint used this word in 1884).

Note: The early rumble followed by a late crescendo to a loud M_1 may be likened to the growl and bark of a dog.

3. Under what circumstances are high frequencies present in a mitral diastolic murmur?

ANS.: High frequencies are present if the velocity of flow across the orifice is increased due to a good circulation time, a strong LV expansion, a strong atrial contraction, or MR.

*Note: The crescendo to the M_1 is usually rich in high frequencies [54]. Therefore, if a wide, rough S_1 is confused with a presystolic crescendo, firm pressure with the diaphragm will bring out the high-pitched crescendo components leading to the M_1. A rough S_1, on the other hand, will separate into split sound components.

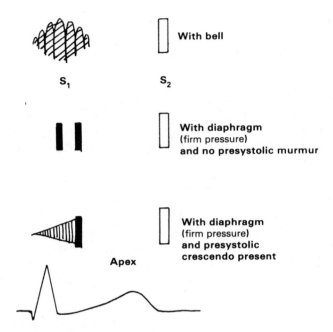

With bell

S_1 S_2

With diaphragm
(firm pressure)
and no presystolic murmur

With diaphragm
(firm pressure)
and presystolic
crescendo present

Apex

A wide, rough first sound due to many low-frequency components can be differentiated from a presystolic murmur of MS plus M_1 by eliminating the low frequencies as much as possible with firm pressure.

Factors That Increase Loudness of Mitral Stenosis Murmurs

1. Besides pushing the stethoscope farther from the heart, why does the MS murmur become softer on inspiration?

   ANS.: Blood is sequestered in the lungs and therefore withheld from the left side of the heart during inspiration. (It is useful to think of the lungs as a sponge that expels its blood into the left atrium during the squeezing effect of expiration and fills with blood from the RV during inspiration.)

2. What factors increase the flow across a moderate to severely obstructed mitral valve at rest, thereby increasing the loudness of the murmur?

   ANS.: a) A high left atrial pressure together with the powerful forces of a healthy LV pull the blood into the LV. (A very dilated left atrium due to severe rheumatic damage can lower the left atrial pressure even with severe MS; this serves to decrease the loudness of the murmur.)

   b) Concomitant MR also increases the loudness of the murmur.

3. What anatomical conditions besides a thin chest wall may bring the LV close to the stethoscope?

   ANS.: a) Anything that enlarges the LV such as MR, aortic regurgitation (AR), or a **cardiomyopathy**.

   Note: A severe cardiomyopathy is least likely to make the mitral diastolic murmur loud because forward flow is poor and because the flow would also be reduced by the decreased diastolic "suction" of a poorly functioning LV.

   b) A large left atrium that pushes the ventricle closer to the chest wall.

   * *Note:* a) Concomitant MR makes the MS murmur louder most effectively because MR not only makes the LV larger and brings the

apex closer to the stethoscope but also elevates the V wave of the left atrial pressure curve during systole. Therefore, there is more pressure forcing blood through the mitral valve in diastole.

b) A grade 4/6 (i.e., with a thrill) mitral diastolic murmur means that there is at least moderate stenosis (in the absence of MR). If, however, it radiates to the base (very unusual), it almost always signifies severe MS. (It also denies systemic levels of pulmonary hypertension [100].)

4. How can you bring out a mitral diastolic murmur that is almost inaudible?

ANS.: a) Bring the LV closer to the stethoscope by turning the patient into the **left lateral decubitus position** and listen during end-expiration over the site where your finger feels the apex beat.

b) Use very light pressure with the largest bell available that will allow a good air seal. Firm pressure can completely obliterate the low frequencies of a faint rumble.

c) Increase the flow across the mitral valve.

5. How can you increase the flow across the mitral valve?

ANS.: a) Have the patient cough a few times, or listen after a **Valsalva** strain during the release phase. In the post-Valsalva release phase, the obstructed vena caval venous flow floods the lungs and pours into the left atrium a few seconds later. There is a more pronounced post-Valsalva rise of pressure in the left atrium in MS than in the normal heart [9].

b) If the heart rate is fast, listen after digitalis or a beta blocker has slowed the rate and increased the volume of diastolic flow into the LV. (Digitalis may also increase the force of LV expansion or "suction.")

c) Listen when the patient is squatting or during a handgrip maneuver. Cardiac output is increased for a few beats after squatting. During handgrip the mitral diastolic gradient has been shown to increase as a result of both the increase in cardiac output and the increase in heart rate [26].

d) Ask the patient to exercise. (Merely turning the patient into the left lateral decubitus position may be sufficient, and you should listen immediately, before the effect of the exertion is lost.) The maximum effective duration for the supine straight leg-raising exercise beyond which there is probably not much increase in cardiac output is, at the most, 3 minutes, i.e., physiologists consider 3 minutes of moderate exercise sufficient to reach a steady state. The more vigorous the exercise, the longer it takes to reach a steady state.

e) Administer amyl nitrite. See page 327 for an explanation of how amyl nitrite increases venous return and cardiac output.

Factors that Make the Mitral Stenosis Murmur Softer

1. What can make MS diastolic murmurs soft besides mild MS, obesity, or emphysema?

ANS.: a) Low flow.

b) A large right ventricle (RV) pushing the LV posteriorly. The RV is an anterior chamber, and if it enlarges, as it often does in MS, it pushes the LV away from the anterior chest wall.

*c) A coincidental atrial septal defect (ASD) [35].

2. What besides the mitral obstruction itself can cause a low flow in MS?

ANS.: a) Severe pulmonary hypertension. This causes an additional obstruction to flow for which RV hypertrophy and a rise in RV pressure do not compensate completely.

b) Other valves causing obstruction, i.e., tricuspid or aortic stenosis.

c) A cardiomyopathy, usually on either a rheumatic or a coronary basis.

d) Atrial fibrillation. Atrial fibrillation often causes too fast a ventricular rate for good diastolic flow through the mitral obstruction, but even when the heart rates are slow, the loss of atrial contraction reduces flow. It has been shown that a well-placed atrial contraction can increase cardiac output by about 25 percent in significant MS [41].

Note: In atrial fibrillation, the murmur of MS may disappear at the end of a long diastole for two opposite reasons:

a) There may be such *mild* MS that the gradient disappears by the end of diastole.

b) There may be such *severe* MS that although the gradient is still high at the end of a long diastole, the flow is too low to permit a murmur to be heard. If the diastolic murmur is heard at the end of a long diastole, both a high gradient and a fair flow are likely to be present.

3. What is peculiar about the site of some soft MS murmurs that may make them difficult to hear?

ANS.: They may occasionally be so localized that the murmur may disappear a few millimeters away from the exact area. You should palpate the apex beat with the patient in the left lateral decubitus position and place the stethoscope bell exactly at the area of the apex beat.

*4. What anatomical factors have been thought to correlate with completely silent MS, i.e., no apical diastolic rumble at any time even when the patient is not in failure?

ANS.: Any one or a combination of the following:

a) An almost completely immobile mitral valve, usually with adhesions, thickening, and shortening of the chordae that cause a second area of stenosis below the valve [93].

b) A posteromedially deviated mitral valve orifice [93].

c) A large left atrial thrombus deviating the stream away from the apex [73, 93].

d) A large ASD (Lutembacher's syndrome) [35].

Note: If there is a large ASD, left atrial blood will cross the ASD rather than the obstructed mitral valve, thus diminishing the MS murmur.

Etiology and Differential Diagnosis

1. What is the usual etiology of MS?

ANS.: Rheumatic fever, which causes a chronic process of valvular fibrosis, fusion, and calcification, together with shortened, thickened chordae tendineae.

*2. What are some unusual causes of MS?

ANS.: a) A left atrial myxoma.

Note: A left atrial myxoma may have a grade 4/6 diastolic murmur, i.e., with a thrill. If a piece of the myxoma embolizes, the murmur may disappear.

b) Congenital MS. Ninety percent of such patients die by age 2 if not treated surgically. Even the exceptional patients who live until adolescence are in heart failure from infancy [84]. In one case report the patient had only fatigue until age 18, probably because an anomalous pulmonary venous connection prevented high left atrial pressures [1].

   Note: The leaflets in one form of congenital MS, known as a "parachute" mitral valve (a single papillary muscle sending chordae to fused, thickened, and fibrosed leaflets), may function normally or even be purely regurgitant [36].

c) A calcified bacterial vegetation, as large as 2 cm in diameter, obstructed the mitral valve in a patient who had only MR prior to the infective endocarditis [6].

   Note: Verrucous endocarditis (Libman-Sacks valvulitis of disseminated lupus) does not usually cause enough mitral obstruction to produce even a diastolic murmur [48].

d) Mitral ring constriction due to localized constrictive pericarditis of the atrioventricular ring (very rare).

3. What may imitate the MS diastolic murmur despite no significant diastolic gradient across the mitral valve?

   ANS.: a) A diastolic flow murmur due to excessive flow across the mitral valve, as in severe MR or **ventricular septal defect** (VSD).

   b) The Austin Flint murmur.

   c) Hypertrophic subaortic stenosis (HSS). The reason is unknown [79].

   *d) A diastolic murmur across a porcine valve may be due to deflection of the blood flow through the valve toward the septum or posterior ventricular wall rather than toward the apex. It can be heard in about half the patients with normally functioning porcine valves [55A]. Fluttering of the respective walls can be seen on echocardiography [33].

4. What auscultatory clues indicate that a mitral diastolic rumble may not be due to true MS?

   ANS.: MS is not likely if

   a) An S_3 precedes a short murmur. Only rarely does a true S_3 precede any MS murmur [34A].

   b) There is no good presystolic crescendo.

   c) There is no loud S_1 or opening snap.

The Austin Flint Murmur Versus the Mitral Stenosis Murmur

1. What is the Austin Flint murmur?

   ANS.: It is an apical diastolic rumble imitating the murmur of organic MS but is due to an AR stream that prevents the mitral valve from opening fully.

   *Note: Right-sided Austin Flint murmurs due to pulmonary regurgitation secondary to pulmonary hypertension have been recorded [38]. They have inspiratory and presystolic accentuation [45].

2. What is the most plausible theory explaining the mechanical cause of the Austin Flint murmur?

   ANS.: The aortic regurgitant stream may impinge on the undersurface of the anterior leaflet of the mitral valve and push it up, creating a relative MS. Support for this theory is found in the following facts:

a) A yellow plaque has been seen on the septal surface of the anterior mitral leaflet of some patients with the Austin Flint murmur. This may be a jet lesion [22A, 61, 92].

b) When an Austin Flint murmur is present, the amplitude of opening of the mitral anterior leaflet is reduced on echocardiograms.

   *Note: Echocardiograms often show fluttering of the anterior mitral leaflet in patients with Austin Flint murmurs. This was once thought to be the cause of the murmur, but some patients with the vibrating leaflets have no Austin Flint murmur, and some with the Austin Flint murmur have no leaflet vibrations.

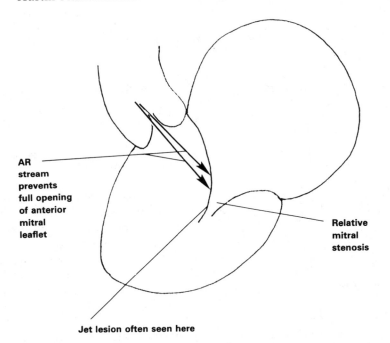

AR
stream
prevents
full opening
of anterior
mitral
leaflet

Relative
mitral
stenosis

Jet lesion often seen here

The aortic regurgitant stream holds the anterior leaflet up in a semi-closed position. This accounts for the mitral diastolic rumble mimicking mitral stenosis and for the attenuated opening snap in patients with both mitral stenosis and aortic regurgitation.

*3. What suggests that the apical diastolic murmur in severe AR is at least sometimes due to transmission of the low-frequency components of the AR murmur to the apex?

ANS.: a) It sometimes starts with the S_2, i.e., before the mitral valve has had a chance to open.

b) If the AR is severe, its murmur is rich in low frequencies, which can be transmitted downstream to the apex. (The low-frequency components of murmurs tend to be best transmitted downstream.)

*4. What was Austin's explanation for the apical diastolic rumble in AR? Why is this theory untenable?

ANS.: The increased ventricular volume due to double filling (from both the normal mitral flow and AR flow) floats the mitral valves upward into the nearly closed position, producing a relative MS [27]. However, this theory requires the LV pressure to become higher than the left atrial pressure, in which case the valves would close completely, as in sudden, severe AR (see p. 388). The Austin Flint murmur would then disappear [70]. Austin Flint's theory also requires the development of a high LV pressure early in diastole, and this does not occur.

*5. How did Austin Flint describe the quality and position of this murmur in diastole? Why?

ANS.: He described it as a "blubbering presystolic murmur." The timing and quality sounded to him exactly the same as the murmur of MS. Since he thought that the atrium contracted just after the early filling phase, he considered almost all of diastole to be "presystolic" except for this very early filling phase. He recommended that all MS diastolic murmurs also be called presystolic [26A].

Note: a) In one study, a definite presystolic accentuation of the Flint murmur was not demonstrable in any patient in an entire series of 17 patients [61]. In another study, a presystolic component was completely absent in 2 of 15 patients with an Austin Flint murmur [92]. The pre-M_1 accentuation of the Austin Flint murmur, even when present, is often a subtle finding and does not have marked crescendo to the S_1 heard in a patient with MS [92].

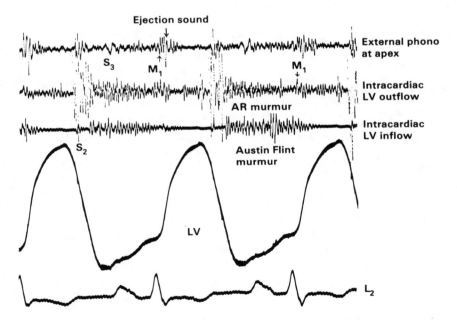

Phonocardiograms and LV pressure tracing from a 45-year-old man with marked orthopnea who had an Austin Flint murmur due to severe AR resulting from a previous infective endocarditis. Note that the diastolic rumble at the apex begins even before the S_3 was recorded externally. Note also the absence of a presystolic crescendo and the soft M_1.

b) In severe AR, there is often a reversal of the pressure gradient across the mitral valve in late diastole [29]. Because angiograms in such patients have shown late diastolic MR, the presystolic component of the Austin Flint murmur in severe AR has been said to be due to this late diastolic mitral regurgitation [52]. Intracardiac phonocardiograms, however, have shown that although a reversed gradient can produce a recordable presystolic murmur in the left atrium, this murmur cannot be recorded either on a chest surface or LV inflow tract phonocardiogram.

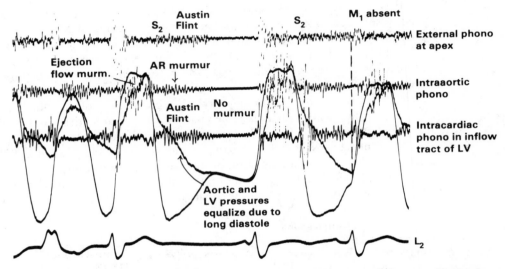

Phonocardiograms, aortic and LV pressure tracings from a 51-year-old man who had severe AR with dyspnea on exertion and paroxysmal nocturnal dyspnea following infective endocarditis two months prior to this tracing. He had a grade 3/6 aortic ejection murmur due to excessive forward flow, a grade 3/6 aortic diastolic blowing murmur at the left sternal border, and a grade 3/6 diastolic rumble (Austin Flint murmur) at the apex. Note the sudden pause (due to sinus suppression secondary to a premature ventricular contraction with retrograde conduction) that allowed the LV pressure to rise as high as aortic pressure. The Austin Flint murmur stopped, even though the LV pressure must have exceeded left atrial pressure; i.e., late MR is not the cause of any part of the Austin Flint murmur. Note also how the amount of AR is limited by the rapid rise of pressure in the LV. This is why, with sudden, severe AR, the diastolic murmur may be short.

6. How can you differentiate an Austin Flint murmur from the murmur of MS by auscultation?

ANS.: a) If there is no OS, the chances that MS is present are diminished. But remember that AR can attenuate or eliminate an OS.

b) If an S_3 is heard, it is more likely to be an Austin Flint murmur. But remember that an S_3 can occasionally introduce an MS murmur [34A].

c) If there is no obvious presystolic crescendo to the S_1 despite short diastoles, it is more likely to be an Austin Flint murmur.

d) Amyl nitrite will produce a louder MS murmur after about 20 sec, whereas an Austin Flint murmur immediately becomes softer or even disappears. The reason for this is that in AR there are two outlets for the blood in the aorta during diastole; one outlet backward into the LV, the other forward into the peripheral arteries. If you lower the resistance in one outlet, blood will tend to flow preferentially toward that outlet. Amyl nitrite lowers peripheral resistance, thus increasing the peripheral runoff and therefore decreasing the amount of AR. (In the presence of severe congestive failure, amyl nitrite may have no effect [78]).

7. When can the detection of an Austin Flint murmur be clinically useful?

ANS.: a) It may be the only auscultatory clue to the presence of at least a moderate degree of AR if there is only a soft AR murmur [64, 67].

*b) It tells you that there is probably a high left atrial mean pressure and a high LV end-diastolic pressure [61, 64].

Mitral Diastolic Flow Murmurs (Inflow Murmurs)

1. What is meant by a mitral diastolic inflow murmur?

ANS: This murmur is a low-pitched rumble heard over the apex area that is produced by a relative MS, i.e., by an excessive flow through a normal mitral valve.

2. List some common causes of excessive flow through a mitral valve that can produce a diastolic flow murmur besides severe MR and hyperkinetic states such as thyrotoxicosis.

ANS.: a) A very slow ventricular rate with a healthy heart, e.g., congenital complete **atrioventricular block** [4, 65].

b) A left-to-right shunt, e.g., a VSD or **persistent ductus arteriosus** with the shunt having a ratio of at least 2:1, i.e., at least twice as much blood flows through the pulmonary artery per minute as through the aorta.

Note: The advantage of hearing a flow murmur in a VSD with findings of pulmonary hypertension is that it is a sign that the condition is operable, i.e., the pulmonary hypetension is not fixed (no pulmonary vascular disease) but is caused instead by an excessive flow into the pulmonary arterioles (hyperkinetic vasospastic pulmonary hypertension).

3. In which way does a mitral diastolic flow murmur differ from the murmur of MS?

ANS.: A flow murmur usually starts with an S_3, is short, and has no late diastolic or presystolic component. (See figure on p. 327.)

* *Note:* An S_3 plus an S_4 close together can mimic a mid-diastolic flow murmur [88].

4. Why does the diastolic flow murmur not start exactly with the onset of opening of the mitral valve?

ANS.: The mitral valve in its immediate opening probably makes too large an orifice for a murmur to be produced. Echocardiograms have shown that immediately after the initial opening movement of the mitral valve, the valve moves rapidly into a semiclosed position, probably as a result of eddy currents. At the time of the S_3, the mitral cusps are moving up and are rapidly becoming more opposed to one another; a murmur then occurs while rapid flow is still continuing for a short time. The murmur is thus probably due to the increasing velocity of flow as a result of a dynamically narrowing mitral orifice, much like the effect of narrowing the nozzle of a hose.

*5. What is meant by a Carey Coombs murmur?

ANS.: It is the diastolic inflow murmur usually ushered in by an S_3, heard in subjects with cardiomegaly and MR due to acute rheumatic fever [15, 16].
Note: Many writers tend to ignore the MR and imply that the inflow murmur is a special type of mitral murmur caused by the valvulitis itself rather than a flow murmur heard commonly in any patient with substantial MR and torrential flow through the valve. Carey Coombs thought that it was due to dilatation of the LV.

TRICUSPID DIASTOLIC FLOW MURMURS

1. What is the site of the tricuspid inflow murmur?
    ANS.: Anywhere over the RV area. This includes all the lower right and left parasternal area as well as the epigastrium. When the RV is very large, the entire left lower chest area can also become the RV area.
2. List the common causes of increased flow through the tricuspid valve.
    ANS.: a) Shunt flows, e.g., ASD and **anomalous pulmonary venous connection** or drainage into a right atrium.
    b) Tricuspid regurgitation (TR).
3. How can a tricuspid inflow murmur be exaggerated besides by exercise or deep inspiration?
    ANS.: a) By holding the legs up or bending the knees toward the chest with the subject supine.
    b) By panting, rapid respirations.
    c) By amyl nitrite inhalation, which opens up arteriovenous communications and constricts veins by means of sympathetic reflexes.
*4. How does an ASD tricuspid diastolic flow murmur differ in timing from a VSD mitral diastolic flow murmur?
    ANS.: In an ASD the murmur starts earlier, at about the time of the opening of the tricuspid valve, and is not preceded by an S_3 [58]. It may occasionally be presystolic as well [25]. In a VSD, it not only starts later but is almost always initiated by an S_3.

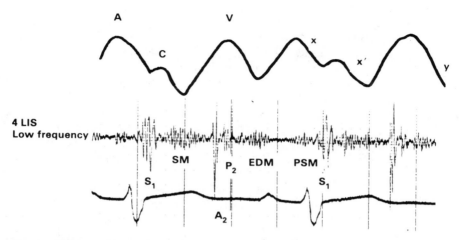

Phonocardiogram and jugular pulse tracing from a teenaged girl with an ostium primum ASD. The presystolic murmur (PSM) is unusual in ASDs, but, when present, is crescendo-decrescendo and not crescendo to the first sound, as in MS. Note that the Y descent in the jugular tracing is almost equal to the combination of X + X' descents. This is due to the high V wave, which results from the addition to the right atrium of blood from some additional source, i.e., not only from the venae cavae but here also from the left atrium and even from the LV because of MR, which is expected with primum defects.

> *Note:* If an ASD has an anomalous pulmonary venous connection with the right atrium, then even when pulmonary hypertension is high enough to markedly decrease the shunt through the ASD, a tricuspid flow murmur may persist, probably because the pulmonary venous pressure remains higher than the right atrial pressure and maintains an increased flow into the right atrium [66].

*5. With what is a tricuspid inflow murmur confused?

ANS.: The murmur of tricuspid stenosis (TS).

> *Note:* In the presence of a normal sinus rhythm, the TS murmur is almost always only presystolic and has many high frequencies in it. The tricuspid inflow murmur usually has only low frequencies and occurs at about the time that an S_3 would occur.

TRICUSPID STENOSIS DIASTOLIC MURMURS

1. Where is the TS murmur heard on the chest wall?

ANS.: In the same place as the tricuspid inflow murmur, i.e., the RV area.

2. How does the TS murmur differ from the MS murmur?

ANS.: a) In sinus rhythm it is only a presystolic murmur but has no presystolic crescendo to the S_1, i.e., the presystolic murmur is nearly always a short crescendo-decrescendo murmur, and it sounds like an S_4 murmur. Only if atrial fibrillation is present is there a delayed early diastolic murmur [23].

> *Note:* In MS a presystolic murmur may also be crescendo-decrescendo if there is a long P-R interval.

b) It always increases with inspiration, often markedly, whereas the MS murmur characteristically decreases with inspiration.

c) The MS murmur is louder in the left lateral decubitus position. The TS murmur is accentuated in the right lateral decubitus position [49].

d) The MS murmur is usually predominantly low-pitched and rumbling; the TS presystolic murmur is often scratchy.

* e) The presystolic TS murmur begins about 60 msec after the onset of the P wave. Because the left atrium contracts later than the right atrium, the MS presystolic murmur begins about 120–200 msec after the P.

* Note: a) Rheumatic TS is probably never present without MS, even though on rare occasions the TS may be the dominant lesion [56]. Therefore, if no MS can be diagnosed, a presystolic murmur at the left sternal border should make you suspect either a right atrial myxoma, an ASD, or carcinoid stiffening of the tricuspid valve [3].

b) One study has shown that presystolic crescendo-decrescendo murmurs with high-pitched components can be recorded in about one-fifth of normal subjects as well as in some patients with ASD, HSS, or a variety of other conditions [43]. Another study showed that such murmurs were present in patients with ischemic heart disease, and they were heard best at the left lower sternal border [72].

3. Does the TS murmur increase with moving inspiration, as when checking for a split S_2, or does it increase with held inspiration?

ANS.: It increases both during moving inspiration and during inspiratory apnea. (An inadvertent Valsalva maneuver during the apnea will make the TS murmur softer.)

* 4. Why does the TS murmur become louder on inspiration?

ANS.: Interestingly, it does not appear to be due to an increase in right atrial pressure alone, because right atrial pressure has been shown to rise relatively little during inspiration with TS. Inspiration increases inflow into the right heart, and because RV inflow is restricted by the TS, the volume in the RV is not increased as much as it is in the right atrium, where venous inflow is unrestricted [101]. The mean right atrial pressure tends to remain unchanged with inspiration, whereas RV pressure falls and the relatively higher pressure in the right atrium increases the gradient across the tricuspid valve [23].

* 5. What should you consider besides rheumatic TS if either a mid-diastolic inflow murmur or a presystolic murmur increases with inspiration?

ANS.: Ebstein's anomaly (which often has both TS and TR), an ASD with large flow, or a right atrial myxoma [87, 97].

Note: a) Some patients with a right atrial myxoma and a mid-diastolic inflow murmur also have a murmur between the M_1 and the second component of a widely split S_1 [6, 46]. The second component is probably the tricuspid component of the S_1. This short murmur may be due to TR with upward movement of the tumor through the tricuspid valve before the valve closes.

b) Constrictive pericarditis can occasionally cause a localized constriction around the tricuspid annulus and produce the gradient and murmur of TS [75].

DIASTOLIC SEMILUNAR VALVE MURMURS

Aortic Regurgitation Murmurs

Causes of Aortic Regurgitation

1. What are the commonest causes of severe AR (a) in the child and (b) in the adult?
   ANS.: a) In the young child, a VSD with aortic valve prolapse may be the commonest cause of severe AR.
   b) In the adult, rheumatic heart disease, endocarditis, or paraprosthetic valve leaks are probably equally common as causes of severe AR.

2. What is the commonest cause of mild AR in the adult? Why?
   ANS.: Severe hypertension. In one series of severe hypertensive patients, 60 percent had AR [53]. In another series of hypertensive patients, 6 percent had AR, all trivial. Those with AR had diastolic blood pressures of at least 110 [68]. When the diastolic pressure is reduced below 115 mm Hg, the AR may disappear [68]. Two causes have been suggested:
   1) Dilatation of the aortic ring.
   2) High pressure above a bicuspid or fenestrated aortic valve. Fenestrations are common in both aortic and pulmonary valves. In one autopsy study, 82 percent of all semilunar valves had fenestrations [31].
   Note: a) Bicuspid aortic valves occur in about 2 percent of males and 1 percent of females.
   *b) In one report of 4 patients with severe AR no etiology for the AR was found at surgery or at autopsy. The patients did, however, have hypertension [96].

*3. List some rare causes of AR (a) with arthritis and (b) without arthritis.
   ANS.: a) With arthritis:
   1) Ankylosing spondylitis. (The cusps are shortened and thickened by fibrous tissue, and occasionally this produces AR a few years before the symptomatic spondylitis, although x-ray evidence of spondylitis may be seen and tissue typing with the antigen HLA–B27 may be positive [24]. However, the incidence rises with the duration of the arthritis [8].
   2) Reiter's syndrome. AR may be found from 1 to 20 years after diagnosis, and it occurs in about 5 percent of patients with this syndrome.
   3) Rheumatoid or psoriatic arthritis [57].
   4) Disseminated lupus erythematosus.
   5) The arthritis associated with ulcerative colitis.
   b) Without arthritis:
   1) Syphilis (luetic aortitis).
   2) Osteogenesis imperfecta. The AR here is due to dilatation of the aortic root [19].
   3) Marfan's syndrome. The AR is due to dilatation of the aortic root and myxomatous degeneration of the cusps [71].
   Note: Although both males and females with Marfan's syndrome may have MR, only males (usually under age 40) develop AR. When a patient has only some but not all of the features of Marfan's syndrome (forme fruste), cystic medial necrosis of

the aorta with or without a dissecting aneurysm is usually an associated lesion [69]. Although myxomatous transformation of the aortic valve is characteristic of Marfan's syndrome, it can occur without Marfan's syndrome; when it does, it can result in rupture of an aortic cusp [62].

4) Dissecting aneurysm of the ascending aorta.

5) Supravalvular AS. The AR here is due either to fusion of a cusp with the supravalvular membrane or to the valve leaflets adhering to the aortic wall [85].

6) Uremia. (See below for explanation.) If the early diastolic murmur is localized to the apex and disappears or decreases with sitting, an atypical friction rub and not AR may be the cause [7].

7) Aortic arch syndrome, or Takayasu's disease (pulseless disease). The AR here is due to dilatation of the aortic ring [94].

8) Rupture of a sinus of Valsalva.

9) Giant cell arteritis [42].

4. What should make you suspect by auscultation that a bicuspid aortic valve is the cause of the AR?

ANS.: In the presence of mild AR, an ejection click followed by an early ejection murmur that is loudest in the second right interspace.

*Note: The following theory may explain the incompetence of a bicuspid aortic valve. If the valve edges were straight between their attachments, the valves would be obstructive as they opened. Obstruction is avoided if at least one of the leaflets has a voluminous or redundant (and pleated) free-edge length that is greater than the straight-line distance between its attachments to the aortic wall. This redundant valvular tissue may allow free forward flow in systole but may prolapse downward during diastole, producing at least mild regurgitation, especially if only one leaflet has the extra diameter [22].

*5. Why may uremia mimic AR?

ANS.: The accentuated diastolic component of a loud venous hum may be transmitted down to the base of the heart.

6. Why may AR be present in a patient with uremia?

ANS.: AR correlates, not with the level of uremia, but with the presence of at least two of the three conditions commonly seen in uremia: severe anemia, volume overload, and diastolic pressure of 120 mm Hg or more [2, 55, 86]. It is not always due to the effect of hypertension on a bicuspid or rheumatic valve because it can occur when the blood pressure has been made normal by dialysis and when the valve is found to be normal at autopsy.

Timing and Shape

1. When in the cycle does the AR murmur begin, and what is its shape?

ANS.: It begins with the aortic component of the second sound (A_2). In general, it is decrescendo.

*Note: There is often a very early and very short crescendo-decrescendo to the murmur. This crescendo-decrescendo is due to the shape of the aortoventricular gradient and flow, which increases in early diastole as ventricular pressure drops precipitously below aortic pressure to nearly zero while aortic pressure falls slowly. A good dicrotic wave to the aortic pressure curve may also be partly responsible for this crescendo-decrescendo. Because the presence of a good dicrotic wave in AR suggests mild or, at the most, moderate AR, a marked crescendo-decrescendo effect in the early part of the murmur probably suggests that the AR is not severe.

Note: The dicrotic wave is thought to be caused by a "rebound" effect of the aortic leaflets immediately after their abrupt closure in early diastole. If true, then a good dicrotic wave would be expected only when the valve is least insufficient.

Systolic and diastolic murmurs

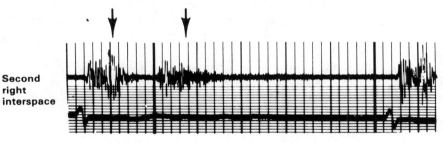

Second right interspace

To-and-fro murmurs

This murmur was due to mild syphilitic AR. It was loudest at the second and third right interspaces. Note the slight early crescendo-decrescendo. A systolic murmur due to blood going in one direction, together with a diastolic murmur due to blood going in the opposite direction, is called a to-and-fro murmur.

*2. What is the auscultatory effect of the short and early crescendo-decrescendo?

ANS.: The murmur appears to start after a short silent period following the A_2. (The peak of the crescendo occurs about 50–200 msec after the A_2.) The background rhythm effect is as follows:

1––––2–HAaaaaaa–1––––2–HAaaaaaa–

3. What is the significance of a pandiastolic murmur in comparison with the short one that finishes before the end of diastole?

ANS.: A pandiastolic murmur suggests that the AR is at least moderate in severity, provided that the heart rate is not so fast that even a short diastolic murmur would be pandiastolic.

Quality and Loudness

1. What is the dominant frequency or pitch of the usual AR murmur? Why?

ANS.: The dominant frequency is high. If the AR is mild, then the murmur will be due more to a large gradient than to flow, i.e., there will be a small but high-velocity regurgitant jet, and the murmur will therefore be purely high-pitched. If the AR is moderate, the murmur will be due to a greater flow as well as to a high-velocity jet, and it will have mixed frequencies but still be dominantly high. If AR is severe, the murmur may be very rough due to an excess of low and medium frequencies.

Note: Although the more low frequencies there are, the more severe the AR, the reverse is not necessarily true, i.e., a pure high-frequency murmur may be present with moderately severe AR. Presumably the low-frequency components are transmitted to areas not accessible to the stethoscope.

2. How can you best imitate by voice the sound of a typical mild AR murmur, i.e., a purely high-pitched murmur?

ANS.: In Mexico this has been called an "aspirative" AR murmur and is imitated by noisily breathing *in* through the mouth. If you breathe *out* quickly with the mouth open or whisper "ah," you can easily imitate the classic AR murmur.

Note: Because it sounds so much like a breath sound, the patient should hold his breath in expiration to allow you to perceive this murmur better.

3. How can you increase the loudness of the very soft AR murmur?

ANS.: a) You can get the stethoscope closer to the heart by having the patient sit up and lean forward. Then press hard with the diaphragm during held expiration.

b) You can increase peripheral resistance as follows:

1) Ask the patient to squat and auscultate the chest immediately. The increase in venous return for a few beats will also help increase the murmur.

Note: a) Squatting is effective in bringing out a grade 1/6 murmur but has little effect on the murmur of moderate to marked AR [63].

b) Kinking of the arteries is probably unimportant in the effect of squatting on blood pressure because drawing the knees up to the chest in the supine position has little effect on blood pressure. Squatting may be a form of isometric exercise.

2) Have the patient do isometric exercise by means of handgrip. The elevation of systolic blood pressure after 3 minutes of 33 percent maximum handgrip pressure is greater in patients with aortic regurgitation than in normal subjects [39A].

3) Administer a vasopressor drug.

* 4. When is moderate AR especially likely to be associated with a soft murmur, despite a normal chest diameter?

ANS.: In the presence of low flow due to MS.

Note: Even with significant MS, concomitant AR with a soft murmur is probably trivial if the diastolic blood pressure is more than 70 mm Hg and the pulse pressure is less than 40 mm Hg [13].

* Musical AR Murmurs

1. What is the significance of a musical AR murmur?

ANS.: Musical aortic diastolic murmurs often occur in patients with a perforated leaflet as in infective endocarditis, everted leaflets (often luetic), or rupture of an aortic sinus of Valsalva. Ruptures of leaflets are usually secondary to myxomatous transformation or infective endocarditis.

*2. What is the timing and shape of musical AR murmurs?

ANS.: a) The same as that of the usual AR murmur, i.e., pandiastolic decrescendo after the usual initial short crescendo, or

b) The musical parts may occur only in early diastole and are then followed by the usual high-frequency decrescendo murmur for the rest of diastole, or

c) There may be a mid- or late-diastolic crescendo-decrescendo musical component.

Note: The dove-coo musical murmur has a peculiar shape (see diagram) that suggests that it is made by vibrations of the aorta itself. The regurgitant stream acts on the aortic valve, which probably acts like a reed that in turn causes the aorta to vibrate. The shape of the murmur may be due to the effect of the mitral valve, which, when open, allows the aortic posterior wall freedom to resonate. In the semiclosed position, the mitral valve pulls on the aorta and keeps it more rigid, thus muting the vibrations [47].

L. lower sternal border   High frequency

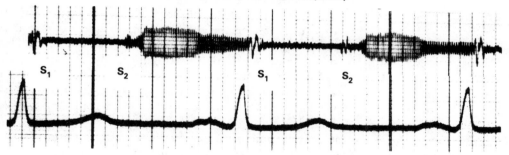

Luetic AR was suspected as the cause of this aortic diastolic murmur. Note the regular vibrations seen in all phonocardiograms of musical murmurs.

Site of AR Murmurs

1. Where, as a rule, is the AR murmur best heard?

ANS.: Over the midsternum or just to the left of the sternum at the level of the third or fourth intercostal space.

2. When is the AR murmur best heard to the *right* of the sternum?

ANS.: In the presence of marked poststenotic dilatation of the aorta (when AS is also present) or when marked atherosclerotic tortuosity pushes the ascending aorta anteriorly and to the right, the murmur may be best heard at the second or third right interspace. However, it is best heard in the *fourth* right interspace only if it is due to nonrheumatic conditions that cause the regurgitant stream to flow in peculiar directions; e.g., when it is secondary to infective endocarditis, an aortic aneurysm, a prolapsed aortic valve, or rupture of a **sinus of Valsalva**.

3. What other unusual murmur radiations are occasionally found in AR?

ANS.: The murmur may be even louder in the high mid-left thorax, at the apex, or in the midaxillary line than at the sternal edge. This has been called the Cole-Cecil murmur [14]. The cause for these unusual radiations is unknown.

Occasionally the murmur may even be heard *only* in the axillary area or at the apex. This may have been one of the reasons why "silent" AR was reported in 16 patients with significant AR on cineangiography [77].

Sudden, Severe Aortic Regurgitation

1. What are the most likely causes of sudden, severe AR?
   ANS.: a) Infective endocarditis.
   b) Rupture of an **aneurysm** of the sinus of Valsalva.
2. What are the auscultatory signs at the apex of sudden, severe AR?
   ANS.: A soft or absent S_1 and a loud S_3 [98].
   Note: a) The soft or absent S_1 in sudden, severe AR is due to the rapid and marked rise of LV pressure in diastole. It is so marked that it rises above the left atrial pressure in mid-diastole, at which time it closes the mitral valve prematurely.
   b) The loud S_3 may be a mid-diastolic S_1, which occurs at the moment that LV pressure becomes higher than left atrial pressure. It may be the result of tensing of the chordae tendineae and papillary muscles by mitral valve closure [98].
   Note: The tachycardia of sudden, severe AR often causes diastole to equal, or even be shorter than, systole, so that it is difficult to tell systole from diastole by auscultation. This occurs because ejection is prolonged by the severe LV volume overload, and the diastolic period may be further shortened by tachycardia. Carotid or apical palpation during auscultation is mandatory to avoid confusing systole with diastole.
*3. Why should an exaggerated atrial hump or A wave occur on the apex cardiogram of some patients with severe chronic AR but disappear in sudden, severe AR?
   ANS.: In severe chronic AR the A wave enlarges, probably because of relative myocardial ischemia. This theory is supported by the finding that dogs with severe chronic AR have high levels of myocardial oxygen extraction, leading to relative ischemia. However, in sudden, severe AR the LV pressure is so high at the end of diastole that it becomes higher than the left atrial pressure and closes the mitral valve, which stays closed despite left atrial contraction.
*4. Why may an AR murmur not be pandiastolic in sudden, severe AR even with diastoles that are shorter than normal?
   ANS.: In sudden, severe AR the LV does not expand as well as it does in chronic AR, i.e., it is less distensible, probably due to the inability of the pericardium to stretch acutely. Indeed, the LV pressure in diastole may rise so high so fast that it may even reach aortic diastolic pressure in mid-diastole. This equalization of aortic and ventricular pressures will limit the amount and duration of AR that can occur. (See figure on page 378.)

Differential Diagnosis

1. What are the common imitators of an AR murmur?
   ANS.: a) A pulmonary regurgitation murmur caused by high pressure in the pulmonary artery (Graham Steell murmur).

*b) High-frequency components of MS murmurs transmitted to the left sternal border.

*2. What are the rare imitators of an AR murmur?

ANS.: a) The diastolic component of a soft, continuous murmur due to a coronary to pulmonary artery fistula [44], or a right coronary to LV fistula, especially if the systolic component is inaudible [34].

b) Inflation of an aortic balloon pump during diastole produces a short, slightly delayed diastolic murmur with a blowing, squirting, or blubbering quality [12].

c) A flail posterior mitral leaflet during the rapid movement from its prolapsed position in the left atrium to its open position in the LV as blood rushes from the left atrium to the LV [32].

d) The soft, AR-like diastolic murmur heard at the second or third left interspace in some patients with moderate obstruction (not more than 50 percent occluded) of the anterior descending coronary artery [11].

*THE MURMUR OF ANTERIOR DESCENDING CORONARY ARTERY STENOSIS

*1. Why is the coronary artery obstruction murmur best heard in diastole?

ANS.: Maximum flow in the coronary arteries occurs in diastole.

*2. What are the characteristics of the diastolic murmur of coronary artery stenosis?

ANS.: a) High-pitched [74].

b) Crescendo-decrescendo, corresponding to the pattern of diastolic coronary flow, which is maximum in the first quarter of diastole [38, 74].

c) Most easily audible when the patient is sitting up.

Note: This murmur has been observed to disappear after infarction and after aortocoronary bypass surgery. It may also appear for the first time after aortocoronary bypass surgery due to slight obstruction at the site of the distal anastomosis. Here it is probably due to retrograde flow across the stenosed native coronary artery. It may increase with either amyl nitrite or dipyridamole [60].

*3. What does the diastolic murmur of coronary artery stenosis suggest about the degree of obstruction?

ANS.: It suggests that the obstruction is not major, i.e., it allows enough flow to produce the turbulence necessary to cause a diastolic murmur. It is not surprising that an obstruction of not more than 50 percent has been found in those cases that have been investigated.

PULMONARY REGURGITATION MURMURS

Murmurs with High Pressure in the Pulmonary Artery (Graham Steell Murmur)

1. Does the pulmonary artery pressure have to be very high to produce a pulmonary regurgitation (PR) murmur?

ANS.: It is usually very high, i.e., at nearly systemic levels. Pulmonary regurgitation murmurs are rarely present with pulmonary artery pressures of below 80 mm Hg systolic unless the main pulmonary artery is markedly dilated.

Note: a) A Graham Steell murmur is a PR murmur that is secondary to pulmonary hypertension, regardless of whether the hypertension is primary or secondary.

*b) A PR murmur with a VSD may occur even with normal pulmonary vascular resistance if the pulmonary pressure reaches about 100 mm Hg.

2. How does the Graham Steell murmur differ from the AR murmur?

ANS.: It may not differ—i.e., both are dominantly high-pitched, may be from grade 1 to 6, may have an early crescendo-decrescendo, and may become louder on expiration [76]. The Graham Steell murmur, however, often increases with inspiration when it is loud.

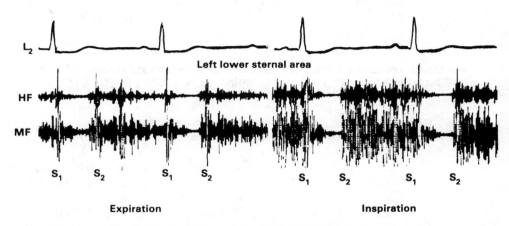

These phonocardiograms are from a patient with a PDA whose pulmonary artery pressure was 145 mm Hg, with an aortic pressure about the same. This loud diastolic murmur (Graham Steell murmur) increased markedly on inspiration. A soft Graham Steell murmur may not increase with inspiration.

Note: A Graham Steell murmur may decrease with inspiration despite the increase in pulmonary artery flow because the PR murmur is usually best heard in the second left interspace, where the effect of inspiration in pushing the stethoscope away from the heart is most marked. Also, inspiration may not increase flow to the lungs in patients with severe pulmonary hypertension if concomitant TR is present.

*3. How can a Valsalva strain help in differentiating a PR from an AR murmur?

ANS.: Immediately on release of the Valsalva strain, the PR murmur will resume its pre-Valsalva loudness. The AR murmur will return to its normal intensity only after four or five beats.

Note: a) In patients with a dilated pulmonary artery there may be an early, short diastolic decrescendo scratch without AR or PR. Such scratches may result from an extracardiac effect of adhesions between the pulmonary artery and the surrounding lung.

b) The hypoxemia produced by 10 percent oxygen plus 90 percent nitrogen inhalation will cause pulmonary arteriolar constriction and therefore will increase a PR murmur within 5–15 minutes, helping to differentiate it from the murmur of AR, which may even diminish [20].

    c) The Graham Steell murmur was once erroneously thought to be common in patients with MS because the murmur of AR was misinterpreted as being due to PR.

*4. When can a PDA with pulmonary hypertension produce a loud diastolic murmur that is produced at the ductus and not by the pulmonary regurgitation?

    ANS.: There are reports of grade 4 or more diastolic murmurs that are due to such a rapid drop in pulmonary artery pressure because of PR that aortic to pulmonary flow through the ductus occurs in diastole. Because the pulmonary artery pressure in diastole may drop faster than the aortic pressure, the murmur may even be crescendo to the first sound [102]. In every one of these patients who died, necropsy showed an unusually short and wide ductus.

Pulmonary Regurgitation Murmurs with Normal Pressure in the Pulmonary Artery (Primary Pulmonary Regurgitation)

1. List three causes of primary PR murmurs.

    ANS.: 1. Idiopathic dilatation of the pulmonary artery. (In some series, about a third of patients with idiopathic dilatation have PR.)

    *2. Congenital absence of the pulmonary valve.

      Note: A patient with tetralogy of Fallot with PR almost invariably has no pulmonary valve, and the pulmonary obstruction is due to a constricted valve ring.

    *3. Surgery for pulmonary stenosis. Pulmonary valvotomy invariably leaves some degree of PR.

      *Note: a) The occasional PR in patients with an ASD might really be another instance of coincidental idiopathic dilatation of the pulmonary artery. In one series of patients with uncomplicated ASDs, a small number had an early basal diastolic murmur that was recorded externally and only in the outflow tract of the RV by internal phonocardiography [25]. In another series of patients with uncomplicated ASDs who were over age 20, 4 percent had a grade 2/6, medium-frequency, diastolic decrescendo murmur that increased on inspiration, was of maximum loudness at the second left interspace, and radiated to the lower right sternal border [51].

      b) A diastolic murmur at the left lower sternal border that begins with the P_2 in some ASD patients with normal pulmonary artery pressures has been shown to sometimes be the diastolic component of a continuous murmur at the ASD caused by a high left atrial pressure due to MR, plus a small to moderate-sized ASD [81].

2. How do the shape, length, and pitch of a primary PR murmur differ from those of the Graham Steell murmur?

    ANS.: With high pressures in the pulmonary artery, the shape, length, and pitch of the PR murmur are the same as those of AR. In the murmur of PR with *normal* pressures in the pulmonary artery, there is sometimes a slight delay after the P_2 before any murmur is heard. However, even if it starts with the P_2, the murmur tends to be short and rough, due to dominant medium and low frequencies.

* *Note:* When the PR is mild, the murmur may have characteristics that are between those of the Graham Steell murmur and the primary PR murmur; i.e., it may start earlier, last longer, and have higher frequencies than the more severe primary PR murmur [59].

One intracardiac phonocardiogram study showed no pause between the P_2 and the murmur [28]. But in one other such study the PR murmur was markedly delayed [10].

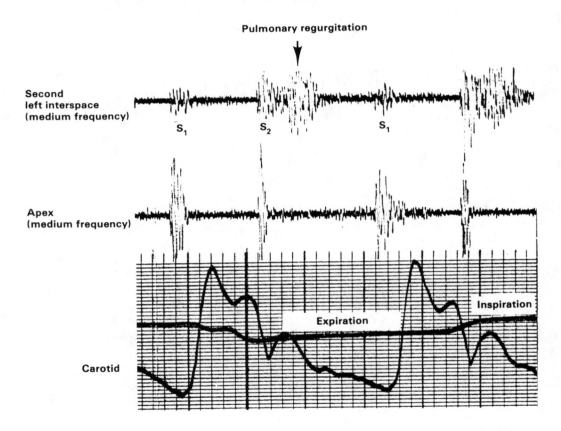

Pulmonary regurgitation

Second left interspace (medium frequency)

S_1 S_2 S_1

Apex (medium frequency)

Inspiration

Expiration

Carotid

Primary PR

This murmur of primary PR in a teenaged boy was early diastolic and had many low and medium frequencies in it. It did not increase with inspiration at the second left interspace because too much air was interposed between heart and stethoscope in that area. The murmur was softer at the left lower sternal border, where, however, it did become louder with inspiration.

* 3. Why is the primary PR murmur short?

ANS.: Diastolic pressure in the pulmonary artery falls rapidly because it begins with a normal pressure at the pulmonary incisura and has diastolic runoff in two directions, so that pulmonary artery and RV pressure rapidly equalize.

PERICARDIAL FRICTION RUBS

Pericarditis

1. What is the mechanism that causes friction rubs?

    ANS.: It is usually assumed that the rub sounds are caused by the two roughened pericardial membranes (the visceral and parietal pericardia) sliding over one another. When the overlying pleura is also involved, perhaps the noises are caused by the pleura rubbing against the outer layer of pericardium. The rub then would be a pleuro-pericardial friction rub.

    Note: The three commonest causes of generalized pericarditis are viral pericarditis, disseminated lupus, and uremia.

2. What is the commonest cause of a localized pericarditis?

    ANS.: Acute myocardial infarction.

    Note: If there has been neither infarction nor trauma to the heart (including radiation to the chest), then consider a metastatic tumor involving the heart.

How to Recognize a Pericardial Friction Rub

1. What adjectives and analogies have been used to describe the quality of friction rubs?

    ANS.: They usually sound crunching, scraping, creaking, grating, crackling, or scratching. They often sound like squeaky shoes or like two pieces of sandpaper rubbed against one another. Occasionally, however, they sound no different from any mixed-frequency murmur. They often sound surprisingly superficial, and increased stethoscope pressure seems to make them unexpectedly louder.

2. How many components are heard in most friction rubs?

    ANS.: Three: one systolic and two diastolic.

3. At what time in diastole do the two diastolic rubs occur?

    ANS.: a) In early diastole, near the end of early rapid expansion of the ventricle, at the time when an S_3 would occur.

    b) At the end of diastole, when atrial contraction produces sudden ventricular expansion. This is the moment when an S_4 would occur.

4. Where in systole may a systolic rub occur?

    ANS.: Anywhere. It may replace the first or second heart sound or occur only in midsystole. There is therefore the possibility that three rubs may occur in systole.

5. If one major rub replaces the first heart sound (the commonest occurrence) and two rubs occur in diastole, what is the cadence of a friction rub that is heard as a background rhythm even if the components are not distinctly separate?

    ANS.: The cadence is the same as that of a quadruple rhythm due to a double gallop, i.e., "ch-DUP-sh-sh——––ch-DUP-sh-sh."

    Note: Because the systolic rub may replace both the S_1 and the S_2, it is common to hear the rhythm as "CH-sh-sh––CH-sh-sh." When one of the diastolic rubs is absent, it is usually the S_3, i.e., an S_4 rub is the last to disappear, probably because the heart is maximally distended at the end of diastole, tending to bring the inflamed pericardial surfaces into contact.

6. Is the friction rub usually louder during inspiration or expiration? Why?

ANS.: In about a third of patients, it increases during inspiration [21, 82]. This may be due to several possible causes:

1) The downward pull of the diaphragm on the pericardium may draw the pericardium more tautly over the heart. The diaphragm is attached to the pericardium, and it is conceivable that a small amount of fluid between the visceral and parietal pericardia could be squeezed out by the tightening of the two layers with inspiration.

2) It may be a pleuropericardial rub. Even when there is a pericardial effusion, there may still be a pericardial rub, and this may be accounted for either by the squeezing out of a small amount of fluid by inspiration or by the expanded lung pressing on the pericardium during inspiration, especially if it is a pleuropericardial rub.

3) There may be greater expansion of the RV during inspiration than expansion of the LV during expiration. This would stretch the pericardium more during inspiration.

7. Of the three major rub components, which one is almost always present? Which is the next commonest component?

ANS.: The systolic component is almost always present. The atrial systolic component is next in frequency of occurrence, but rarely does an atrial systolic rub occur alone as the only rub sound. It almost always occurs together with at least a systolic rub.

*Note: A systolic rub alone (rare) is more likely to occur in atrial fibrillation than in sinus rhythm [40].

8. Where are most friction rubs best heard?

ANS.: Near the left sternal border, at about the third or fourth left interspace.

9. When is the friction rub transient?

ANS.: During the course of acute myocardial infarction, when it may last only a few hours.

*Note: In the **postmyocardial infarction syndrome** (Dressler's syndrome) it may last for weeks.

*10. What can imitate a friction rub?

ANS.: A noisy left-sided pneumothorax. A shallow pneumothorax at the left lung apex (occasionally seen, only on a film taken on full expiration) can apparently cause air pockets on the medial aspect of the lung. The contraction of the LV against these bubbles of air may produce sounds at the apex that are synchronous with systole and diastole [78]. They have been described as grinding, clicking, and crunching, and may be heard at a distance from the patient. They do not occur with a right-sided pneumothorax and seem to occur almost entirely in young males.

Note: a) A mixture of fluid and air in the pericardium, as when a few milliliters of air are introduced into the pericardium to replace the fluid withdrawn, produces a metallic tinkle that is synchronous with systole. A large amount of injected air can produce a churning, splashing sound (mill wheel murmur) [83].

b) Temporary transvenous pacemakers have been associated with friction rubs thought to be caused by contact of the pacing wire with the inner surface of the myocardium, i.e., they may be endocardial friction rubs, although occasionally they are a sign of perforation [37].

REFERENCES

1. Aldridge, H. E., and Wigle, E. D. Partial anomalous pulmonary venous drainage with intact interatrial septum associated with congenital mitral stenosis. *Circulation* 31:579, 1965.
2. Alexander, W. D., and Polak, A. Early diastolic murmurs in end-stage renal failure. *Br. Heart J.* 39:900, 1977.
3. Ashman, H., Zaroff, L. I., and Baronofsky, I. Right atrial myxoma. *Am. J. Med.* 28:487, 1960.
4. Ayers, C. R. Boineau, J. P., and Spach, M. S. Congenital complete heart block in children. *Am. Heart J.* 72:381, 1966.
5. Bardet, J., and Bardet, A. Phonocardiographie du retrecissement mitral. *Arch. Mal. Coeur* 59:917, 1966.
6. Barlow, J., Fuller, D., and Denny, M. A case of right atrial myxoma. *Br. Heart J.* 24:120, 1962.
7. Barratt, L. J., et al. The diastolic murmur of renal failure. *N. Engl. J. Med.* 295:121, 1976.
8. Benisch, B. M. Mitral stenosis and insufficiency: A complication of healed bacterial endocarditis. *Am. Heart J.* 82:39, 1971.
9. Bjork, V. O., and Malmstrom, G. Simultaneous left and right atrial pressure curves during Valsalva's experiment. *Am. Heart J.* 50:742, 1955.
10. Brayshaw, J. R., and Perloff, J. K. Congenital pulmonary insufficiency complicating idiopathic dilatation of the pulmonary artery. *Am. J. Cardiol.* 10:282, 1962.
11. Burg, J. R., et al. Disappearance of coronary artery stenosis murmur after aortocoronary bypass. *Chest* 63:440, 1973.
12. Clements, S. D., Jr., et al. Phonocardiographic study of sounds produced by a circulatory assist device. *Arch. Intern. Med.* 137:1619, 1977.
13. Cohn, L. H., et al. Preoperative assessment of aortic regurgitation in patients with mitral valve disease. *Circulation* 34 (Suppl. 31):76, 1966.
14. Cole, R., and Cecil, A. B. The axillary diastolic murmur in aortic insufficiency. *Bull. Johns Hopkins Hosp.* 19:353, 1908.
15. Coombs, C. F. *Rheumatic Heart Disease.* Bristol, England: Wright, 1924. P. 203.
16. Coombs, C. F. Rheumatic myocarditis. *Quart. J. Med.* 2:26, 1908.
17. Criley, J. M., and Hermer, A. J. The crescendo presystolic murmur of mitral stenosis with atrial fibrillation. *N. Engl. J. Med.* 285:1284, 1971.
18. Criley, J. M., Blaufuss, A. H., and Hermer, A. J. Presystolic murmur in atrial fibrillation. *Circulation* 56:133, 1977.
19. Criscitiello, M. G., et al. Cardiovascular abnormalities in osteogenesis imperfecta. *Circulation* 31:255, 1965.
20. Curiel, R., et al. The cardiovascular effects of acute hypoxemia as a diagnostic aid. *Chest* 81:159, 1982.
21. Dressler, W. Effect of respiration on the pericardial friction rub. *Am. J. Cardiol.* 7:130, 1961.
22. Edwards, J. E. The congenital bicuspid aortic valve. *Circulation* 23:485, 1961.
22A. Edwards, J. E. and Burchell H. B. Endocardial and intimal lesions (jet impact). *Circul.* 18:946, 1958.
23. El-Sherif, N. Rheumatic tricuspid stenosis: a haemodynamic correlation. *Br. Heart J.* 33:16, 1971.
24. Eversmeyer, W. H., Rosenstock, D., and Biundo, J. J., Jr. Aortic insufficiency with mild ankylosing spondylitis in black men. *J.A.M.A.* 240:2652, 1978.
25. Feruglio, G. A., and Sreenivasan, A. Intracardiac phonocàrdiogram in thirty cases of atrial septal defect. *Circulation* 20:1087, 1959.
26. Fisher, M. L., et al. Haemodynamic response to isometric exercise (handgrip) in patients with heart disease. *Br. Heart J.* 35:422, 1973.
26A. Flint, A. *Diseases of the Heart.* 2nd ed. New York: Macmillan, 1870, P. 206.
27. Flint, A. On cardiac murmurs. *Am. J. Med. Sci.* 44:29, 1862.
28. Fontana, M. E., and Wooley, C. F. The murmur of pulmonic regurgitation in tetralogy of Fallot with absent pulmonic valve. *Circulation* 57:986, 1978.
29. Fortuin, N. J., and Craige, E. On the mechanism of the Austin Flint murmur. *Circulation* 45:558, 1972.
30. Fortuin, N. J., and Craige, E. Echocardiographic studies of genesis of mitral diastolic murmurs. *Br. Heart J.* 35:75, 1973.

31. Foxe, A. N. Fenestrations of the semilunar valves. *Am. J. Pathol.* 5:179, 1929.
32. Fuchs, R. M., and Achuff, S. C. Auscultatory findings of mitral prolapse mimicking aortic stenosis and regurgitation. *Am. Heart J.* 101:351, 1981.
33. Futamata, H., et al. The diastolic rumble and fluttering of the ventricular wall after atrioventricular valve replacement with the Hancock xenograft. *J. Cardiography* 11:371, 1981.
34. Galioto, F. M., Jr., et al. Right coronary artery to left ventricle fistula. *Am. Heart J.* 82:93, 1971.
34A. Gamble, W. H., and Reddy, P. S. Preservation of the third heart sound in mitral stenosis. *N. Engl. J. Med.* 309:498, 1983.
35. Garbagni, R., Angelino, R., and Tartara, D. Lutembacher's syndrome: Clinical and hemodynamic studies before and after operation. *Arch. Mal. Coeur* 54:511, 1961.
36. Glancy, D. L., et al. Parachute mitral valve. *Am. J. Cardiol.* 27:309, 1971.
37. Glassman, R. D., et al. Pacemaker-induced endocardial friction rubs. *Am. J. Cardiol.* 40:811, 1977.
38. Green, E. W., Agruss, N. S., and Adolph, R. J. Right-sided Austin Flint murmur. *Am. J. Cardiol.* 32:370, 1973.
39. Gregg, D. E. *Coronary Circulation in Health and Disease* London: Kimpton, 1950.
39A. Gumbiner, C. H., and Gutgesell, H. P. Response to isometric exercise in children and young adults with aortic regurgitation. *Am. Heart J.* 106:540, 1983.
40. Harvey, W. P. Auscultatory findings in disease of the pericardium. *Am. J. Cardiol.* 7:15, 1961.
41. Heidenreich, F. P., et al. Left-atrial transport in mitral stenosis. *Circulation* 40:545, 1969.
42. How, J., and Strachan, R. W. Aortic regurgitation as a manifestation of giant cell arteritis. *Br. Heart J.* 40:1052, 1978.
43. Ide, Y., et al. A study of atrial presystolic murmurs. *J. Cardiography* 8:505, 1978.
44. Ishikawa, T., et al. A case of coronary artery-pulmonary artery fistula presented diastolic blowing murmur. *J. Cardiogr.* 6:169, 1976.
45. Kambe, T., et al. Clinical study on the right-sided Austin Flint murmur using intracardiac phonocardiography. *Am. Heart J.* 98:701, 1979.
46. Kaufmann, G., Rutishauser, W., and Hegglin, R. Heart sounds in atrial tumors. *Am. J. Cardiol.* 8:350, 1961.
47. Kohno, K., Hiroki, T., and Arakawa, K. Aortic regurgitation with dove-coo murmur with special reference to the mechanism of its generation using dual echocardiography. *Jap. Heart J.* 22:861, 1981.
48. Kong, T. O., Kellum, R. E., and Haserick, J. R. Clinical diagnosis of cardiac involvement in systemic lupus erythematosus. *Circulation* 26:7, 1962.
49. Laake, H. Rheumatic tricuspid stenosis. *Acta Med. Scand.* 161:109, 1958.
50. Lakier, J. B., et al. Haemodynamic and sound events preceding first heart sound in mitral stenosis. *Br. Heart J.* 34:1152, 1972.
51. Liberthson, R. R., Buckley, M. J., and Boucher, C. A. Pulmonary regurgitation in large atrial shunts without pulmonary hypertension. *Circulation* 54:966, 1976.
52. Lochaya, S., Igarashi, M., and Shaffer, A. B. Late diastolic mitral regurgitation secondary to aortic regurgitation: Its relationship to the Austin Flint murmur. *Am. Heart J.* 74:161, 1967.
53. Luisada, A. A., and Argano, B. The phonocardiogram in systemic hypertension. *Chest* 58:598, 1970.
54. Luisada, A. A., and diBartole, G. High-frequency phonocardiography. *Am. J. Cardiol.* 8:51, 1961.
55. Matalon, R., et al. Functional aortic insufficiency—a feature of renal failure. *N. Engl. J. Med.* 285:1522, 1972.
55A. Mirro, M. J., et al. Auscultatory and phonocardiographic features of normally functioning porcine mitral valves. *Circulation* 55 & 56 (Suppl. III):69, 1977.
56. Morgan, J. R., et al. Isolated tricuspid stenosis. *Circulation* 44:729, 1971.
57. Muna, W. F., et al. Psoriatic arthritis and aortic regurgitation. *J.A.M.A.* 244:363, 1980.
58. Nadas, A. S., and Ellison, R. C. Phonocardiographic analysis of diastolic flow murmurs in secundum atrial septal defect and ventricular septal defect. *Br. Heart J.* 29:684, 1967.
59. Nemickas, R., et al. Isolated congenital pulmonic insufficiency. *Am. J. Cardiol.* 14:456, 1964.
60. Nozawa, T., et al. Two cases with the heart murmur originated from aortocoronary bypass: The diagnostic use of dipyridamole. *J. Cardiography* 11:825, 1981.
61. O'Brien, K. P., and Cohen, L. S. Hemodynamic and phonocardiographic correlates of the Austin Flint murmur. *Am. Heart J.* 77:603, 1969.

62. O'Brien, K. P., et al. Spontaneous aortic cusp rupture associated with valvular myxomatous transformation. *Circulation* 37:273, 1968.
63. O'Donnell, T. V., and McIlroy, M. D. The circulatory effects of squatting. *Am. Heart J.* 64:347, 1962.
64. Parker, E., Craig, E., and Hood, W. P., Jr. The Austin Flint murmur and the A wave of the apexcardiogram in aortic regurgitation. *Circulation* 43:349, 1971.
65. Paul, M. H., Rudolph, A. M., and Nadas, A. S. Congenital complete atrioventricular block: Problems of clinical assessment. *Circulation* 18:183, 1958.
66. Perloff, J. K. Auscultatory and phonocardiographic manifestations of pulmonary hypertension. *Progr. Cardiovasc. Dis.* 9:303, 1967.
67. Pridie, R. B., Benham, R., and Oakley, C. M. Echocardiography of the mitral valve in aortic valve disease. *Br. Heart J.* 33:296, 1971.
68. Puchner, T. C., Huston, J. H., and Hellmuth, G. A. Aortic valve insufficiency in arterial hypertension. *Am. J. Cardiol.* 5:758, 1960.
69. Read, R. C., Thal, A. P., and Wendt, V. E. Symptomatic valvular myxomatous transformation (the floppy valve syndrome). *Circulation* 32:897, 1965.
70. Reddy, P. S., et al. Sound pressure correlates of the Austin Flint murmur. An intracardiac sound study. *Circulation* 53:210, 1976.
71. Rosenthal, T., and Kariv, I. A pathognomonic murmur of "atypical" patent ductus arteriosus. *Chest* 56:350, 1969.
72. Sagara, T., et al. The clinical significance of the presystolic murmur in ischemic heart disease. *CV Sound Bull.* 4:471, 1974.
73. Saksena, F. B., Kroll, G., and Boer, A. Massive left atrial thrombus: A case report. *Cardiology* 61:298, 1976.
74. Sangster, J. F., and Oakley, C. M. Diastolic murmur of coronary artery stenosis. *Br. Heart J.* 35:840, 1973.
75. Schire, V., Gotsman, M. S., and Beck, W. Unusual diastolic murmurs in constrictive pericarditis and constrictive endocarditis. *Am. Heart J.* 76:4, 1968.
76. Schwab, R. H., and Killough, J. H. The phonocardiographic differentiation of pulmonic and aortic insufficiency. *Circulation* 32:352, 1965.
77. Segal, B. L., Likoff, W., and Kasper, A. J. "Silent" rheumatic aortic regurgitation. *Am. J. Cardiol.* 14:628, 1964.
78. Semple, T., and Lancaster, W. M. Noisy pneumothorax. *Br. Med. J.* 1:1342, 1961.
79. Shabetai, R., and Davidson, S. Asymmetrical hypertrophic cardiomyopathy simulating mitral stenosis. *Circulation* 54:37, 1972.
80. Silverman, J., Olwin, J. S., and Graettinger, J. S. Cardiac myxomas with systemic embolization. *Circulation* 26:99, 1962.
81. Somerville, J., and Resnekov, L. The origin of an immediate diastolic murmur in atrioventricular defects. *Circulation* 32:797, 1965.
82. Spodick, D. H. Pericardial friction. *N. Engl. J. Med.* 278:1204, 1968.
83. Spodick, D. H. Acoustic phenomena in pericardial disease. *Am. Heart J.* 81:114, 1971.
84. Starkey, G. W. B. Surgical experiences in the treatment of congenital mitral stenosis and mitral insufficiency. *J. Thorac. Cardiovasc. Surg.* 38:336, 1959.
85. Starr, A., Dotter, C., and Griswold, H. The supravalvular aortic stenosis: Diagnosis and treatment. *J. Thorac. Cardiovasc. Surg.* 41:134, 1961.
86. Storstein, O., and Orjavik, O. Aortic insufficiency in chronic renal failure. *Acta Med. Scand.* 203:175, 1978.
87. Tai, A., Gross, H., and Siegelman, S. S. Right atrial myxoma and pulmonary hypertension. *N.Y. State J. Med.* 70:2996, 1970.
88. Taquini, A. C., Massell, B. F., and Walsh, B. J. Phonocardiographic studies of early rheumatic mitral disease. *Am. Heart J.* 20:295, 1940.
89. Thompson, M. E., et al. Sound, pressure and motion correlates in mitral stenosis. *Am. J. Med.* 49:436, 1970.
90. Toutouzas, P., Velimezis, A., and Avgoustakis, D. Double diastolic murmur in mitral stenosis with atrial fibrillation and complete heart block. *Br. Heart J.* 43:92, 1980.
91. Toutouzas, P., et al. Mechanism of diastolic rumble and presystolic murur in mitral stenosis. *Br. Heart J.* 36:1096, 1974.
92. Ueda, H., et al. The Austin Flint murmur. *Jap. Heart J.* 6:294, 1965.

93. Ueda, H., et al. "Silent" mitral stenosis. *Jap. Heart J.* 6:206, 1965.
94. Ueda, H., et al. Aortic insufficiency associated with aortitis syndrome. *Jap. Heart J.* 8:107, 1967.
95. Van Der Spuy, J. C. The functional and clinical anatomy of the mitral valve. *Br. Heart J.* 20:471, 1958.
96. Waller, B. F., et al. Severe aortic regurgitation from systemic hypertension (without aortic dissection) requiring aortic valve replacement. *Am. J. Cardiol.* 49:473, 1982.
97. Waxler, E. B., Kawai, N., and Kasparian, H. Right atrial myxoma: Echocardiographic, phonocardiographic, and hemodynamic signs. *Am. Heart J.* 83:251, 1972.
98. Wigle, E. D., and Labrosse, C. J. Sudden, severe aortic insufficiency. *Circulation* 32:708, 1965.
99. Wood, P. An appreciation of mitral stenosis. I. Clinical features. *Br. Med. J.* 1:1051, 1954. Classic article.
100. Wood, P. An appreciation of mitral stenosis. II. Investigation and results. *Br. Med. J.* 1:1113, 1954. Classic article.
101. Wooley, C. F., et al. Intracardiac sound and pressure events in man. *Am. J. Med.* 42:248, 1967.
102. Wunsch, C. M., and Tavel, M. E. Patent ductus arteriosus and pulmonary valve insufficiency: Unusual clinical manifestations. *Chest* 57:572, 1970.

16. *Abdominal Murmurs*

1. List the common causes of abdominal murmurs.
   ANS.: a) Normal arterial and venous flow murmurs, usually heard only in young people.
   b) Renal artery stenosis.
   c) Hepatic malignancies, alcoholic hepatitis and portal-systemic vein anastomoses in portal hypertension [4].
   d) Splenic artery aneurysms or stenosis.
   e) Aortic atheromatous obstruction [5].
   f) Superior mesenteric or iliac artery stenosis [4].

NORMAL ABDOMINAL MURMURS

1. How common are abdominal murmurs in normal subjects?
   ANS.: They occur in almost half of subjects under age 25 but in only about 5 percent of those over age 50. (Thus, an abdominal murmur in an older adult should probably be considered abnormal [2, 7].)
2. Where are normal abdominal murmurs heard?
   ANS.: Normal murmurs are heard in the epigastrium or over the inferior vena cava, where a venous hum is heard in about 5 percent of normal subjects [2].
   Note: In very thin patients, the murmur may radiate to the left lower sternal border of the chest and may be confused with a cardiac murmur.
*3. How can amyl nitrite inhalation indicate the degree of stenosis producing the arterial murmur?
   ANS.: With moderate stenosis, the arterial murmur is intensified by increasing the flow through the stenotic area. With severe stenosis, on the other hand, the murmur may soften, because amyl nitrite can dilate collateral vessels to the area beyond the obstruction, and the blood escapes via these collaterals [3].

RENAL ARTERY STENOSIS MURMURS

1. What is the pitch and timing of the stenosing renal vascular lesion murmur?
   ANS.: It is high-pitched. It is sometimes a to-and-fro murmur with systolic accentuation, sometimes only a short systolic murmur, and sometimes continuous.
   *Note: The kind of renal artery lesion that is likely to have an arterial murmur is fibromuscular dysplasia.
2. Where are the best sites for hearing renal vascular murmurs?

* Material marked with an asterisk is for reference and for advanced students in cardiology.

399

ANS.: a) Beneath the costal margin anteriorly, lateral to the aorta and lumbar spine.

b) Just above the umbilicus, usually to the left of the midline.

*Note: In a hypertensive patient a murmur over a femoral artery due to atherosclerosis suggests the presence of renal artery stenosis.

MISCELLANEOUS ABDOMINAL MURMURS

1. What does a venous hum over the abdominal wall suggest?

   ANS.: If it is not the normal venous hum in a young person, it suggests portal hypertension and an anastomosis between the portal and systemic veins.

   Note: A continuous murmur means either an arteriovenous fistula of the portal system or renal artery stenosis.

2. What should a systolic murmur in the left hypochondrium suggest?

   ANS.: a) An aneurysmal or tortuous and calcified splenic artery, a huge spleen, a traumatized spleen, or compression of the splenic artery by carcinoma of the pancreas.

   b) Renal artery stenosis.

   *Note: a) A friction rub over the splenic area suggests splenic infarction.

   b) An epigastric murmur is more likely to be due to celiac artery compression than to renal artery stenosis [1].

REFERENCES

1. McLoughlin, M. J., Cotapinto, R. F., and Hobbs, B. B. Abdominal bruits. *J.A.M.A.* 232:1238, 1975.
2. Rivin, A. U. Abdominal vascular sounds. *J.A.M.A.* 221:688, 1972.
3. Ueda, H., et al. Quantitative assessment of obstruction of the aorta and its branches in "aortitis syndrome": The value of functional phonoarteriography using vasoactive drugs. *Jap. Heart J.* 7:3, 1966.
4. Zoneraich, S., and Zoneraich, O. Diagnostic significance of abdominal arterial murmurs in liver and pancreatic disease. *Angiology* 22:197, 1971.
5. Zoneraich, S., and Zoneraich, O. Value of auscultation and phonoarteriography in detecting atherosclerotic involvement of the abdominal aorta and its branches. *Am. Heart J.* 83:620, 1972.

17. *Prosthetic Valve Sounds*

NORMAL BALL VALVE SOUNDS AND RHYTHMS

1. Does a Starr–Edwards ball valve produce a sound both on opening and closing?

   ANS.: Yes. When it opens, it strikes the cage struts to produce an opening click (OC). When it closes, it strikes the ring to produce a closing click (CC).

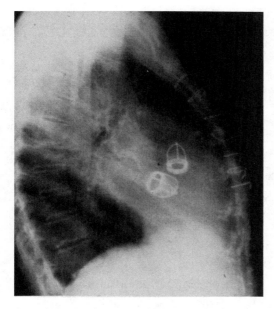

The lower larger cage is mitral. The balls, or poppets, are not radiopaque enough to tell their position.

2. Which *normal* heart sounds are heard in the presence of (a) an aortic ball valve and (b) a mitral ball valve?

   ANS.: a) With an aortic prosthesis, the M_1 will be the only normal heart sound not replaced by an aortic OC and CC.

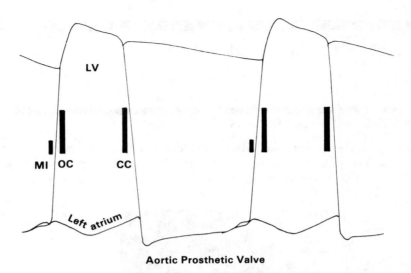

Aortic Prosthetic Valve

The aortic prosthetic valve will sound like a normal heart that has a loud ejection click and loud S_2.

b) With a mitral prosthesis, the S_2 will be the only normal heart sound.

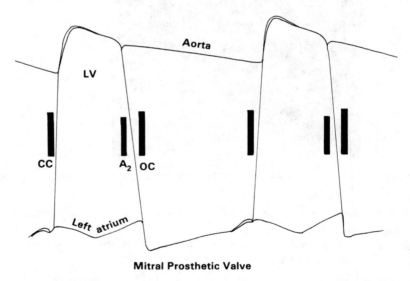

Mitral Prosthetic Valve

The only normal sound expected with a mitral prosthetic valve is the S_2. Any aortic component of the S_1 would be masked by the loud CC. The rhythm with the OC is exactly like that heard in mitral stenosis with an opening snap.

3. What is the rhythm or cadence produced by the OC plus the CC of an aortic prosthetic ball valve together with the normal M_1 included?

ANS.: The order of sounds is M_1–OC-----CC. Therefore, the rhythm is duCLICK----CLICK............duCLICK----CLICK

Note: With an aortic prosthetic valve, the M_1 is rarely well heard away from the apex area, perhaps because most patients with a prosthetic aortic valve have some myocardial damage, thus producing a softer M_1.

4. What is the rhythm or cadence of a mitral ball valve together with the normal S_2?
   ANS.: The order of sounds is CC----S_2-OC. Therefore, the rhythm is CLICK----duCLICK............CLICK----duCLICK.

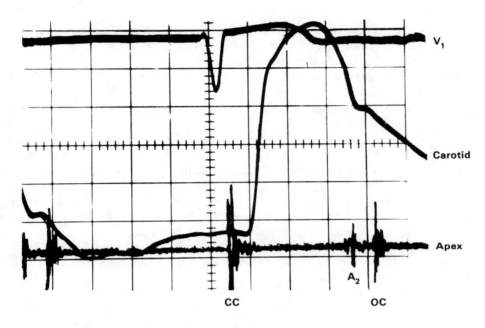

Mitral Prosthesis

With a mitral prosthetic valve, the first sound is replaced by the CC, but the second sound is the patient's own (at the apex it is only an A_2). The opening of the prosthetic valve (OC) will be heard at the same time as would an opening snap.

Note: a) This is a very important rhythm to recognize because it is the same as the rhythm of mitral stenosis with an opening snap, i.e., S_1----S_2-OS.

*b) A mitral CC, unlike the loud M_1 of mitral stenosis, is sometimes louder at the left lower sternal border than at the apex [12].

5. What extra sounds are commonly heard with a normal ball valve?
   ANS.: a) The ball often bounces and strikes the cage several times. This may produce from one to three multiple clicks, trailing off after the major click.

   Note: If the extra clicks disappear, it may be a sign of early ball valve swelling if a Silastic ball is present, or of thrombus on the cage.

   b) An early systolic crunchy murmur following the OC may be heard normally with an aortic prosthesis.

   *c) A presystolic click due to atrial contraction may be heard at the apex; by causing either eddy currents or a **Bernoulli effect,** it may raise the ball high enough to strike the ring.

---

*Material marked with an asterisk is for reference and for advanced students in cardiology.
Boldface type indicates that the term is explained in the Glossary.

PROSTHETIC VALVE ABNORMALITIES

Aortic Prosthetic Valve Abnormalities

* 1. What is meant by "ball valve variance"?

   ANS.: It refers to the deformation of a Silastic ball by swelling or cracking [6, 7, 8]. This does not occur with the metallic balls now in use.

2. What can make the OC softer than normal?

   ANS.: The OC may be muffled, i.e., less than 50 percent of the loudness of the CC on a phonocardiogram

   a) If there is a clot on the cage that cushions the impact of the ball as it strikes the cage, or

   b) If there is a cardiomyopathy, with resultant poor myocardial contractility [4].

3. How can you tell that a metallic (titanium or "stellite") ball is malfunctioning owing to clot formation?

   ANS.: A normal metallic ball valve produces multiple systolic clicks (like the rapid firing of a machine gun) owing to fluttering of the ball. When these clicks disappear, metallic ball valve malfunction is probable.

   Note: Plastic balls do not produce multiple clicks as a rule.

4. What can cause an aortic prosthetic valve to become regurgitant?

   ANS.: A paravalvular (suture line) leak.

   Note: a) Small aortic paravalvular leaks occur in at least 15 percent of such valves [13] and usually produce regurgitant murmurs.

   * b) When *severe* aortic regurgitation occurs with a prosthetic aortic valve, there has usually been a heavily calcified valve preoperatively, involving the valve ring, which does not hold sutures well.

   * c) When an aortic prosthesis becomes detached and has a rocking motion as it hangs only by a hinge of sutures (usually at the site of the former posterior noncoronary cusp), the detached prosthesis may push up the anterior mitral leaflet during diastole, resulting in a relative stenosis. This can cause a mid-diastolic murmur [13]. The abnormal rocking motion can usually be detected by fluoroscopy.

5. What is the major difference in the OC and CC of a disc valve and those of a ball valve?

   ANS.: The OC of a disc valve is normally softer than the CC and therefore sounds like an abnormal ball valve.

Mitral Prosthetic Valve Abnormalities

1. How can you diagnose mitral ball valve abnormalities?

   ANS.: There is a ball valve abnormality if

   a) The OC becomes muffled or disappears.

   b) A mitral diastolic murmur indicative of prosthetic valve stenosis is heard [9].

   c) The A_2–OC interval varies without regard to cycle length [10].

   d) The A_2–OC interval is greater than 150 msec.

   e) The A_2–OC is less than 70 msec. This suggests that the ball valve is either too small or is obstructed by clot and is producing significant stenosis [15].

* *Note:* a) If the OC is less than 35 percent of the amplitude of the CC at the apex or left sternal border, either interference with the prosthetic ball or disc or a paravalvular leak should be suspected [14]. (Severe LV failure may also soften the OC.)

b) An OC of the mitral valve (disc or ball) can disappear with marked valve ring detachment because ventricular filling then takes place preferentially through the paravalvular leak, and flow through the prosthetic valve may not be sufficient to cause the ball to produce a sound [2].

c) An Austin Flint murmur (diastolic rumble at the apex) due to aortic regurgitation that interferes with mitral valve opening may occur even in the presence of a prosthetic mitral ball valve [9].

2. How does the murmur of a paravalvular prosthetic mitral valve leak differ from that of native valve regurgitation?

ANS.: a) A systolic apical murmur due to a paravalvular leak is often not audible even when severe [14].

b) It may be audible only in unexpected places, such as the posterior chest wall.

Note: The development of unexplained heart failure in a patient with a prosthetic mitral valve should always raise the suspicion of silent, severe mitral regurgitation due to a paravalvular leak.

* 3. When can a mitral ball valve close even before the ventricle contracts?

ANS.: a) In sinus rhythm, when there is a long P–R interval. This will produce a very soft CC [3, 5].

b) In atrial fibrillation, when there is a long R–R interval [5].

c) In sudden, severe aortic regurgitation, when the diastolic pressure in the LV exceeds left atrial pressure in mid-diastole [1].

PORCINE HETEROGRAFTS

1. Which valve is taken from the pig's heart to be used for mitral valve replacement? Why?

ANS.: The aortic valve. An aortic valve does not require chordae tendineae or papillary muscles.

2. What proportion of normally functioning porcine heterografts in the mitral position have (a) an OS (b) a "mitral" diastolic rumble?

ANS.: a) About two-thirds.

b) About one-half [11].

REFERENCES

1. Agnew, T. M., and Carlisle, R. Premature valve closure in patient with a mitral Starr-Edwards prosthesis and aortic incompetence. *Br. Heart J.* 32:436, 1970.

2. Aravanis, C., Toutouzas, P., and Stavrou, S. Disappearance of opening sound of Starr-Edwards mitral valve due to valvular detachment. *Br. Heart J.* 34:1314, 1972.
3. Brown, D. F. Decreased intensity of closure sound in a normally functioning Starr-Edwards mitral valve prosthesis. *Am. J. Cardiol.* 31:93, 1973.
4. Delman, A. J. Aortic ball variance. *Am. Heart J.* 83:291, 1972.
5. Hamby, R. I., Aintablian, A., and Wisoff, G. B. Mechanism of closure of the mitral prosthetic valve and the role of atrial systole. *Am. J. Cardiol.* 31:616, 1973.
6. Hylen, J. C., et al. Phonocardiographic diagnosis of aortic ball variance. *Circulation* 38:90, 1968.
7. Hylen, J. C., et al. Sound spectographic diagnosis of aortic ball variance. *Circulation* 38:849, 1969.
8. Hylen, J. C., et al. Aortic ball variance: Diagnosis and treatment. *Ann. Intern. Med.* 72:1, 1970.
9. Leachman, R. D., and Cokkinos, D. V. P. Absence of opening click in dehiscence of mitral valve prosthesis. *N. Engl. J. Med.* 281:461, 1969.
10. Schaefer, R. A., et al. Diastolic murmurs in the presence of Starr-Edwards mitral prosthesis. *Circulation* 51:402, 1975.
11. Schluger, J., Mannix, E. P., Jr., and Wolf, R. E. Auscultatory and phonocardiographic sign of ball variance in a mitral prosthetic valve. *Am. Heart J.* 81:809, 1971.
12. Shah, P. M., McCanon, D. M., and Luisada, A. A. Spread of the "mitral" sound over the chest: A study of five subjects with the Starr-Edwards valve. *Circulation* 28:1102, 1963.
13. Smith, N. D., Raisada, V., and Abrams, J. Auscultation of the normally functioning prosthetic valve. *Ann. Intern. Med.* 95:5, 1981.
14. Sutton, G. C., and Wright, J. E. C. Major detachment of aortic prosthetic valves. *Br. Heart J.* 337, 1970.
15. Willerson, J. T., et al. Non-invasive assessment of prosthetic mitral paravalvular and intravalvular regurgitation. *Br. Heart J.* 34:561, 1972.
16. Wise, J. R., Jr., Webb-Peploe, M., and Oakley, C. M. Detection of prosthetic mitral valve obstruction by phonocardiography. *Am. J. Cardiol.* 28:107, 1971.

18. *Systolic Time Intervals*

DEFINITIONS AND METHODS OF MEASUREMENTS

1. What are the systolic time intervals (STIs)?
   ANS.: They are the left ventricular (LV) ejection time (ET) and the preejection period (PEP).
2. What is the advantage of learning how to record and interpret STIs?
   ANS.: Measuring and interpreting STIs is probably the most simple and accurate noninvasive method of evaluating myocardial function because they reveal not only the degree of ejection but also the heart's ability to undergo isovolumic contraction.
3. What is meant by "left ventricular ET"? How is it measured?
   ANS.: It is the time between the opening and closing of the aortic valves. It can be measured directly from an echocardiographic study of aortic valve motion. It can also be measured indirectly as the interval between the upstroke and the dicrotic notch of an external carotid pulse tracing. The external carotid tracing is obtained by applying a funnel or other pulse pickup over the carotid artery. The pulse pickup is connected to a pressure transducer amplifier, and recorder. (See page 141 for explanation of transducer.)

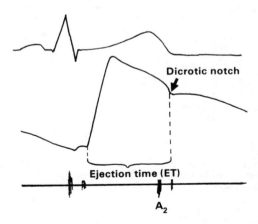

The ET is measured from the upstroke of the carotid to the dicrotic notch. A slight hump is often seen preceding the first sharp upstoke. This probably represents isovolumic contraction time and should not be included in the ET. The ET is often called the LVET, but the LV seems redundant, since we assume that we are dealing with left-sided events unless told otherwise.

4. What is meant by the "PEP"?
   ANS.: It is the time between the beginning of electrical activation of the heart (the onset of the Q or R wave of the QRS) and the opening of the aortic valve (indirectly measured by the onset of the rise in carotid pressure on the pulse

tracing). Because it is mostly dependent on LV **isovolumic contraction** time, changes in isovolumic contraction time are reflected in changes in PEP [54].

*Note: a) The PEP actually consists of three intervals:

1) Beginning of QRS to onset of LV contraction (electromechanical interval).
2) Onset of LV contraction to closure of mitral valve (M_1) (preisovolumic contraction).
3) M_1 to onset of aortic ejection (isovolumic contraction). Most changes in PEP are due to changes in the isovolumic contraction period [51].

b) There is a delay of 10–40 msec between the actual opening of the aortic valve and the time of the upstroke of the carotid pulse because it takes time for the pulse wave to travel from the aortic valve to the carotid and then from the pulse pickup on the neck through the rubber tubing to the transducer. There is a similar delay between the A_2 and the dicrotic notch. (The A_2 and the central aortic incisura have been found to be simultaneous when corrected for delays of transmission.) Since the delay is equal for the events

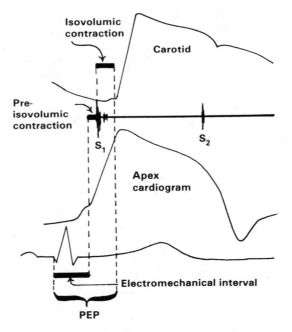

The PEP consists of 3 intervals; Q to onset of ventricular contraction, onset of ventricular contraction to M_1, and M_1 to aortic opening intervals. However, the M_1 to aortic opening (isovolumic contraction) is the major determinant of the PEP.

describing the ET, no correction is required for ET measurements. However, the PEP is defined by the QRS and the carotid upstroke, i.e., if the PEP were taken from the QRS to the onset of the carotid

---

Boldface type indicates that the term is explained in the Glossary.
* Material marked with an asterisk is for reference and for advanced students in cardiology.

upstroke without correction for pulse wave delay, the PEP would be falsely long.

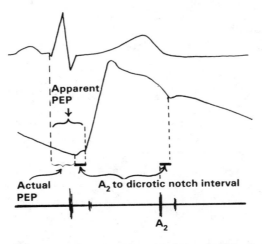

Apparent PEP

Actual PEP

A₂ to dicrotic notch interval

A₂

The A₂ to dicrotic notch interval is due to the delay that occurs when the pulse wave travels from the aortic root in the middle of the chest and through the rubber tubing of the pulse unit to the neck. The duration of the A₂ to notch delay is the same as that which occurs at the onset of the carotid upstroke.

5. How is the PEP measured and corrected for the delay in carotid upstroke?

   ANS.: You can correct the PEP for the delay in carotid upstroke by using the fact that the delay of the carotid upstroke is the same as the delay between the A₂ and the dicrotic notch [51]. The Q–A₂ (total electromechanical systole) is measured and the ET is subtracted. This gives you the PEP corrected for the pulse wave delays.

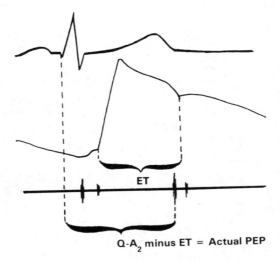

ET

Q-A₂ minus ET = Actual PEP

The Q–A₂, or total electromechanical systole, minus the ejection time will give you the PEP without the delays in pulse transmission.

Note: Accurate measurement of STIs can be obtained only by taking the following precautions:

a) The true initial electrical activation must show on the ECG lead that you use for the QRS. Therefore, it must show a septal vector, i.e., either a qR or an rS. The V_1 has been shown to represent the earliest deflection most accurately if it has a rS configuration [26, 92].

b) The upstroke of the carotid must not be measured from the beginning of any hump preceding the onset of the steepest slope. Such early humps are likely to occur during LV isovolumic contraction. The major cause of interobserver variation is the determination of the exact point of carotid upstroke [40].

c) The pulse tracing should be taken toward the end of expiration when the LV contains its maximum volume.

d) The patient must be supine. Only in severe congestive failure will the STIs not be affected by tilting the chest up, presumably because the failing ventricle responds very poorly to small changes in filling pressure. After administration of diuretics, however, the STIs may be affected by tilting the patient up even in heart failure [78].

e) Although the absolute Q–aortic opening time and ET can be read off directly from an M mode echocardiogram, the ET on echocardiograms tends to be longer and the PEP tends to be shorter than by the carotid and phonocardiogram method [20, 64].

PHYSIOLOGICAL CHANGES IN SYSTOLIC TIME INTERVALS

1. How are the STIs affected by (a) heart rate, (b) sex, (c) age, and (d) active occupation?

   ANS.: a) The faster the heart rate, the shorter the STI (both PEP and ET are shortened).

   b) Women have slightly longer STIs than men, due mainly to a prolongation of the ET. This difference begins at puberty [33].

   * c) Children have slightly shorter STIs than adults. Older subjects have slightly longer PEPs and ETs. (The ET increases by about 2 msec (0.002 sec) per decade, so that by age 80, it is about 10–20 msec (0.01–0.02 sec) longer than normal by the usual regression equation that corrects for heart rate.)

   * d) Active people have been found to have shorter PEPs than those who are sedentary [100].

   Note: If atrial pacing or atropine is used to change the heart rate, the PEP will not decrease with faster rates [22, 23, 75]. Sympathetic stimulation shortens both the ET and the PEP [16].

2. How can you correct the STIs for heart rate and sex?

   ANS.: Three methods are used.

   a) Read off the upper and lower limits of normal for rate and sex from graphs made from established linear regression equations. The graphs use one standard deviation as the limits [95].

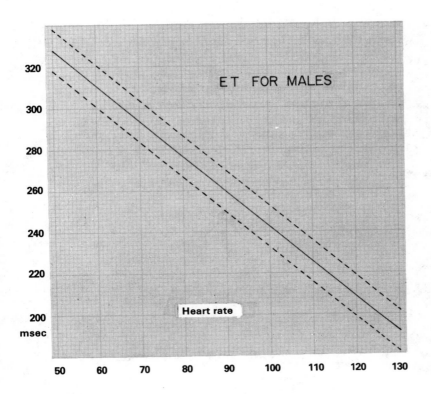

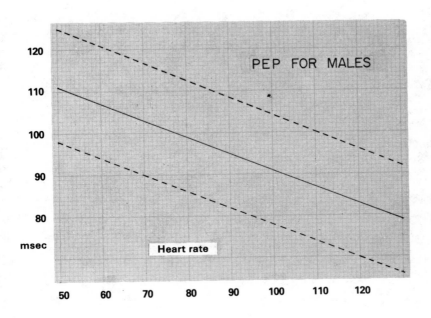

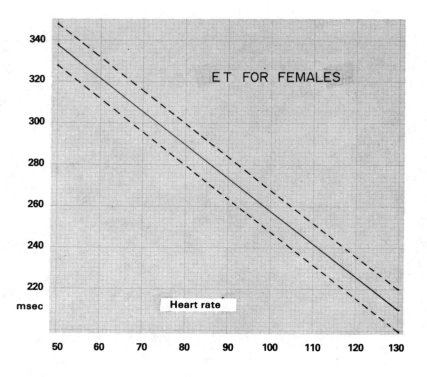

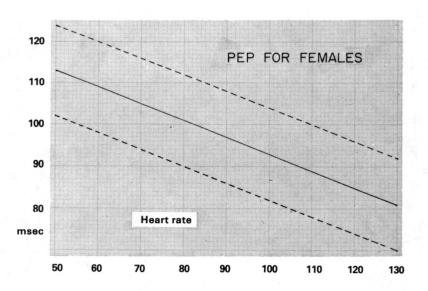

b) Use a single number calculated from the regression equation. This is the STI index [48, 94]. It offers a convenient expression for studying serial changes and for comparing patients.

*Note: The ET index for males is the ET plus 1.7 times the heart rate. The normal index is 413 ± 10 msec. For females, use 1.6, and the normal index is 418 ± 11 msec. The PEP index for males and females is the PEP plus 0.4 times the heart rate. The normal PEP index for males is 131 ± 10; for females, 133 ± 10.

c) Use the ratio of PEP/ET in order to ignore heart rate and sex.

*Note: a) PEP/ET ratios are unrelated to age or heart rates from age 1 month to 15 years, when the mean is 0.31 (S.D. = 0.05) [74]. For adults, the mean is 0.34 (S.D. = 0.04). Adolescents have a PEP/ET ratio between that of children and adults because although both PEP and ET increase with age, the PEP lengthens slightly more than does the ET [16, 91]. The upper normal for adults should therefore be considered to be 0.42, i.e., two standard deviations.

b) These regression equations cannot be used for STIs performed *during* exercise, although they can be used for the immediate post-exercise state [50].

c) A linear relation may be accepted in the normal adult between the ET and heart rate for heart rates of between 50 and 120 [99]. In children the linear relation is acceptable up to heart rates of 140 [17].

*3. How does a change in volume of the LV affect the STI?

ANS.: Although the increased Starling effect of increased volume tends to shorten the PEP, the volume effect lengthens the ET. (The $Q-S_2$ is scarcely affected.) Conversely, the decreased Starling effect of a decreased volume to the LV, such as occurs with diuretics, raising the chest, or standing, lengthens the PEP and shortens the ET. If the chest is raised to 45 degrees, the PEP/ET is 28 ± 0.03 [58]. If the chest is raised to 60 degrees, there is almost a 25 percent decrease in return of blood to the heart and lungs.

Note: a) In the seventh or eighth month of pregnancy, at the time of maximum expansion of blood volume (20–100 percent increase), the PEP is shortened and the ET is prolonged, as expected [61].

b) Athletes tend to have lengthened STIs, but especially the PEP, so that their PEP/ET tends to be 0.38 ± 0.08 [84]. This is presumably the effect of their increased cardiac volume, bradycardia, and physiological hypertrophy.

EFFECT OF MYOCARDIAL DAMAGE ON THE SYSTOLIC TIME INTERVALS

1. How does total time for contraction of a piece of muscle from a subject in heart failure compare with normal muscle?

ANS.: Surprisingly, the total time for contraction is *unchanged,* i.e., if it takes 300 msec (0.30 sec) for total contraction time before failure, it will take about 300 msec after heart failure [73].

2. How has it been shown that the entire LV also takes the same time for total contraction after heart failure as before it went into failure?
   ANS.: The Q–S$_2$ (PEP + ET) is the same in patients with and without failure.
3. Does the heart in failure take a longer or shorter time to raise pressure to open the aortic valve, i.e., how is isovolumic contraction time affected?
   ANS.: Isovolumic contraction time is prolonged (which is the same as saying that the PEP is prolonged.)
4. If the PEP is prolonged in heart failure, and the total contraction time is unchanged, what must happen to the ET in heart failure?
   ANS.: The ET must shorten.
*5. How is the PEP/ET ratio affected by heart failure?
   ANS.: Since the PEP lengthens and the ET shortens, the ratio increases with increasing failure.
   Note: The PEP/ET ratio can be used in a regression equation for **ejection fraction** in the formula $1.125 - (1.25 \times PEP/ET)$ with a standard deviation of 0.08.

   This formula was obtained from a study of mitral valve disease (with and without atrial fibrillation), coronary and idiopathic cardiomyopathies, hypertrophic subaortic stenosis, aortic regurgitation, and acute pericarditis [30]. The r value was 0.90, with a p value of less than 0.01. Another study of patients with pure coronary disease, with and without previous infarction, showed a good PEP/ET correlation with the angiographic ejection fraction (r value of 0.84) [77]. The poor correlation obtained in some studies between ejection fraction and STIs in patients with coronary disease may be explained by methodology [8, 77]. Prolongation of PEP has been shown to correlate closely with incoordinate LV wall movement during isovolumic contraction.

*HYPERTENSION AND SYSTOLIC TIME INTERVALS

*1. How does chronic hypertension without failure affect the STIs?
   ANS.: If the diastolic blood pressure is 90 or more, the PEP is prolonged. If the systolic pressure is 140 or more, the ET is prolonged [39].
   Note: a) In the elderly the ET increases by about 1.3 msec for each 10 mm Hg increment in systolic blood pressure [101].
   b) The prolonged PEP in a hypertensive patient may be entirely due to a prolonged Q–1 and not to a prolonged isovolumic contraction time [86]. The reason is unknown.
   c) If a hypertensive patient has a high catecholamine level, the PEP and PEP/ET ratio are normalized [24].
   d) If the hypertension is due to renal artery stenosis, the PEP is shorter than it is in essential hypertension [86]. (This has been studied only in women.)
*2. How are the STIs affected by a transient (a) increase in blood pressure and (b) decrease in blood pressure?
   ANS.: A transient increase in blood pressure prolongs the PEP, but the effects on the ET are variable.

Note: Raising the blood pressure of young healthy men with a vasopressor agent prolongs the ET [71].

EFFECT OF CORONARY ARTERY DISEASE (WITHOUT FAILURE) ON STIs

* 1. How does ischemic heart disease without heart failure affect the $Q–S_2$ (total contraction time) and the STIs? Why?

   ANS.: It shortens the $Q–S_2$. This has been attributed to a hyperadrenergic state. (See Question 3, below.) One study in patients with triple coronary disease showed that this hyperadrenergic state primarily shortens the ET [16]. The isovolumic contraction time was prolonged but was counterbalanced by a shortening of the $Q–M_1$ interval [13].

   Note: In heart failure due to ischemic coronary disease the PEP is prolonged by both isovolumic contraction time and $Q–M_1$ prolongation.

* 2. How do STIs change immediately after exercise in patients with coronary disease?

   ANS.: If the ET is taken with the patient supine immediately after about 4 minutes of moderate exercise, it is prolonged by more than 10 msec, and the maximum prolongation occurs about 30 sec postexercise. After vigorous exercise (**Bruce protocol** treadmill test), the maximum effect occurs about 4 minutes after exercise [47, 60].

   Note: a) This prolongation of ET has allowed identification of coronary disease when the exercise ECG was negative for ischemia. A coronary patient participating in an exercise program three to five times a week for a year will not have a prolonged ET after exercise [102].

   b) The ET prolongation after exercise does not necessarily occur in hypertensives without coronary disease [13].

   c) With diazepam or beta blockade, the ET may be prolonged with supine exercise even in normal subjects [11, 49, 53].

   d) In patients with heart failure from any cause the postexercise PEP is prolonged more than the slight increase in ET, and therefore the PEP/ET is prolonged (82).

   e) The ET is also prolonged after exercise in some patients with the prolapsed mitral valve syndrome even when there are only clicks and no murmurs [46].

   f) The ET divided by the external isovolumic contraction time, i.e., the ET/EICT ratio, measured immediately after 3 minutes of exercise, correlates well with the ejection fraction. (The external isovolumic contraction time is calculated by subtracting the ET from the $M_1–A_2$ interval.)

   If the ET/EICT ratio is 5.7 or less, the ejection fraction is less than 50 percent. If the ratio is 5.8 or more, the ejection fraction is more than 50 percent. In normal men without angina or a history of infarction, the ratio after exercise is over 6 [5].

   g) Patients with asymptomatic coronary disease have an increased PEP/ET ratio 5 minutes after smoking two cigarettes. Normal subjects have a decreased PEP/ET ratio in the same situation [42].

* 3. Why is the ET prolonged with exercise in subjects with coronary disease?

ANS.: The increased volume that returns to the heart in the immediate postexercise state can be ejected in a normal time by normal heart beats because of the effect of catecholamines. The ischemic heart may have a decreased ability to respond to catecholamines, perhaps because it is already hyperadrenergic, even at rest.

* 4. What happens to the STIs in the first few days after acute myocardial infarction in the absence of clinical heart failure? Why?

ANS.: In the first few days all the STIs are shortened. The shortened PEP is due presumably to the effect of excess catecholamines [88, 89]. However, the shortened ET cannot be correlated with catecholamine secretion and probably reflects a true decrease in stroke volume [66].

Note: a) This means that a "normal" PEP at this time is actually too long, i.e., under the influence of catecholamines, the PEP should be short [48].

5. How can STIs be used in angina pectoris patients to indicate prognosis?

ANS.: In one study, a PEP/ET ratio of 0.5 or more predicted a 50 percent chance of dying within 10 months [32]. In another study, the cumulative 5-year survival rate after a myocardial infarction for patients with a normal PEP/ET (0.42 or less) was 93 percent and with an abnormal ratio was 57 percent. This was a more potent prognostic indicator than was the extent of coronary disease by angiography [95A].

6. When will the PEP/ET ratio correlate with the echocardiographic LV ejection fraction in the presence of coronary disease?

ANS.: This correlation is found if the patient has had at least one acute myocardial infarction in the past and the septal echos moved normally [76].

* Note: a) In asymptomatic postinfarction patients the PEP/ET ratio is prolonged almost entirely via the PEP [70].

b) After nitroglycerin administration, the PEP is prolonged more in patients with ischemic heart disease (without failure) than in normal subjects [69].

EFFECT OF VALVULAR HEART DISEASE ON STIs

1. Why does aortic stenosis (AS) prolong the ejection time?

ANS.: It takes the LV longer than normal to drop from its high systolic pressure to a low aortic closing pressure. Post-stenotic dilatation will lower impedance. The PEP is shortened, i.e., becomes "supernormal" partly because the LV starts to contract from a high end-diastolic pressure.

Note: a) In **hypertrophic subaortic stenosis** (HSS) the STIs are the same as they are in valvular AS. There is a fair correlation between the outflow gradient in HSS and the PEP/ET, so that if the ratio is 0.25 or less, the gradient is 60 or more. If the ratio is 0.2 or less, the gradient is 120 or more [80].

b) If the ET is not prolonged, the cross-sectional area of the valve is not reduced enough to require surgery [6].

c) The ET is progressively prolonged with increasing obstruction as long as LV function is normal [45]. When an AS patient is in failure, the STIs may become normal, i.e., the ET and PEP may be at the upper limit of normal [9].

d) When LV failure develops in valvular AS, the ET index never decreases below two standard deviations from normal (<398) [48].

e) If the ET/isovolumic contraction time (M_1–aortic upstroke) is 5 or more, the gradient is 90 or more [38].

f) Although in both HSS and valvular AS the ET may be prolonged by exercise [21], only in HSS will a "pointed-finger" carotid be produced by exercise or amyl nitrite (midsystolic dip and late, low end-systolic shoulder). (See figure on page 43.)

g) In one study on HSS, the degree of prolongation of ET in a postextrasystolic beat was (in the absence of failure) indicative of the gradient produced by the postextrasystolic potentiation. The prolongation of the ET varied from 0 to 85 msec [79]. With valvular AS, the ET was never prolonged more than 20 msec [99].

2. How does aortic regurgitation (AR) affect STIs?

ANS.: The increased end-diastolic volume causes a Starling effect that shortens the PEP. The increased volume to be ejected through only one outlet prolongs the ET.

*Note: Significant AS or AR tends to make the dicrotic notch on a carotid tracing disappear, so that the ET becomes impossible to measure. You can measure an ET even if the dicrotic notch is missing by using a transducer that is no longer useful for pulse tracings because it has developed a short time constant, thus changing it into a differential transducer that will show any change in velocity of movement as a sharp notch. The onset of the carotid first derivative upstroke and the final nadir correlate highly with the undifferentiated carotid tracing, even though both points come slightly earlier [55] than these points on a simultaneous ordinary carotid pulse tracing. This could make the PEP appear slightly shorter than it does with a normal pulse transducer.

3. How does mitral stenosis affect the STIs?

ANS.: If myocardial function is normal and the ejection fraction is normal, the STIs may be almost normal even with significant mitral stenosis except for a slightly long PEP, which does not, however, extend beyond the upper limits of normal [63, 83]. If, however, the ejection fraction is decreased, the PEP will be lengthened beyond normal and the ET will be shortened, as expected.

4. How does mitral regurgitation affect the STIs?

ANS.: The STIs remain normal or the PEP shortens unless there is at least moderate LV disease or moderate to severe MR [29]. Then an increase in PEP and a shortened ET occur [90].

*Note: a) After prosthetic valve replacement, the STIs that may have been normal preoperatively may become abnormal postoperatively. As the heart shrinks during the months following the operation, the STIs tend to return to normal.

b) In the presence of marked MS or MR, the prolonged ET of patients with significant AS can be reduced to normal [44].

c) Although the PEP/ET ratio is no different in patients with acute versus chronic MR, acute MR has shorter PEP and ET intervals, i.e., a shorter total electromechanical interval [10].

---

*EFFECT OF CONSTRICTION AND TAMPONADE ON STIs

*1. How can respiratory changes in STIs help diagnose tamponade?

ANS.: The normal maximum respiratory variation in ET is about 10 msec with slightly deeper respirations than normal. In tamponade, the ET may vary as much as 40 msec with respiration, even in the absence of any pulsus paradoxus [18].

Note: Even without tamponade, the greater the pericardial effusion, the higher the PEP ratio [41].

*2. How does chronic constrictive pericarditis (with markedly elevated venous pressure) affect the STIs?

ANS.: The ejection fraction is usually normal by the STI formula (see p. 413) [42]. A normal cardiac index at rest is usually found in such patients. Therefore, in a patient in heart failure, constriction should be suspected if he has an ejection fraction of more than 45 percent, an ET of more than 380 msec, or a PEP of less than 155 msec [4, 31].

Note: a) The PEP/ET ratio in constrictive pericarditis is usually normal or about 0.41 ± 0.07; in restrictive cardiomyopathy it is usually abnormal and is more likely to be 0.62 ± 0.08 [31, 43].

b) Conditions in which changes in diastolic duration do not affect LV filling, such as constrictive pericarditis or ASDs (blood shunted to the right side during long diastoles), do not change STIs with heart rate [67].

EFFECT OF CONDUCTION DEFECTS AND ARRHYTHMIAS ON STIs

1. How does left bundle branch block (LBBB) affect STIs? Why?

ANS.: It prolongs the PEP. Although in 2 studies only isovolumic contraction was prolonged [14], in other studies the prolonged PEP was occasionally due only or in addition to a delay in onset of ventricular contraction (a long electromechanical interval) [7, 34, 98, 103]. If marked left axis deviation is present with the LBBB, then isovolumic contraction time is almost always prolonged [57].

Note: In one study with intermittent RBBB, the STIs were not affected significantly by the block [59].

*2. How does anterior divisional block affect STIs?

ANS.: Anterior divisional block (marked left axis deviation) may prolong the PEP slightly. If RBBB is also present, the PEP is significantly prolonged, due both to a delay in the onset of LV contraction and to prolongation of isovolumic contraction time.

*3. How does atrial fibrillation affect the STIs?

ANS.: As the R–R becomes shorter and shorter, the decrease in LV filling pressure prolongs the PEP and shortens the ET. However, at long R–R intervals that would give a rate of less than 75 (cycle length 80 msec or more), the STIs appear much as if the patient were in sinus rhythm; you can then judge how the heart would function in sinus rhythm, although the "atrial kick" is absent, i.e., there will be a slightly depressed myocardial function [87].

*Note: In patients in atrial fibrillation and with mitral stenosis, AR, or severe failure from any cause, the ET remains linearly related to the heart rate [9, 87].

* 4. Why will a fast heart rate caused by atrial pacing or atropine not cause a short PEP, as in sinus tachycardia?

ANS.: Atrial pacing or atropine does not produce the positive inotropic effect of increased sympathetic discharge that usually accompanies sinus tachycardia. It merely shortens the diastolic filling period and reduces the Starling effect on the ventricles.

EFFECT OF DRUGS, HORMONES, AND MANEUVERS ON STIs

* 1. How does 15 sec of amyl nitrite inhalation affect the STIs in normal and ischemic hearts?

ANS.: Amyl nitrite inhalation in normal subjects decreases ET by about 25 msec and the PEP by about 30 msec. In patients with ischemic heart disease, the ET decreases by about 50 msec and the PEP by only about 20 msec [68]. When there is a less than 30 percent increase in the ET/PEP ratio after amyl nitrite inhalation, coronary artery disease can be diagnosed with a sensitivity of about 90 percent, a specificity of 85 percent, and a predictive value of 90 percent.

2. What is the effect of propranolol on STIs in a normal heart and in a heart subject to catecholamine stimulation?

ANS.: 10 mg of propranolol given intravenously (a large dose) will prolong a normal person's PEP by only 10–15 msec, but a catecholamine-shortened PEP will be prolonged much more.

Note: The effect of propranolol on the STIs of patients with angina and normal intervals at rest is sometimes surprising. In one study the ET was slightly prolonged or not affected and the PEP did not change, i.e., the negative inotropic effect of propranolol did not significantly prolong the PEP or shorten the ET [27]. However, another study showed the expected increase in PEP (but no change in ET) with increasing doses of propranolol [28]. In a study in which elevated levels of circulating and urinary catecholamines were found in patients with angina, propranolol lengthened the $Q–S_2$ more than it did in patients without coronary disease [97].

3. How does digitalis affect the STIs of (a) normal hearts and (b) hearts in failure?

ANS.: a) In normal hearts both the PEP and the ET are shortened.

b) In the failing heart the PEP is shortened to as much as the upper limit of normal, whereas the ET may either be shortened or stay the same, or, if a marked increase in stroke volume occurs, it may even be lengthened [35, 96].

Note: The effects of heart failure rarely are completely reversed by digitalis, so that an abnormal PEP/ET ratio is usually still evident even with large doses of digitalis.

4. How does the afterload and preload reduction of prazosin and nitrates affect STIs in patients with heart failure?

ANS.: The ET is prolonged, but the PEP is unaffected except by hydralazine, which shortens it. Therefore, there is little apparent positive inotropic effect on isovolumic contraction unless hydralazine is used.

*EFFECT OF SHUNTS ON STIs

*1. What happens to the isovolumic contraction time in children with (a) an uncomplicated VSD or (b) persistent ductus arteriosus (PDA)?

ANS.: Normal children have isovolumic contraction times of 29 ± 9 msec, with VSD 34 ± 8 msec, and with PDA, 18 ± 7 msec (all three groups were measured at heart rates of about 105). The PDA isovolumic contraction time was probably decreased by the low peripheral resistance. Therefore, PEPs should be short in PDAs but normal or prolonged in VSDs [81].

*2. What is the relationship between STIs and ASD shunt flows?

ANS.: The larger the shunt, the longer the PEP index, presumably because the larger the shunt, the less the volume of blood flowing into the LV. The ET tends to be shorter than normal but does not correlate with shunt size. The regression equation is

$$\frac{Q\,P}{Q\,S} = (0.077 \times \text{the PEPI}) - 8.48\ [93].$$

*3. How does a VSD shunt with normal pulmonary artery pressure correlate with STIs?

ANS.: In adults, if the PEP/ET ratio is normal, the pulmonary to systemic flow ratio is not more than 1.5:1. A markedly shortened ET suggests a shunt of at least 2:1 [56].

Note: This may not be true for children. The PEP increase does not correlate well with shunt flows in children.

4. How can STIs be used to predict adriamicin toxicity?

ANS.: If the PEP/ET ratio increases to more than 0.5 there is a danger that heart failure will develop [19].

5. What is the effect of (a) quinidine and (b) phenothiazines on STIs?

ANS.: a) Therapeutic doses of quinidine prolong the PEP and shorten the ET.

b) Phenothiazines have no effect on STIs [65].

6. What is the effect of uncontrolled diabetes on STIs?

ANS.: The PEP is shorter than expected, presumably due to increased adrenergic stimulus. This becomes normal when blood sugar is controlled by oral antidiabetic agents [85].

7. How are the STIs affected by (a) hypothyroidism and (b) hyperthyroidism?

ANS.: a) In hypothyroidism the PEP is prolonged and the ET is shortened [25, 35]. The severity of myocardial dysfunction varies with the severity of the hypothyroidism [12].

b) In hyperthyroidism, the PEP is shortened and the ET remains normal or is shortened slightly [3, 14, 59]. This suggests an effect of excess catecholamines [35, 85]. Propranolol lengthens the short PEP in thyrotox-icosis but not to normal values [52].

MISCELLANEOUS CONDITIONS AND STIs

1. How does chronic obstructive pulmonary disease (COPD) affect STIs?
   ANS.: Severe COPD patients have longer PEPs and shorter ETs than normal. The reason is unknown [37].
2. What is the effect on STIs if anemia is present but no heart failure?
   ANS.: If the anemia is under 7 grams, the PEP may be shortened and the ET lengthened if there is a high output state [1]. When anemia was due to sickle cell disease in adults, an abnormal PEP/ET ratio was seen in one study [85].
*3. What is the effect on STIs of Cushing's disease in patients treated with large doses of corticosteroids for prolonged periods?
   ANS.: The PEP/ET ratio is markedly increased [2].

REFERENCES

1. Abdullah, A. K., Siddiqui, M. A., and Tajuddin, M. Systolic time intervals in chronic anemia. *Am. Heart J.* 94:287, 1977.
2. Akatsuka, N., Yamaguchi, T., and Matsuda, M. Long-term effect of corticosteroids on cardiac function. *Jap. Heart J.* 15:443, 1974.
3. Amidi, M., et al. Effect of the thyroid state of myocardial contractility and ventricular ejection rate in man. *Circulation* 38:229, 1968.
4. Armstrong, T. S., Lewis, B. S., and Gotsman, M. S. Systolic time intervals in constrictive pericarditis and severe primary myocardial disease. *Am. Heart J.* 85:6, 1973.
5. Aronow, W. S., Bowyer, A., and Kaplan, M. A. External isovolumic contraction times and left ventricular ejection time/external isovolumic contraction time ratios at rest and after exercise in coronary heart disease. *Circulation* 43:59, 1971.
6. Bache, R. J., Wang, Y., and Greenfield, J. C., Jr. Left ventricular ejection times in valvular aortic stenosis. *Circulation* 47:527, 1973.
7. Baragan, J., et al. Chronic left complete bundle-branch block. *Br. Heart J.* 30:196, 1968.
8. Basilico, F. C., et al. Non-invasive measurement of left ventricular function in coronary artery disease. *Br. Heart J.* 45:369, 1981.
9. Bonner, A. J., Jr., and Tavel, M. E. Systolic time intervals. *Arch. Intern. Med.* 132:816, 1973.
10. Boudoulas, H., et al. Abbreviation of systolic time intervals in acute mitral regurgitation: Effect of prosthetic mitral valve replacement. *Am. J. Cardiol.* 44:595, 1979.
11. Boudoulas, H., et al. Effect of propranolol on postexercise left ventricular ejection time index. *J. Am. Cardiol.* 48:357, 1981.
12. Bough, E. W., et al. Myocardial function in hypothyroidism. *Arch. Intern. Med.* 138, 1476, 1978.
13. Bowlby, J. R. Effects of exercise on left ventricular ejection in patients with hypertension or angina pectoris. *Am. Heart J.* 97, 348, 1979.
14. Braunwald, E., and Morrow, A. G. Sequence of ventricular contraction in human bundle branch block. *Am. J. Med.* 23:205, 1957.
15. Burckhardt, D., et al. The systolic time intervals in thyroid dysfunction. *Am. Heart J.* 95:187, 1978.
16. Buyukozturk, K., Kimbiris, D., and Segal, B. L. Systolic time intervals. *Am. J. Cardiol.* 28:183, 1971.
17. Cantor, A., et al. Systolic time intervals in children: Normal standards for clinical use. *Circulation* 58:1123, 1978.

18. Carter, W. H., McIntosh, H. D., and Orgain, E. S. Respiratory variation of left ventricular ejection time in patients with pericardial effusion. *Am. J. Cardiol.* 29:427, 1972.
19. Chaudron, J-M, et al. Adriamycin cardiotoxicity, prognostic value of the systolic time intervals. World Congress Cardiology, Tokyo, 1978.
20. Chilton, R. J., et al. Echocardiographic systolic time intervals: Left ventricular performance in coronary artery disease. *Arch. Intern. Med.* 140:240, 1980.
21. Cohn, K. E., Flamm, M. D., and Hancock, E. W. Amyl nitrite inhalation as a screening test for hypertrophic subaortic stenosis. *Am. J. Cardiol.* 21:681, 1968.
22. Cokkinos, D. V., et al. Influence of heart rate increase on uncorrected pre-ejection period/left ventricular ejection time (PEP/LVET) ratio in normal individuals. *Br. Heart J.* 38:683, 1976.
23. Conrad, K. A. Effects of atropine on diastolic time. *Circulation* 63:371, 1981.
24. Cousineau, D., Lapointe, L., and de Champlain, J. Circulating catecholamines and systolic time intervals in normotensive and hypertensive patients with and without left ventricular hypertrophy. *Am. Heart J.* 96:227, 1978.
25. Crowley, W. F., et al. Noninvasive evaluation of cardiac function in hypothyroidism. *N. Engl. J. Med.* 296:1, 1977.
26. Danzig, M. D., et al. Earlier onset of QRS in anterior precordial ECG leads. *Circulation* 54:447, 1976.
27. Frankl, W. S., Smith, W. K., and Orr, P. The effect of propranolol on left ventricular function in angina pectoris as measured by systolic time intervals. *Res. Commun. Chem. Pathol. Pharmacol.* 4:77, 1972.
28. Frishman, W., et al. Noninvasive assessment of clinical response to oral propranolol therapy. *Am. J. Cardiol.* 35:635, 1975.
29. Fujiki, A., et al. Noninvasive assessment of left ventricular performance and grade of regurgitation in mitral insufficiency. *J. Cardiography* 10:521, 1980.
30. Garrard, C. L., Jr., Weissler, A. M., and Doge, H. T. The relationship of alterations in systolic time intervals to ejection fraction in patients with cardiac disease. *Circulation* 42:455, 1970.
31. Ghose, S. K., Mitra, S. R., and Chhetri, M. K. Differential diagnosis between constrictive pericarditis and cardiomyopathy. *Br. Heart J.* 38:47, 1976.
32. Gillilan, R. E., et al. The prognostic value of systolic time intervals in angina pectoris patients. *Circulation* 60:268, 1979.
33. Golde, D., and Burstin, L. Systolic phases of the cardiac cycle in children. *Circulation* 42:1029, 1970.
34. Haft, J. I., Herman, M. V., and Gorlin, R. Left bundle branch block. *Circulation* 42:279, 1971.
35. Hillis, W. S., et al. Systolic time intervals in thyroid disease. *Clin. Endocrinol.* 4:617, 1975.
36. Hoeschen, R. J., and Cuddy, T. E. Dose-response relation between therapeutic levels of serum digoxin and systolic time intervals. *Am. J. Cardiol.* 35:469, 1975.
37. Hooper, R. G., and Whitcomb, M. E. Systolic time intervals in chronic obstructive pulmonary disease. *Circulation* 50:1205, 1974.
38. Ibrahim, M., et al. Systolic time intervals in valvular aortic stenosis and idiopathic hypertrophic subaortic stenosis. *Br. Heart J.* 35:276, 1973.
39. Inoue, K., et al. Left ventricular function in essential hypertension. *Am. J. Cardiol.* 32:264, 1973.
40. Ishikawa, K., et al. Intra- and interobserver variations in the measurement of systolic time intervals. *Chest* 81:341, 1982.
41. Ito, M., et al. Echocardiography, phonocardiography and carotid artery pulse wave in patients with pericardial effusion, with special reference to echocardiographic evaluation of left ventricular function. *J. Clin. Cardiol.* (Jap.) 5:15, 1976.
42. Jain, A. C., et al. Left ventricular function after cigarette smoking by chronic smokers: Comparison of normal subjects and patients with coronary disease. *Am. J. Cardiol.* 39:27, 1977.
43. Khullar, S., and Lewis, R. P. Usefulness of systolic time intervals in differential diagnosis of constrictive pericarditis and restrictive cardiomyopathy. *Br. Heart J.* 38:43, 1976.
44. Kligfield, P., et al. Effect of additional valve lesions on left ventricular ejection time in aortic stenosis. *Br. Heart J.* 39:1259, 1977.
45. Kligfield, P., and Okin, P. Effect of ventricular function on left ventricular ejection time in aortic stenosis. *Br. Heart J.* 42:438, 1979.

46. Kraus, M. E., and Naughton, J. Effect of exercise on left ventricular ejection time in patients with prolapsing mitral leaflet syndrome. *Chest* 69:484, 1976.
47. Lewis, R. P., et al. Enhanced diagnostic power of exercise testing for myocardial ischemia by addition of post-exercise left ventricular ejection time. *Am. J. Cardiol.* 39:767, 1977.
48. Lewis, R. P., et al. A critical review of the systolic time intervals. *Circulation* 56:146, 1977.
49. Lopez-Arostegul, F., et al. Effect of beta-adrenergic receptor blockade on response of systolic time intervals to exercise. *Circulation* 43 & 44 (Suppl. II):II-196, 1971.
50. Maher, J. T., et al. Systolic time intervals during submaximal and maximal exercise in man. *Am. Heart J.* 87:334, 1974.
51. Martin, C. E., et al. Direct correlation of external systolic time intervals with internal indices of left ventricular function in man. *Circulation* 44:419, 1971.
52. Mazzaferri, E. L., et al. Propranolol as a primary therapy for thyrotoxicosis. *Arch. Intern. Med.* 136:50, 1976.
53. McConahay, D. R., Martin, C. M., and Cheitlin, M. D. Resting and exercise systolic time intervals. *Circulation* 54:592, 1972.
54. Metzger, C. C., et al. True isovolumic contraction time; Its correlation with two external indexes of ventricular performance. *Am. J. Cardiol.* 25:434, 1970.
55. Nandi, P. S., and Spodick, D. H. Determination of systolic intervals utilizing the carotid first derivative. *Am. Heart J.* 80:495, 1973.
56. Nesje, O. A. Systolic time intervals in isolated ventricular septal defect in the adult. *Circulation* 62:609, 1980.
57. Nezuo, S., et al. Polygraphic analysis of the left ventricular function and systolic time intervals in cases of bundle-branch blocks. *Kawasaki Med. J.* 2:61, 1976.
58. Northover, B. J. Left ventricular systolic time intervals in patients with acute myocardial infarction. *Br. Heart J.* 43:506, 1980.
59. Parisi, A. F., et al. The short cardiac pre-ejection period. *Circulation* 49:900, 1974.
60. Pouget, J. M., et al. Abnormal responses of the systolic time intervals to exercise in patients with angina pectoris. *Circulation* 43:289, 1971.
61. Rubler, S., Schneebaum, R., and Hammer, N. Systolic time intervals in pregnancy and the postpartum period. *Am. Heart J.* 86:182, 1973.
62. Sabbah, H. N., et al. The aortic closure sound in pure aortic insufficiency. *Circulation* 56:859, 1977.
63. Sakamoto, T., et al. Systolic time intervals as a noninvasive quantitation of left ventricular function in mitral stenosis: Pre- and post-operative analysis of fifty-five cases. *Cardiovasc. Sound Bull.* 3:253, 1973.
64. Sakamoto, T., Matsuhisa, M., and Hayashi, T. Echocardiographic and phonocardiographic measurement of systolic time intervals. *Cardiovasc. Sound Bull.* 5:63, 1975.
65. Samet, J., and Surawicz, B. Chronic phenothiazine intake. *J. Clin. Pharmacol.* 174:588, 1974.
66. Samson, R. Changes in systolic time intervals in acute myocardial infarction. *Br. Heart J.* 32:839, 1970.
67. Sawayama, T., et al. Noninvasive evaluation of diastolic filling patterns in patients with atrial fibrillation by ejection time and preceding cycle length. *Am. J. Cardiol.* 45:1005, 1980.
68. Sawayama, T., et al. Influence of amyl nitrite inhalation on the systolic time intervals in normal subjects and in patients with ischemic heart disease. *Circulation* 40:327, 1969.
69. Sawayama, T., et al. Polygraphic studies on the effect of nitroglycerin in patients with ischaemic heart disease. *Br. Heart J.* 35:1234, 1973.
70. Schlesinger, Z., Ingber, A., and Stryjer, D. A comparative study of systolic time intervals in asymptomatic post-myocardial infarction patients versus "non-coronary" individuals. World Congress Cardiology, Tokyo, 1978. P. 1349.
71. Shaver, J. A., et al. The effect of steady-state increases in systemic arterial pressure on the duration of left ventricular ejection time. *J. Clin. Invest.* 47:217, 1968.
72. Shaw, D. J., et al. The effects of age and blood pressure upon the systolic time intervals in males aged 20–89 years. *J. Geron.* 28:133, 1973.
73. Spann, J. F., et al. Contractile state of cardiac muscle. *Circ. Res.* 21:341, 1967.
74. Spitaels, S., et al. The influence of heart rate and age on the systolic and diastolic time intervals in children. *Circulation* 49:1107, 1974.
75. Spodick, D. H. Systolic time intervals and impedance cardiography. *Br. Heart J.* 41:253, 1979.

76. Stack, R. S., et al. Left ventricular performance in coronary artery disease evaluated with systolic time intervals and echocardiography. *Am. J. Cardiol.* 37:331, 1976.

77. Stack, R. S., Sohn, Y. H., Weissler, A. M. Accuracy of systolic time intervals in detecting abnormal left ventricular performance in coronary artery disease. *Am. J. Cardiol.* 47:603, 1981.

78. Stafford, R. W., Harris, W. S., and Weissler, A. M. Left ventricular systolic time intervals as indices of postural circulatory stress in man. *Circulation* 41:485, 1970.

79. Stefadouros, M. A., et al. Postextrasystolic changes in systolic time intervals in the assessment of hypertrophic cardiomyopathy. *Br. Heart J.* 47:261, 1982.

80. Stefadouros, M. S., et al. Internally recorded systolic time intervals in hypertrophic subaortic stenosis. *Am. J. Cardiol.* 40:700, 1977.

81. Stopa, A., et al. The left isovolumic contraction time in left to right shunts. *Am. J. Cardiol.* 39:266, 1977.

82. Sugimoto, T., and Inasaka, T. The measurement of systolic time intervals in assessment of left ventricular performance. *Cardiovasc. Sound Bull.* 3:241, 1975.

83. Sutton, R., Hood, W. P., and Koch, G. G. Noninvasive assessment of left ventricular function in chronic heart disease. *Am. Heart J.* 93:289, 1977.

84. Suzuki, H., et al. The study of isometric contraction time and isometric relaxation time of left ventricle in athletes. World Congress Cardiology, Tokyo, 1978. P. 1343.

85. Sykes, C. A., et al. Changes in systolic time intervals during treatment of diabetes mellitus. *Br. Heart J.* 39:255, 1977.

86. Tarazi, R. C., Frohlich, E. D., and Dustan, H. P. Left atrial abnormality and ventricular preejection period in hypertension. *Dis. Chest* 55:214, 1969.

87. Tavel, M. E., et al. Left ventricular ejection time in atrial fibrillation. *Circulation* 46:744, 1972.

88. Val-Mejias, J., et al. Left ventricular performance during and after sickle cell crisis. *Am. Heart J.* 97:585, 1979.

89. Waagstein, F., Hjalmarson, A. C., and Wasir, H. S. Apex cardiogram and systolic time intervals in acute myocardial infarction and effect of practolol. *Br. Heart J.* 36:1109, 1974.

90. Wanderman, K. L., et al. Left ventricular performance in mitral regurgitation assessed with systolic time intervals and echocardiography. *Am. J. Cardiol.* 38:831, 1976.

91. Wanderman, K. L., et al. Systolic time intervals in adolescents, *Circulation* 63:204, 1981.

92. Wanderman, K. L., et al. Choice of electrocardiographic leads for recording the earliest QRS onset in noninvasive measurements. *Circulation* 63:933, 1981.

93. Wanderman, K. L., Ovsyshcher, I., and Gueron, M. Left ventricular performance in patients with atrial septal defect: Evaluation with noninvasive methods. *Am. J. Cardiol.* 41:487, 1978.

94. Weissler, A. M., and Garrard, C. L., Jr. Systolic time intervals in cardiac disease (1) *Mod. Concepts Cardiol. Dis.* 40:1, 1971.

95. Weissler, A. M., Harris, W. S., and Schoenfeld, C. D. Systolic time intervals in heart failure in man. *Circulation* 37:149, 1968.

95A. Weissler, A. M., et al. Prognostic significance of systolic time intervals after infarction. *Am. J. Cardiol.* 48:995, 1981.

96. Weissler, A. M., and Schoenfeld, C. D. Effect of digitalis on systolic time intervals in heart failure. *Am. J. Med. Sci.* 259:4, 1970.

97. Welch, T. G., and Lewis, R. P. Hyperadrenergic state in coronary artery disease. *Clin. Res.* 22:155, 1974.

98. Wennemark, J. R., Blake, D. F., and Keyde, P. Cardiodynamic effect of experimental bundle branch block in the dog. *Circ. Res.* 10:280, 1962.

99. White, C. W., and Zimmerman, T. J. Prolonged left ventricular ejection time in the post-premature beat: A sensitive sign of idiopathic hypertrophic subaortic stenosis. *Circulation* 52:306, 1975.

100. Whitsett, T. L., and Naughton, J. The effect of exercise on systolic time intervals in sedentary and active individuals and rehabilitated patients with heart disease. *Am. J. Cardiol.* 27:252, 1971.

101. Willems, J. L., et al. The left ventricular ejection time in elderly subjects. *Circulation* 42:37, 1970.

102. Winter, W. G., Leaman, D. M., and Anderson, R. A. The effect of exercise on intrinsic myocardial performance. *Circulation* 48:50, 1973.

103. Wong, B., et al. Effect of intermittent left bundle branch block on left ventricular performance in the normal heart. *Am. J. Cardiol.* 39:459, 1977.

Glossary

aneurysm Localized dilatation of either a blood vessel or a heart chamber. The commonest cause of an aterial aneurysm is atherosclerosis. In the aorta, an atherosclerotic aneurysm may be found in any part of the vessel where atrophy of the media (muscular layer) deep to an atherosclerotic plaque results in either a saccular or a fusiform (spindle-shaped) dilatation. The commonest site is the abdomen distal to the renal arteries. Syphilis (lues) used to be the commonest cause of thoracic aortic aneurysms, usually in the ascending aorta. When infection destroys a local area of any artery to cause a local dilatation, a mycotic aneurysm is said to have formed.

dissecting aneurysm In the correct pronunciation the "diss" rhymes with "kiss." Localized aortic dilatation that results from separation of the layers of the aortic wall by hemorrhage into the media secondary to degeneration of the media (cystic medial necrosis). In some patients it may begin with an intimal tear. It usually dissects distally, but when it dissects proximally, it may involve the aortic valve and produce aortic regurgitation, or it may dissect into the pericardial space, producing a fatal tamponade.

ventricular aneurysm A dilated segment of LV. It is commonly caused by myocardial infarction, but trauma has also caused it. These aneurysms vary in size from a few centimeters in diameter to a size one-half that of the LV. They rarely ever rupture but are likely to be the cause of mild to severe heart failure, or they may become the source of an embolus due to a thrombus that may completely fill the aneurysm. If the aneurysm is empty, it will usually bulge during systole (paradoxical motion or dyskinesis). Sometimes a large area of damaged myocardium fails to show any motion during systole, and this also is sometimes called an aneurysm. However, it is better to call this an area of akinesis, and, if the movement is slight but normal in direction, it may be called an area of hypokinesis.

anomalous pulmonary venous connection or drainage Drainage of one or more pulmonary veins, usually into the right atrium, superior vena cava, or inferior vena cava. In partial anomalous pulmonary venous return, if one or more of the pulmonary veins from the right lung have the anomalous connection, they empty into one of the following: azygos vein, superior or inferior vena cava, or right atrium. More rarely, a vein (or veins) from the left lung empties into the innominate vein, a left vertical vein, or the coronary sinus. The anomalous connection results in a left-to-right shunt with the same chambers overloaded as in an **atrial septal defect**. In *total anomalous pulmonary venous return* all of the pulmonary veins may enter any one of the following: a left vertical vein, the innominate vein, the coronary sinus, the right atrium, the superior or inferior vena cava, or the portal vein. An atrial septal defect is essential for survival. The hemodynamics are similar to those of a large atrial septal defect.

aortic sclerosis See **calcific aortic sclerosis**

aortic stenosis   Obstruction to LV outflow. This may occur at valvular, supravalvular, or subvalvular levels. The subvalvular obstruction may occasionally be due to a congenital fibrous ring just below the aortic valve (discrete subvalvular AS), but usually it is due to a hypertrophied septum impinging on the anterior leaflet of the mitral valve during systole (hypertrophic subaortic stenosis). See figure on page 98. The supravalvular type is associated with a characteristic facies. See page 33.

Aortic valvular stenosis without any other valves involved is almost always congenital, and about half of these are due to calcification of a bicuspid aortic valve. The acquired ones are usually due to rheumatic valvulitis and are associated with some mitral valve disease. In subjects over age 70, degenerative calcification of the aortic valve may be the commonest cause of aortic stenosis, especially in women.

arteriosclerosis   1. Atherosclerosis (the progressive laying down of lipid in the intima of an artery, starting with a fatty streak and ending with fibrosis and calcium and finally in a plaque). 2. Medial sclerosis (fibrosis of the media or muscular layer of arteries, which may end in "pipestem" arteries). Medial sclerosis affects only the larger peripheral arteries; i.e., the aorta and coronary arteries are subject to atherosclerosis, but not to medial sclerosis. Arterioles are not usually affected either by medial sclerosis or by atherosclerosis.

atrial myxoma   Tumor made up of soft, loose, friable tissue that is usually on a pedicle (pendunculated) attached to the atrial septum in the region of the fossa ovalis. It is almost twice as common in the left atrium as in the right atrium. It can protrude through its respective atrioventricular valve in diastole to produce a partial obstruction that imitates mitral or tricuspid stenosis and occasionally causes syncope. It may merely prevent complete closure of the valve, resulting in various degrees of mitral or tricuspid regurgitation. If the tumor becomes calcified, it may act like a wrecking ball and completely destroy the atrioventricular valve, producing severe regurgitation. Emboli from the friable tumor are among the commonest causes of clinical manifestations. For unknown reasons, the tumor acts as an inflammatory agent and commonly produces a high sedimentation rate and intermittent fevers, which, together with the occasional **clubbing,** mimic infective endocarditis. It may even produce reactions of an allergic type, resulting in puzzling skin and joint manifestations.

atrial septal defect   Opening between the atria, which may occur at three possible levels. The lower one is called a *primum* defect, the middle one is a *secundum* defect, and the upper one is called a *sinus venosus* defect. By far the commonest is the secundum, or fossa ovalis defect.

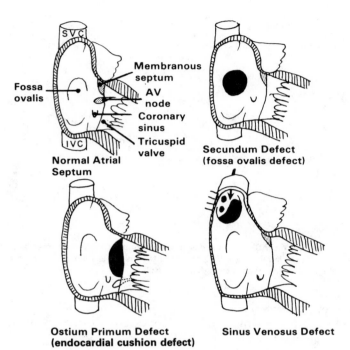

Normal Atrial Septum

Fossa ovalis

Membranous septum

AV node

Coronary sinus

Tricuspid valve

Secundum Defect (fossa ovalis defect)

Ostium Primum Defect (endocardial cushion defect)

Sinus Venosus Defect

The three levels of atrial septal defects are, in general, low, middle, and high. It may help your memory if you think of the lower two levels as the "first floor," or primum defect, and the "second floor," or secundum defect. The sinus venosus defect then remains and thus must be the "top floor," or high defect. The sinus venosus is the embryological site of the pacemaker of the heart, or the sinoatrial node. If you keep in mind that the sinoatrial node is at the junction of the superior vena cava and right atrium, it will be easy for you to remember that the sinus venosus defect is the high one. When the inferior wall of the fossa ovalis acts like a flap valve, it is called a patent foramen ovale. There will then be flow from the right to left atrium only if the pressures rises abnormally high in the right atrium. The flap is normally closed by the higher pressure in the left atrium relative to that in the right atrium. Note that in the sinus venosus defect, pulmonary veins are shown draining into the superior vena cava.

primum defect (incorrectly pronounced "preemum")   An atrial septal defect that is part of a possible spectrum of abnormalities caused by maldevelopment of the endocardial cushions, which are the dorsal and ventral tissues in the center of the fetal heart that give rise to

a) The inferior part of the atrial septum above.
b) The upper part of the ventricular septum below.
c) The medial (anterior) leaflet of the mitral valve to the left.
d) The septal leaflet of the tricuspid valve to the right.

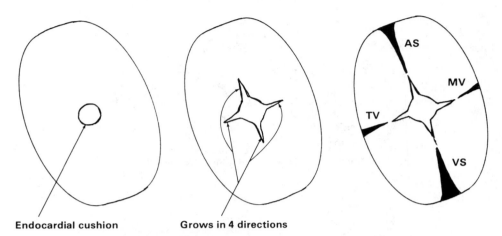

Endocardial cushion   Grows in 4 directions

If the lower part of the atrial septum (AS) does not develop, an ostium primum ASD results. If the upper part of the ventricular septum (VS) is missing, a VSD results. If the medial cushion parts of the mitral or tricuspid valves are missing, a cleft mitral or tricuspid leaflet results.

Any permutation or combination of endocardial cushion defects may occur. When defects in all four of the above structures are present, the condition is called a *complete atrioventricular canal*.

A left axis deviation on ECG is so common with endocardial cushion defects and so rare with atrial septal defects at higher levels that clinical differentiation of the primum from the secundum and sinus venosus defects by electrocardiogram is quite helpful.

sinus venosus defect   A high atrial septal defect that is always associated with an anomalous drainage of one or two right pulmonary veins into the superior vena cava. (See **anomalous pulmonary venous drainage**.)

The shunted blood in atrial septal defects travels from the left to the right atrium, from the right atrium to the right ventricle, from the right ventricle to the pulmonary artery, from the pulmonary artery to the pulmonary arterioles and veins, and from the pulmonary veins to the left atrium. Therefore, the right atrium, right ventricle and pulmonary vessels all have a volume overload. The left atrium, however, serves only as a conduit and does not become enlarged except under exceptional circumstances.

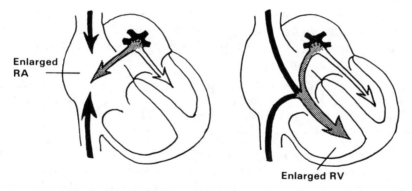

Enlarged
RA

Enlarged RV

Note that with an atrial septal defect, the right atrium and ventricle receive blood from two sources. They are volume-overloaded at the expense of blood to the left ventricle. An increase in total blood volume is the compensatory mechanism by which the left ventricle receives a normal volume for average physiological needs. When an atrial septal defect or any other left-to-right shunt is closed surgically, the total blood volume of the body decreases by the exact amount of the shunt.

atrioventricular block (AV block)   Conduction delay anywhere from the AV node to the ending of the bundle branches in the ventricle; i.e., the delay may occur in the AV node, the bundle of His, or the bundle branches. A first-degree AV block is recognized on an ECG by seeing a long P–R interval. Second-degree AV block refers to intermittent complete AV block in which a dropped QRS occurs periodically. If the AV block is complete, the atria and ventricles are dissociated and an independent pacemaker for the ventricles occurs either at or below the bundle of His. To use the term "heart block" to refer specifically to AV block should be avoided since all conduction defects are heart blocks. Also, "heart block" is a terrifying term to a patient.

atrioventricular dissociation   A condition in which the atria and ventricles have independent pacemakers. The lower pacemaker may be in the junctional area or deep in a ventricle. AV dissociation implies that atrial contraction has varying relationships to ventricular contraction; i.e., if the atria are in sinus rhythm, the P–R interval will be continually changing in a haphazard manner.

base of the heart   The upper part of the heart or **semilunar valve** area. The term implies that the heart looks like an inverted cone in the chest. The base of the cone is in the upper chest area.

beriberi heart disease   The effect on the heart of total body capillary dilatation caused by a deficiency of vitamin B_1 (thiamine). In order to fill the enlarged vascular bed, a marked hyperkinetic state is produced, with a high venous pressure, tachycardia, cardiomegely, peripheral edema, and rapid **circulation time**. In the occident, it is seen almost entirely in alcoholic persons who resort to an enormous intake of beer. An acute, fulminant, nonedematous form characterized by cardiovascular collapse and death within hours or days has been called Shoshin beriberi. (*Sho* is Japanese for "damage," and *shin* means "heart.")

Bernheim effect   Encroachment on the right ventricular cavity by the interventricular septum, which is bowed to the right by a dilated left ventricle, as described by the pathologist Bernheim in 1915 [1]. The enlargement of the left ventricle in diastole prevents diastolic filling of the right ventricle but does not interfere with right ventricular outflow; i.e., it is not a kind of infundibular outflow obstruction but an obstruction to inflow. Such a large left ventricle is usually due to severe, chronic mitral regurgitation.

Bernoulli effect The drop in pressure on the surface of any structure caused by a flow over that structure. This tends to pull the structure toward the stream. An instrument utilizing the Bernoulli effect to measure flow is called a Venturi meter. The Bernoulli effect on the wings of an airplane raises it and keeps it airborne.

calcific aortic sclerosis or **aortic sclerosis** The infiltration of the aortic valve with fibrous tissue and often also with enough calcium to stiffen it and create turbulent flow but not enough to produce a significant pressure gradient across the valve. It is due to an unknown aging process. The term may also refer to atherosclerotic plaques in the aortic root, that are possibly responsible for some ejection murmurs in the elderly. Without calcium the condition is simply aortic sclerosis.

carcinoid heart disease Accumulation of grossly whitish-yellow fibrous tissue on the inner surface of the right ventricle or atrium, as well as on the undersurface of the tricuspid and pulmonary valves (rarely, of the mitral valve). It can hold the tricuspid or pulmonary valve in the semiclosed position and so cause tricuspid or pulmonary stenosis and regurgitation. Carcinoid heart disease is usually associ-

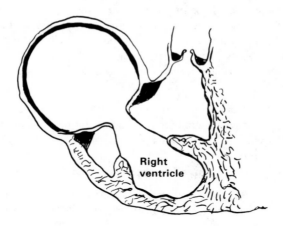

Carcinoid deposits tend to form on the undersurface of the tricuspid valves and the upper surface of the pulmonary valves and so hold them in a rigid, semiclosed position. The compliance of the right atrium can be reduced by a lining of carcinoid material, thus raising its pressure conspicuously.

ated with a carcinoid tumor of the bowel and with metastases to the liver. Bronchospasm, diarrhea, and various types of flushing (general redness, bright red patches or violaceous cyanosis) are all part of the carcinoid syndrome.

cardiomyopathy Myocardial damage from any cause. Therefore, it should have an adjective preceding it, e.g., idiopathic cardiomyopathy (often called primary myocardial disease), amyloid cardiomyopathy, or coronary or ischemic cardiomyopathy [3, 4, 11]. In the past, the term meant specifically only an idiopathic cardiomyopathy or primary myocardial disease.

Cheyne-Stokes respiration The periodic breathing characterized by a gradually increasing depth of respiration, culminating in a period of apnea that may last from a few seconds to as long as a minute. The commonest associated condition for the cardiologist is severe low-output due to heart failure. The neurologist more commonly sees it as a result of cerebral disease. Because it is exaggerated when dozing, and the hyperpneic phase can cause enough cerebral stimulation to prevent sleep, it is a possible cause of insomnia in a patient with heart failure.

circulation time The time it takes for a marker material to travel from the site of injection to the site of appearance, usually after it passes through the lungs or lesser circulation. The term has fallen into disuse because the usual injected materials, such as 5 ml of 20 percent Decholin (dehydrocholic acid) or 20 percent calcium gluconate, have caused occasional serious reactions and because comparison with objective methods (fluorescein) has shown many false prolongations of circulation time [13, 16]. The normal range is 10–18 sec.

clubbing A condition in which soft tissue of the terminal phalanges of the fingers or toes becomes hypertrophied and the nail finally curves excessively, giving a drumstick appearance. (See page 27 for method of eliciting.) In cardiac patients, clubbing is usually associated with **cyanosis,** but if not, it should suggest the presence of acute **infective endocarditis** that has been present for a few weeks, suppurative lung lesions, anoxic **cor pulmonale,** or metastatic lung cancer. More rarely, it is caused by chronic diarrhea with ulcerative colitis or may even be familial. In cardiac patients, the commonest causes of clubbing are tetralogy of Fallot and transposition of the great vessels. When clubbing and cyanosis are greater in the toes than in the hands, the condition is called differential cyanosis (see p. 351) and clubbing. (See figure on page 27.)

Note: Because the flow rate through clubbed digits is higher than normal and the venous blood from the arm appears brighter than the blood of a normal person, one of the possible causes of clubbing is patent arteriovenous anastomoses that bypass the capillaries, resulting in oxygen deficit and tissue hypertrophy [18].

coarctation Localized or diffuse narrowing of the aorta. The degree of constriction varies from slight to severe; rarely, it is complete. It is usually seen around the isthmus, which is the area just beyond both the left subclavian artery and the ductus arteriosus. It can occur proximal to the left subclavian artery and occasion-

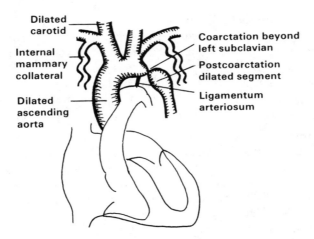

Dilated carotid

Internal mammary collateral

Dilated ascending aorta

Coarctation beyond left subclavian

Postcoarctation dilated segment

Ligamentum arteriosum

Localized narrowing of the aorta most often occurs at the junction of the aortic arch and the descending aorta distal to the ductus arteriosus. When on rare occasions it occurs proximal to the ductus, the narrowing is often diffuse and for some unknown reason associated with severe pulmonary hypertension and therefore with differential cyanosis.

ally even in the abdominal aorta. Collateral circulation to the vessels beyond the coarcted site is from arteries proximal to the coarctation, so that with the usual site of coarctation, collateral vessels develop through the internal mammary and shoulder girdle arteries to the intercostal arteries and can become very large and even palpable. In all the vessels proximal to the coarctation, there is hypertension and increased pulse pressure as well as dilatation. There is a very low systolic pressure and pulse pressure beyond the coarctation.

The aortic valve is commonly bicuspid and regurgitant, but is occasionally stenotic.

Preductal coarctation is commonly associated with diffuse narrowing of the aortic arch, pulmonary hypertension, and an **Eisenmenger syndrome,** as well as with differential cyanosis (see p. 27). This is sometimes known as the infantile type because patients rarely live beyond infancy.

compliance   Elastic resistance or stiffness of a structure, e.g., the stiffer the left ventricle, the less the compliance. To physicists it is change of volume/change of pressure. Generally, a thick ventricle is a noncompliant or stiff ventricle. Chronically volume-overloaded ventricles due to shunt or regurgitant flows are generally compliant. Pressure-overloaded ventricles are noncompliant.

constrictive pericarditis   Thickening of the pericardium by dense, fibrous tissue that may calcify. It results primarily in restriction of expansion of the heart but also often causes a slight restriction of systole as well, especially if the duration of the constriction is long enough to allow much infiltration of the epicardium by the fibrous tissue. Although both ventricles and atria are almost always involved simultaneously, inflow into the atria is not affected. The commonest cause is idiopathic, but the commonest *known* cause is tuberculosis. It has occasionally followed bacterial or viral pericarditis, radiotherapy of the chest, and the hemopericardium resulting from trauma. It is sometimes known as "Pick's disease" for no very good reason, since Pick was not the first to describe it.

cor pulmonale Right ventricular hypertrophy secondary to a lung abnormality. The term *cor pulmonale* does not require that the patient be in right ventricular failure. The pulmonary problem is usually chronic obstructive pulmonary disease (formerly known as emphysema) or arteriolar obstruction due to emboli or idiopathic (primary) pulmonary hypertension. (See checklist, p. 7 for clinical picture.)

corrected transposition Congenitally corrected transposition, or reversal of the great vessels so that the aortic root is anterior to the pulmonary artery, but with reversal or "inversion" of the ventricles as well. There is no physiological disturbance because vena caval blood feeds a right atrium that goes to a ventricle—anatomically, a left ventricle—that gives off the pulmonary artery. The blood from the lungs flows into a left atrium, which passes through a tricuspid valve to a systemic ventricle that is anatomically a right ventricle (trabeculated and with an **infundibulum,** or outflow tract).

Corrigan's pulse Large-volume carotid pulsation seen in patients with severe aortic regurgitation. It refers to what is seen, not what is felt.

cor triatriatum Congenital cardiac anomaly in which all the pulmonary veins join together to form a common chamber and empty into the left atrium through a small opening; i.e., it is a kind of supravalvular mitral stenosis. The common chamber is usually situated inside the left atrium. Its major complication is secondary pulmonary hypertension.

cyanosis Bluish or purplish color imparted to the skin and mucous membranes, usually as a result of at least 5 gm of reduced hemoglobin per 100 ml of blood in the surface capillaries, but occasionally due to an abnormal hemoglobin such as sulfmethemoglobin or methemoglobin. The higher the absolute concentration of circulatory hemoglobin, the more easily will cyanosis be apparent. For example, an 80 percent saturation with 10 gm hemoglobin per 100 ml of blood would produce 2 gm of reduced hemoglobin, whereas the same percentage of saturation in a person with 15 gm of hemoglobin would produce 3 gm of reduced hemoglobin.

central cyanosis A condition in which the arterial blood has a reduced saturation with oxygen. When it is severe and chronic, polycythemia and clubbing accompany it. It can be seen in the warm areas, such as the tongue and inner surface of the lips. Usually the oxygen saturation is 80 percent or less before central cyanosis can be recognized.

differential cyanosis See pp. 10, 27, 351.

peripheral cyanosis Cyanosis in cool areas of the body, which is usually associated with normally saturated arterial blood. It is seen on the nose, ears, cheeks, and fingers. It is due to sluggish blood flow that allows excessive extraction of oxygen in these tissues and can be seen in normal subjects, as when swimming in cold water.

Down's syndrome (trisomy 21 or mongolism) The outstanding findings are mental retardation, hypotonia, medial epicanthus, large (often protruding) fissured tongue, small orbits, gray–white specks in the iris (Brushfield's spots), and a hand with short fingers, a distally displaced axial triradius, and a transverse side-to-side palmar crease (simian crease). The major cardiac abnormalities are some form of endocardial cushion defect (see **atrial septal defect**).

ductus arteriosus See **persistent ductus arteriosus.**

Ebstein's anomaly A downward displaced deformed tricuspid valve. One leaflet is displaced into the right ventricle (RV), so that some RV is in the right atrium [8]. There is commonly tricuspid regurgitation, which can enlarge the **outflow tract** of the RV. The right atrium may be so large that it dominates the ECG (tall peaked P waves) and x-ray picture. A right-to-left shunt through an **atrial septal defect** or patent foramen ovale with resultant cyanosis is common. Atrial arrhythmias or heart failure are the most common complications.

Eisenmenger syndrome or **reaction** Severe pulmonary hypertension due to high and fixed pulmonary arteriolar resistance caused by a large left-to-right shunt due to a ventricular septal defect (VSD), atrial septal defect (ASD), or persistent ductus arteriosus (PDA). The high right ventricular and right atrial pressure result in a right-to-left shunt through the ASD, VSD, or PDA. The right-to-left shunt may be dominant or it may be a balanced shunt, i.e., as much left-to-right as right-to-left. When a VSD is the cause, the term Eisenmenger *complex* is often used, because this is the original lesion described by Eisenmenger in 1897 [9].

The Eisenmenger syndrome begins in infancy when a PDA or VSD is responsible; it begins in the teens or later when the shunt is an ASD. The pulmonary hypertension of the Eisenmenger syndrome with cyanosis is irreversible and prohibits surgical closure of the defect. A patient with the irreversible pathological changes in the lung vessels (plexiform lesions) due to an Eisenmenger reaction is often said to have "pulmonary vascular disease."
Note: An Eisenmenger PDA has occasionally developed in adulthood [10].

ejection fraction Relationship between stroke volume (volume ejected) and end-diastolic volume (volume at the moment of greatest filling of the ventricle at the end of diastole). It is the volume at the end of diastole minus the volume at the end of systole divided by the volume at the end of diastole times 100. (The normal range is 70 ± 10%.)

endocardial cushion defect See **atrial septal defect.**

endocarditis See **infective endocarditis.**

Fallot's tetralogy See **tetralogy of Fallot.**

filling pressure The pressure in the ventricle that distends it, especially toward the end of diastole, so that it is most related to the end-diastolic pressure in the ventricle. The change in volume that produces this diastolic pressure is called the preload. It is controlled on the right side by venous pressure and, in sinus rhythm, also by the power of the right atrial contraction. On the left side it is controlled by the left atrial pressure and, in sinus rhythm, also by the power of left atrial contraction or the "atrial kick."

*Material marked with an asterisk is for reference and for advanced students in cardiology.

frequency   In auscultation, the number of oscillations per second made by a vibrating or sound-producing structure.

gradient   Difference in pressure along a conduit that results in flow from highest to lowest pressure. In cardiology, it usually refers to a difference in pressure across an obstruction, i.e., it is generally caused by a drop in pressure across an obstruction (usually a stenotic artery or valve), so that the pressure is higher proximal than distal to the obstruction. (See figure on page 238.)

Hurler's syndrome (gargoylism)   A rare autosomal recessive metabolic disorder in which abnormal glycoproteins are deposited in most of the organs, resulting in dwarfism, mental retardation, deafness, and **cardiomyopathy.** The heart valves may be thickened.

hypertelorism   Widely set eyes found in such syndromes as pulmonary stenosis with **atrial septal defect,** and supravalvular aortic stenosis.

Hypertrophic subaortic stenosis   Disproportionate hypertrophy of the septum, which causes obstruction in midsystole as the septum draws toward the anterior or septal mitral leaflet in systole. (See figure on page 298 for hemodynamics.) The disproportionate septal hypertrophy has engendered the term *asymmetric septal hypertrophy*. Originally, it was called idiopathic hypertrophic subaortic stenosis in the first extensive report [2]; but the term *idiopathic* seems an unnecessary appendage. *Asymmetric septal hypertrophy* (commonly called ASH) does not necessarily imply obstruction to outflow, since ASH can occur without obstruction. Therefore, *hypertrophic subaortic stenosis* or *hypertrophic obstructive cardiomyopathy* (HOCM) should be used when referring to a patient with obstruction due to asymmetric septal hypertrophy.

infective endocarditis   Infection of the heart valves or of certain congenital defects, usually those that cause regurgitant or retrograde flows, such as **ventricular septal defect** or **patent ductus arteriosus.**

In former years, the infection was nearly always bacterial and thus the condition was called bacterial endocarditis. Because it could last for as long as 2 years before the diagnosis was made, it was known as subacute bacterial endocarditis. Today, fungi and *Rickettsia* are the causative organisms in a significant proportion of infections. Therefore, *infective* is a more embracing term.

The diagnosis used to be considered when there was fever and "changing murmurs." Because a regurgitant murmur is the only murmur likely to develop when a valve is destroyed, the term *changing* should be modified to mean a new or increasing *regurgitant* valvular murmur. (See checklist, page 6, for clinical details.)

inflow and outflow tract of the left ventricle   The inflow tract of the left ventricle is the area just below the mitral valve. The outflow tract is made up of the septum anteromedially and the anterior or septal leaflet of the mitral valve, plus their chordae laterally. (See figure on page 282.)

infundibulum   Outflow tract of the right ventricle, made up mostly of muscle called the crista supraventricularis. It is much like the spout of a teapot, the body of the right ventricle being the pot. (See figure on page 282.)

intermittent claudication   Pain in ischemic working muscle produced by certain metabolites; classically, pain in the legs due to inadequate arterial supply during walking. If the obstruction is high in the aortoiliac area, the pain may be in the hip or buttock. However, the pain may be felt in unusual sites, such as in the thighs or the arch of the foot. When the **ischemia** is due to thrombosis of the lower aorta (chronic aortoiliac occlusion), impotence and leg weakness may occur as well (Leriche's syndrome) [12]. If the celiac or mesenteric arteries are involved, the pain after meals is called "abdominal angina."
Note: Intermittent claudication is not related to the nocturnal leg or foot muscle cramps that occur in bed.

ischemia   (Pronounced is-kē-mi-a) Inadequate blood supply to a part of the body.

isovolumic contraction   The rise in LV pressure between closure of the mitral valve and opening of the aortic valve. This used to be called isometric contraction, but because the measurements of the ventricle change while the volume does not, the term *isovolumic* is more accurate. In some cardiological literature the period from the beginning of ventricular contraction to the opening of the aortic valve is considered isovolumic. This is not the physiologists' definition, and it is not really a proper use of the word *isovolumic,* because the volume is still changing until the mitral valve closes.

isovolumic relaxation   The fall in LV pressure between closure of the aortic valve and opening of the mitral valve. If the opening of the mitral valve is audible, as in mitral stenosis, the A_2-opening snap interval represents the isovolumic relaxation time. (See figure on page 233.) (The term should really be *isovolumic expansion* because it is an active process, i.e., the ventricle is capable of generating a negative pressure or "suction" effect [15].

left lateral decubitus position   Body position in which the subject is horizontal and lying on the left side. (See figure on page 128.)

malpositions of the heart   Abnormal placement of the cardiac chambers. The three commonest cardiac malpositions are situs inversus, dextroversion, and levoversion. *Situs solitus* (*solitus* means "usual") is the term used to denote a normal position of all chambers and vessels of the heart and, when used alone, it implies that the viscera are also normally placed. It specifically means that the descending aorta, left atrium, cardiac apex, and stomach are all on the left. In *situs inversus,* the descending aorta, left atrium, apex, and stomach are all on the right. This is also known as mirror-image dextrocardia. Dextrocardia alone means that the heart and aorta are on the right as in situs inversus but the stomach is on the left, i.e., there is a discordance between the heart and the gut. In *dextroversion,* the aorta and stomach are situated the same place as in situs solitus, but the heart is rotated so that the apex is on the right. In *levoversion,* the aorta and stomach are in the same place as in dextrocardia, but the heart is rotated so that the apex is on the left. The term *levocardia* has been used to refer to situs solitus of the heart but with the viscera inverted (stomach on the right). Dextrocardia and levocardia are almost always associated with other congenital abnormalities.
Note: Kartagener's syndrome is situs inversus with sinusitis and bronchiectasis.

Marfan's syndrome   See pages 24 and 30.

medial sclerosis   See **arteriosclerosis.**

Mueller maneuver   An inspiratory effort against a closed mouth and nose or against a closed glottis that decreases intrathoracic pressure. It is the opposite of a Valsalva maneuver.

neurocirculatory asthenia   A syndrome occurring in some patients with anxiety neurosis and consisting of palpitations and tachycardias, nondescript chest pains, shortness of breath, chronic fatigue, and other signs of sympathetic overactivity. It has been called Da Costa's syndrome (American Civil War), "soldier's heart" (World War I), "effort syndrome," "neurotic heart syndrome," "cardiac neurosis," and "vasoregulatory asthenia" [6]. If these patients are chronic hyperventilators, their breath-holding time will be less than 20 seconds.

Noonan's syndrome   A syndrome comprising the physical characteristics of Turner's syndrome but with no known chromosomal abnormalities (called Ullrich's syndrome in Europe). It has been referred to as "male Turner syndrome," a poor term because it ignores the conditions in females [14]. (See **Turner's syndrome** for physical and cardiac characteristics.)

outflow tract   See **inflow and outflow tract.**

patent ductus arteriosus   See persistent ductus arteriosus.

pectus excavatum   Posterior displacement of the lower sternum. It can be slight or so severe that it not only displaces the heart to the left but also may interfere with cardiac function by raising the right ventricular diastolic pressure and may cause palpitations and dyspnea on strenuous exertion [19]. It is commonly seen in Marfan's syndrome (see p. 436) and in patients with the straight back syndrome (see p. 290). The three degrees of severity have been described as the "saucer," "cup," and "funnel." If the anteroposterior measurement of the adult chest is measured by obstetric calipers and is less than 6½ inches (about 16 cm), the heart is very likely compressed. If the anteroposterior measurement is less than 5 inches (about 11 cm), the entire heart will usually be displaced to the left but is not compressed. The apex beat is almost always displaced to the left, even in saucer depressions.

persistent ductus arteriosus   Usually incorrectly called patent ductus arteriosus. The word ductus itself implies patency [13A]. Opening between the aorta and pulmonary artery in which flow normally occurs between the higher pressure aorta and the lower pressure pulmonary artery. Thus, some of the blood ejected by the LV into the aorta will pass into the pulmonary artery, resulting in a left-to-right shunt. The volume overload and dilatation occur where the shunted blood circulates, i.e., in the pulmonary artery, pulmonary veins, left atrium, and LV. The right-sided chambers should be normal.

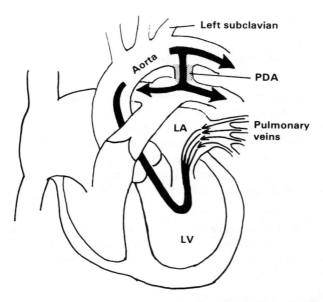

The persistent ductus arteriosus is a slightly left-sided structure that usually connects the junction of the main and pulmonary artery to the aorta just distal to the origin of the left subclavian artery. Since normal aortic pressure (120/80 mm Hg) is usually higher than pulmonary artery pressure (25/10 mm Hg), the shunt flow is normally from aorta to pulmonary artery in both systole and diastole.

A persistent ductus arteriosus represents persistence of the fetal ductus arteriosus that is designed to bypass the lungs in fetal life; i.e., the high pulmonary artery pressure in the fetus forces blood into the aorta through the ductus.

In persistent ductus arteriosus, severe pulmonary hypertension may develop if the fetal arterioles do not involute. When pulmonary hypertension develops, its onset occurs early in infancy or childhood. Then the right ventricle will remain hypertrophied, resulting in an **Eisenmenger syndrome** or **reaction** with right-to-left shunting. If a patient with a large persistent ductus reaches adulthood without developing pulmonary hypertension in infancy, he may go into heart failure with acute pulmonary edema. **Infective endocarditis** can occur as one of the complications of small ductus arteriosus. (See page 10 for explanation of differential cyanosis, which is one of the characteristics of the Eisenmenger reaction in persistent ductus arteriosus.)

postextrasystolic potentiation Increased contractility that occurs in the beat following a premature electrical depolarization of the heart. Although a pause after a premature beat can increase contractility by the long diastole, causing more filling and a **Starling effect,** premature depolarization itself produces increased contractility, i.e., contractility that is independent of the length of diastole. The cause of this increased inotropism is thought to be a calcium flux phenomenon.

postmyocardial infarction syndrome Syndrome consisting of fever, pneumonitis, and painful pericarditis and pleuritis that may occur from about 2–11 weeks after myocardial infarction and is probably an autoimmune response to myocardial necrosis. It is only dangerous in the presence of anticoagulants, when it may produce a bloody effusion and **tamponade.** The syndrome closely resembles the postcardiotomy syndrome and may be recurrent for as long as 2 years. Also called Dressler's syndrome [7].

pressure load   Load on a ventricle caused by resistance to ejection. An increased pressure load may result from such conditions as hypertension, coarctation of the aorta, or aortic stenosis. Also called a systolic load or afterload.

primary pulmonary hypertension   Irreversible pulmonary hypertension of unknown etiology, usually progressing to severe degrees, producing more and more right ventricular hypertrophy and dilatation, as well as main pulmonary artery dilatation and atherosclerosis. The age and sex incidence strongly favors females under age 40. Histologically, the small pulmonary arteries and arterioles usually show intimal fibrosis and proliferation as well as medial thickening.

pulse pressure or volume   Amplitude of a pulse. In palpation, it refers to the distance your fingers are moved between the least and the greatest expansion of a vessel. On an arterial pulse tracing, it refers to the difference between the systolic and diastolic pressures.

Raynaud's phenomenon   Intermittent constriction of small arteries and arterioles of the fingers, resulting in a change of color, usually produced by cooling but also by sympathetic stimulation of any kind. It begins with blanching, progresses to cyanosis, and often ends with a reactive redness (reactive hyperemia) that may be very painful. It is occasionally a precursor of a collagen or other connective-tissue disease. It is called Raynaud's *disease* when it is not secondary to trauma or to neurogenic lesions or other systemic disease.

Note: Acrocyanosis is a persistent blueness and coldness of the distal parts of the extremities, probably due to an abnormality of the small vessels.

right ventricular failure   This is a poor term because it is usually used for a patient with a high venous pressure and peripheral edema due to a low LV cardiac output. It is a poor substitute for the term *peripheral venous congestion* because it suggests that the primary cause of the high venous pressure and peripheral edema is a decrease in RV function even though the RV may be perfectly healthy. In one study of patients with LV failure the RV was shown to have normal contractile function while it was responding to the low output of a damaged LV [17]. The RV cannot put out more than it receives from the LV. If a damaged LV puts out only 30 ml (instead of a normal 60 ml) with each systole, the RV will eventually receive, and therefore also eject, about 30 ml per systole. Because the fibers of the LV are intertwined with those of the RV, the output of the latter is usually mechanically dependent on the action of the LV. Therefore if the LV is in failure, the RV will act the same way in terms of **ejection fraction** and stroke volume. To call this "right ventricular failure" is placing the blame on the wrong ventricle.

Primary right ventricular failure is rare but can occur chronically with severe obstruction to right ventricular outflow, such as occurs in very severe pulmonary stenosis or pulmonary hypertension. Acute RV failure can occur with a massive pulmonary embolism or acute RV infarction.

The high venous pressure and peripheral edema caused by left ventricular failure is better called *peripheral congestive failure.* (See checklist, page 4.) When the LV fails, the high venous pressure is caused as much by the high venous tone and increased blood volume secondary to its low output as it is by the secondary response of the RV. The peripheral edema is caused by salt retention and high venous pressure, both of which can be blamed on the low output of the LV.

semilunar valves The aortic or pulmonary valves. Their leaflets are half-moon-shaped (semilunar).

sinus arrhythmia Increase in heart rate with inspiration and decrease with expiration due to vagal inhibition during inspiration. (Remember "in" for "*in*crease" on inspiration.)

sinuses of Valsalva The three bulges or sinuses at the root of the aorta, two of which give rise to the coronary arteries. They help to prevent the open aortic leaflets from occluding the orifice of the coronary arteries. Occasionally, they may be congenitally weak and rupture into adjacent chambers, or they may become aneurysmal, especially in Marfan's syndrome (see pp. 24, 30), producing any degree of aortic regurgitation.

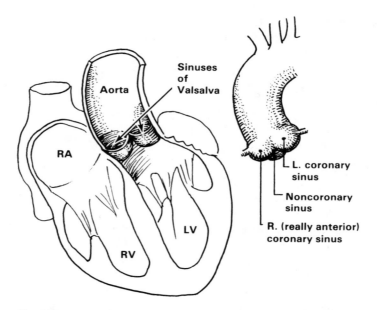

The right coronary sinus is anterior when viewed from above, but it is called the right coronary sinus probably because it gives rise to the right coronary artery.

Starling effect The effect of the Frank–Starling law of the heart, which states that if the heart muscle is stretched before it contracts, it will contract with more energy. This is equivalent to a bow-and-arrow effect; i.e., the more taut the bow, the farther the arrow will go.

Sternal angle, or **angle of Louis** (pronounced Loo-ee) The first protuberance or hump in the sternum below the suprasternal notch. It is at the junction of the manubrium and body of the sternum. It marks the point where the second costal cartilage joins the sternum. Below this cartilage is the second intercostal space.

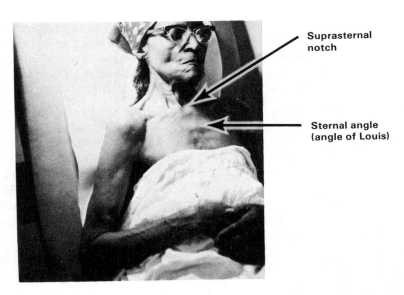

Suprasternal notch

Sternal angle (angle of Louis)

The sternal angle is one of the most important landmarks in cardiology, not only because it is the zero level for jugular pressures but also because it is the only accurate way to find the fourth right interspace in order to place the V₁ electrode for an ECG.

Stokes-Adams attack or **Adams-Stokes attack**   An episode of syncope secondary to complete AV block (see p. 429 of Glossary). Any cerebral symptom secondary to complete AV block may probably also be considered a minor degree of Stokes-Adams attack because it may presage syncope and death. Syncope secondary to any other arrhythmia should probably be called cardiac syncope and not a Stokes-Adams attack.

subclavian steal   Use of a vertebral artery as collateral circulation to feed a subclavian artery beyond an obstruction (usually on the left). Blood from a vertebral artery flows retrogradely into the distal subclavian, thus "stealing" blood from the brain. (See checklist on page 15 for symptoms.)

Tamponade   Restriction of cardiac diastole caused by fluid in the pericardium. Because the pressure in the pericardium is equal to venous pressure, the patient with tamponade must of necessity have a high venous pressure and usually also has peripheral edema when the tamponade becomes severe. Pericardial effusion without a high venous pressure is not tamponade. A combination of fluid and solid pericardial material causing constriction is called "effusive-constrictive pericarditis."

tetralogy of Fallot   Classically, it refers to a large ventricular septal defect, pulmonary stenosis, an overriding aorta, and right ventricular hypertrophy (RVH). Because pulmonary stenosis will always lead to RVH, the latter is a necessary result of the other congenital lesions and not really part of the basic abnormality.

The pulmonary stenosis may be either valvular, infundibular, or both and is the cause of the murmur. The enlargement of the aorta by virtue of receiving blood from both ventricles may contribute to the overriding.

Tetralogy of Fallot is the commonest form of congenital cyanotic heart disease.

thrill Vibratory sensation similar to what is felt when touching the head and neck of a purring cat. A long thrill is merely a palpable murmur and signifies that the murmur is at least grade 4/6 in loudness. A short thrill on the chest wall may be a juxtaposition of split heart sound vibrations. A short thrill felt on a carotid artery may be due to a midsystolic dip or a minor degree of bisferiens pulse.

transposition of the great vessels It is often called "complete" transposition of the great vessels and means that the anteroposterior relationship of the aorta and pulmonary arteries are reversed, i.e., instead of the aortic root being posterior to the pulmonary artery it is anterior (and often to the right). This results in the right ventricle giving rise to the aorta and the left ventricle giving rise to the pulmonary artery. One or more abnormal communications between the systemic and pulmonary circulations must exist for the patient to survive. Mixing may occur through either an atrial septal defect, a ventricular septal defect, a patent ductus, or large bronchial arteries.

Cyanosis is usually present either from birth or within a few days of birth. The commonest cause of cyanosis combined with shunt vascularity in the lungs on x-ray is transposition of the great vessels, especially if it is accompanied by congestive failure in infancy.

Turner's syndrome Female phenotype consisting of short stature, receding chin, webbed neck, low hairline over the back of the neck, broad shield chest resulting in widely separated nipples, exaggerated carrying angle, sparse axillary and pubic hair, lymphedema of the lower extremities (in infancy), and a short fourth metacarpal. It is sometimes simply described as short stature, neck webbing, and sexual infantilism in a female with a sex chromosome abnormality (absence of one of the two sex chromosomes). Coarctation of the aorta is the commonest associated cardiovascular lesion. When patients with such an appearance have normal sex chromosomes and also have hypertelorism with a slight antimongoloid slant to the eyes as well as ptosis of the upper lids and exophthalmos, especially if the above physical characteristics are found in a male, they are likely to have pulmonary stenosis and are said to have **Noonan's syndrome** [14]. Hypertrophic cardiomyopathies and persistent ductus arteriosus have also been associated with Noonan's syndrome.

Valsalva maneuver A forced expiration against a closed glottis. It is used as a simple way to raise the intrathoracic pressure. The patient is asked either to blow up a column of mercury to as close to 40 mm Hg as possible or to push his abdomen against your hand for about 10 sec. The rise in intrathoracic pressure (phase 1) decreases venous return to the heart despite a marked rise in venous pressure, thus causing a gradual decrease in heart size, stroke volume, and pulse pressure. There is a reflex tachycardia and the blood pressure falls (phase 2). On release of the strain there is a further sudden drop of blood pressure for a few beats because most of the blood in the right ventricle is used to fill the almost empty pulmonary venous reservoir (phase 3). The blood that had been dammed up in the venae cavae now pours into the lungs, LV, and aorta. There now occurs a slowing of the heart rate and an excessive rise in blood pressure for a few beats that is due to the reflex sympathetic stimulation caused by the strain that takes a few seconds to be "turned off," plus the effect of the sudden increase in volume distending the carotid baroreceptors.

ventricular aneurysm   See **aneurysm**.

ventricular septal defect   Opening or hole in the ventricular septum. This is the commonest of all congenital lesions and is most usually found in the membranous portion of the ventricle, i.e., in the translucent area, a few centimeters below the aortic valve. It may, however, be found in the muscular septum, in the supracristal area, leading directly into the pulmonary artery (rare), or posterior and superior to the attachment of the tricuspid valve to the membranous septum and therefore may lead directly into the right atrium (Gerbode defect). (See figure on page 340.) Ventricular septal defect shunts that occur during systole are normally from left to right, i.e., left to right ventricle, and produce volume overloads in the right ventricle, pulmonary artery, pulmonary veins, left atrium, and left ventricle.

The defect usually varies from pinpoint size to slightly more than a centimeter in diameter. When it involves the entire septum, a single ventricle is produced. When multiple muscular defects are present, it is known as a *Swiss cheese defect.*

Unless the defect is very large, the hole may close in the first few years of life, often with a membranous septal pouch or **aneurysm.**

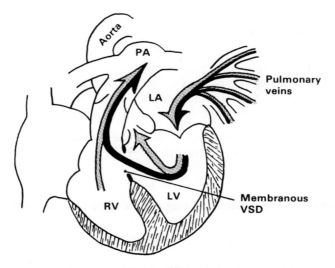

In most ventricular septal defects, only the right atrium is spared the volume overload caused by the left-to-right shunt. In the rare left ventricle-to-right atrium type of ventricular septal defect, however, all cardiac chambers are volume-overloaded. In this figure, the black portion of the arrow represents the shunt flow, and the dotted portion represents the normal flow that comes from the venae cavae.

A dreaded complication of large defects is severe pulmonary hypertension, which may become irreversible. When it becomes severe enough to reverse the shunt, this is known as an Eisenmenger complex (see **Eisenmenger syndrome),** which usually occurs within the first few years of life.

water-hammer pulse   A brisk, sharp, rapidly rising arterial pulse. A water-hammer was a Victorian toy consisting of a tube in which a vacuum was produced and containing water that dropped like a rock with the unopposed gravity when the tube was turned. When the water struck against the vessel, it produces a noise similar to that of a hammer.

Wolff-Parkinson-White (W-P-W) **preexcitation** This refers to an atrioventricular bypass pathway. It is an electrocardiographic phenomenon in which an abnormal conduction pathway between the atrium and ventricle bypasses the atrioventricular node, thus shortening the P-R interval and producing a wide QRS. When this pathway is used to produce a tachycardia, it is called a Wolff-Parkinson-White syndrome.

xanthelasma Flat xanthoma found on or around the eyelid. It is a yellowish, cholesterol-filled plaque, and is often, but not invariably, associated with hypercholesterolemia.

xanthoma Cholesterol-filled nodule found either subcutaneously or over a tendon. *Tuberous xanthomas* are subcutaneous xanthomas on the extensor surfaces of the extremities. They are associated with an increase in serum levels of both cholesterol and triglycerides. They are most commonly found in patients with type III hyperlipoproteinemia but also with predominately type II or IV. They are associated with coronary disease, even before puberty. Since they are under the skin, their yellow pigment is visible. Tendon xanthomas are too deep to impart any change of color to the skin.

eruptive xanthomas Tiny yellowish nodules, 1–2 mm in diameter, on an erythematous base and found all over the body, mostly on pressure areas. They are often transient and vary with the degree of hypertriglyceridemia, with which they are associated. The triglyceride level is usually at least 1,000 mg per 100 ml, no matter what the cause, whether diabetes or pure type 1 hyperlipoproteinemia. There is some correlation with coronary disease.

palmar xanthomas Very small xanthomas found in the palmar crease and probably representing an early stage of the tuberous type.

REFERENCES

1. Bernheim, P. De la stenose ventriculaire droite. *Rev. Gen. Clin. Therap.* (or *J. Pract.*) 20:721, 1915.
2. Braunwald, E., et al. Idiopathic hypertrophic subaortic stenosis: Description based on analysis of 64 patients. *Circulation* 29 (Suppl. 14):1, 1964.
3. Burch, G. E. Ischemic cardiomyopathy. *Am. Heart J.* 79:291, 1970.
4. Burch, G. E., Giles, T. D., and Colcolough, H. L. Ischemic cardiomyopathy. *Br. Heart J.* 79:291, 1970.
5. Corrigan, D. J. On permanent patency of the mouth of the aorta, or inadequacy of the aortic valves. *Edin. Med. Surg. J.* 37:229, 1832.
6. DaCosta, J. M. On irritable heart: A clinical study of a form of functional cardiac disorder and its consequences. *Am. J. Med. Sci.* 61:17, 1871.
7. Dressler, W. The post-myocardial infarction syndrome. *Arch. Intern. Med.* 103:28, 1959.
8. Ebstein, W. Uber einem sehr seltenen Fall von Insufficienz der Valvula tricuspidalis. *Arch. Anat. Physiol. Wissensch Med.* January, 1866.
9. Eisenmenger, V. Die angeborenen Defect de Kammerscheidewand des Herzens. *Ztschr. Klin. Med.* 32:1, 1897.

10. Evans, D. W., and Heath, D. Disappearance of the continuous murmur in a case of patent ductus arteriosus. *Br. Heart J.* 23:469, 1961.

11. Gould, K. L., et al. Left ventricular hypertrophy in coronary artery disease. *Am. J. Med.* 55:595, 1973.

12. Leriche, R., and Morel, A. The syndrome of thrombotic obliteration of the aortic bifurcation. *Ann. Surg.* 127:193, 1958.

13. Mahl, M. M., and Lange, K. Reliabilitiy of subjective circulation time determinations. *Circulation* 17:922, 1958.

13A. Marquis, R. M., and Godman, M. J. Nomenclature of the ductus arteriosus. *Br. Heart J.* 49:288, 1983.

14. Noonan, J. A., and Ehmke, D. A. Associated noncardiac malformations in children with congenital heart disease. *J. Pediatr.* 63:468, 1963.

15. Sabbah, H. N., Anbe, D. T., and Stein, P. D. Negative intraventricular diastolic pressure in patients with mitral stenosis: Evidence of left ventricular diastolic suction. *Am. J. Cardiol.* 45:562, 1980.

16. Selzer, A. Circulation time and venous pressure: Routine tests? *Am. Heart J.* 80:142, 1970.

17. Stein, P. D., et al. Performance of the failing and nonfailing right ventricle of patients with pulmonary hypertension. *Am. J. Cardiol.* 44:1050, 1979.

18. Takaro, T., and Hines, E. A., Jr. Digital arteriography in occlusive arterial disease and in clubbing of the fingers. *Circulation* 35:682, 1967.

19. vanBuchem, F. S. P., and Nieveen, J. Findings with funnel chest. *Acta Med. Scand.* 174:657, 1963.

Index